THE ETHICS OF RESEARCH INVOLVING HUMAN SUBJECTS:
Facing the 21st Century

Edited by

Harold Y. Vanderpool

Frederick 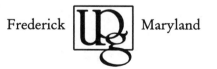 Maryland

University Publishing Group, Inc.
Frederick, Maryland 21701

Copyright 1996 by University Publishing Group.
All rights reserved
Printed in the United States of America

ISBN 1-55572-036-6

Contents

Preface .... *vii*

Acknowledgments .... *ix*

Contributors .... *xi*

1   Introduction and Overview: Ethics, Historical
    Case Studies and the Research Enterprise......................... 1
    Harold Y. Vanderpool

Part I Current Debate Over Research Ethics and Regulations

Introduction to Part I 33
    Harold Y. Vanderpool

2   From Nuremberg Through the 1990s:
    The Priority of Autonomy 45
    Robert M. Veatch

3   The Weight and Weighing of Ethical Principles 59
    Albert R. Jonsen

4   Choosing Between Nuremberg and the National
    Commission: The Balancing of Moral Principles in
    Clinical Research 83
    Terrence F. Ackerman

5   Changing Views of Justice after Belmont:
    AIDS and the Inclusion of "Vulnerable" Subjects 105
    Carol Levine

6   Challenges to IRBs in the Coming Decades 127
    Charles R. McCarthy

Part II Conflicts of Interest

Introduction to Part II 147
    Harold Y. Vanderpool

7   The Promise and Perils of Public Bioethics 155
    John C. Fletcher and Franklin G. Miller

8 Financial Issues and Incentives Related to Clinical
   Research and Innovative Therapies 185
   Stuart E. Lind
9 Physicians' Conflicts of Interest in Post-Marketing
   Research: What the Public Should Know, and Why
   Industry Should Tell Them 203
   John La Puma

Part III Controversy Over Cross-Cultural Research
   Introduction to Part III 223
   Harold Y. Vanderpool
10 International Codes and Guidelines for Research Ethics:
   A Critical Appraisal 235
   Robert J. Levine
11 The Distinction Between Ethical Pluralism and Ethical
   Relativism: Implications for the Conduct of
   Transcultural Clinical Research 261
   Nicholas A. Christakis
12 Medical Research and the Principle of Respect for
   Persons in Non-Western Cultures 281
   Carel B. IJsselmuiden and Ruth R. Faden

Part IV Critical Issues in Specialized Areas
   Introduction to Part IV 305
   Harold Y. Vanderpool
13 The Ethical Analysis of Clinical Trials: New Lessons
   for and from Cancer Research 319
   Benjamin Freedman
14 Ethical Issues in Pediatric Research 339
   William G. Bartholome
15 Fetal and Embryo Research: A Changing Scientific,
   Political, and Ethical Landscape 371
   Constance M. Pechura
16 Respecting Human Subjects in Genome Research:
   A Preliminary Policy Agenda 401
   Eric T. Juengst

Appendices 431

A   *Nuremberg Code,* 1946 431
B   *Declaration of Helsinki* 1964, revised 1975,
    1983, 1989 433
C   *The Belmont Report,* April 1979 437
D   Code of Federal Regulations, Title 45
    U.S. Code of Federal Regulations, Part 46
    (revised 18 June 1991) 449
E   *NIH Guidelines on the Inclusion of Women and
    Minorities as Subjects in Clinical Research,* March 1995 .. 484
F   CIOMS/WHO, *International Ethical Guidelines for
    Biomedical Research Involving Human Subjects,* 1993 501

Index 511

Preface

This book is about the current status and future directions of the ethics of research involving human subjects. Medical researchers, members and administrators of institutional review boards (IRBs) in academia and industry, ethicists, government officials, and informed citizens face a maze of changes and challenges over the ethics and regulation of biomedical research. These are the persons for whom this book is written. Its chapters depict where we are and envision where we are going.

A state-of-the-art understanding of the ethics of research cannot be static. Contemporary research ethics is characterized by change, change more akin to a story or film than a snapshot. This change manifests itself as ever-continuing debate and turmoil over the ethical principles and officially adopted guidelines for research. Change also appears as newly surfacing topics over scientific advancements and biomedical innovations.

Powerful interests fuel changes past and at present--the stability and reputations of academic and private medical institutions; high-stake interests of pharmaceutical, medical device, and biotechnology industries; the careers and ambitions of individual researchers; the laws of constitutional democracies; and long-standing commitments to ethical principles and inquiry.

As its primary objective, this book seeks to make sense of an almost overwhelming body of literature and regulation on research ethics. Each of the book's contributors is a leader in his or her field of inquiry. Each author deals with a critical feature of contemporary research ethics.

To meet the needs of many readers, the book's first chapter explains what ethics is, gives case studies on research ethics's checkered past, depicts the extensiveness of present day research on human subjects, and surveys the chapters to come. The first sections of this chapter are especially designed for readers searching for an initial or mid-level acquaintance with ethics and research ethics. The chapter's expansive notes and later sections are for the experienced and inexperienced alike. Chapters 2 through 16 are arranged in four major parts: current debate over research ethics and regulations, conflicts of interest, controversies over cross-cultural research, and critical issues in specialized areas of research. For the sake of clarity and comprehension, each part is introduced with a "road map" essay that places each of its author's essays in the context of current debate and discussion.

To capture current trends, many of the essays are arranged in a debate-like format. Different points of view are juxtaposed, and at points the authors of this volume address or oppose the positions of their fellow authors. On the one hand, this accurately reflects the nature of contemporary research ethics as the subject of controversy and change. On the other, this arrangement is designed to draw professionals and students inside current debates so as to stimulate understanding and increase competency of judgment and decision making.

Finally, this book serves as a bibliographical and document resource. Each chapter and introduction points to pivotal sources and background discussions. Each references the latest literature in its field of inquiry. The appendices contain critically important documents in the ethics and regulations of past and present research involving human subjects.

HAROLD Y. VANDERPOOL

Acknowledgments

This book is the product of several years of research conducted in collaboration with, or perhaps more accurately, in conversation with, many persons. Each of its authors contributes to the national and international conversation represented in these pages. Other contributing conversants are identified in notes that give the dates of our exchanges. Still others, who are identified through their publications, personally shared their musings and convictions. Over time, I discovered an incalculable fund of knowledge in the mind of Robert J. Levine, with whom I consulted on many occasions.

My interest in these topics began with service on the University of Texas Medical Branch's (UTMB) Institutional Review Board. When I decided to develop projects regarding the ethics of research involving human subjects at a national and international level, I received personal and financial support from many sources. I thank Ronald A. Carson, the Director of UTMB's Institute for the Medical Humanities, for his unflagging encouragement and counsel. And I thank my humanities and clinician colleagues and graduate students for their insights and questions.

Three years ago, leading scholars of research ethics were convened in a national-international conference hosted by UTMB and entitled The Ethics of Clinical Research on Human Subjects. UTMB's President, Thomas N. James, M.D., its Dean, George T. Bryan, M.D., its Vice Dean, Walter J. Meyer, III, M.D., and the Chairman of its Institutional Review Board, Courtney M. Townsend, Jr., M.D., provided outstanding support for that endeavor. Each of these individuals deserves special praise for suggestions arising from underlying commitments to the benefits of biomedical research. Concurrently, the able planning and administrative assistance of Sharon Goodwin added to the conference's success.

Further financial support was provided by the Harris and Eliza Kempner Fund, the National Institutes of Health's Office for Protection from Research Risks, the Jesse H. Jones Research Endowment in the Medical Humanities, the John P. McGovern Fund for the Behavioral Sciences, as well as Pfizer, Incorporated, the Johnson and Johnson Family of Companies, the Wyeth-Ayerst Research Division of American Home Products, Abbott Laboratories, and Smithkline Beecham.

As revised manuscripts of conferees, as well as manuscripts from a number of additional authors, were received, excellent editorial and secretarial assistance was provided by four persons to whom I owe special thanks: Stacey Gottlob, Beverly Claussen, Dorothy Karilanovic, and my research assistant, Dr. Sara J. Clausen. I also thank Leslie LeBlanc of the University Publishing Group for her valuable support and editorial suggestions.

Respecting personal recognition, I praise these five: Bill Bartholome for exchanges that began when we were Kennedy Fellows at Harvard and for modeling perseverence in the face of ultimate tests to body and will; my deceased son Jay with whom I shared unwritten covenants exceeding the power of codes; my son Jon and daughter Katherine for legacies lived and living; and my wife Jan for a mastery of English literature and a relish of fine writing and sharing.

Contributors

Terrence F. Ackerman, Ph.D., is Professor of Medical Ethics and the Chairman of the Department of Human Values and Ethics, College of Medicine, University of Tennessee, Memphis.

William G. Bartholome, M.D., M.T.S., is Professor of Pediatrics in the Department of the History and Philosophy of Medicine, University of Kansas Medical Center.

Nicholas A. Christakis, M.D., M.P.H., M.A., is Assistant Professor of Medicine and Sociology, University of Chicago.

Ruth R. Faden, Ph.D., M.P.H., is Professor in the Department of Health Policy and Management in the School of Hygiene and Public Health, Johns Hopkins University, Baltimore, Maryland.

John C. Fletcher, Ph.D., is Kornfeld Professor of Biomedical Ethics and the Director of the Center for Biomedical Ethics, School of Medicine, University of Virginia, Charlottesville.

Benjamin Freedman, Ph.D., is Professor in the McGill Centre for Medicine, Ethics and Law, McGill University, and a Clinical Ethicist in the Jewish General Hospital in Montreal, Province Quebec.

Carel B. IJsselmuiden, M.D., M.P.H., D.P.H., is Senior Lecturer in the Department of Community Health, Medical University of Southern Africa, and a Senior Epidemiologist in the South African Research Council.

Albert R. Jonsen, Ph.D., is Professor of Ethics in Medicine and the Chairman of the Department of Medical History and Ethics, School of Medicine, University of Washington, Seattle.

Eric T. Juengst, Ph.D., is Associate Professor of Biomedical Ethics in the Center for Biomedical Ethics, Case Western Reserve University School of Medicine, Cleveland, Ohio.

John La Puma, M.D., is Clinical Associate Professor of Medicine at University of Chicago Hospital and Clinics, and a Consultant in clinical ethics and a general internist in Chicago.

Carol Levine is the Executive Director of the Orphan Project, the Fund for the City of New York.

Robert J. Levine, M.D., is Professor of Medicine and Lecturer in Pharmacology in the School of Medicine, Yale University, New Haven, Connecticut.

Stuart E. Lind, M.D., is in the Department of Medicine, Evanston Hospital and Northwestern University Medical School, Evanston, Illinois.

Charles R. McCarthy, Ph.D., is a Senior Research Fellow in the Joseph and Rose Kennedy Institute of Ethics, Georgetown University, and the former Director of the Office for Protection from Research Risks, National Institutes of Health, Bethesda, Maryland.

Franklin G. Miller, Ph.D., is Assistant Professor of Biomedical Ethics and Medical Education, School of Medicine, University of Virginia, Charlottesville.

Constance M. Pechura, Ph.D., is the Director of the Division of Biobehavioral Sciences and Mental Disorders, Institute of Medicine, National Academy of Sciences, Washington, D.C.

Harold Y. Vanderpool, Ph.D., Th.M., is Professor of the History and Philosophy of Medicine, Institute for the Medical Humanities, University of Texas Medical Branch at Galveston.

Robert M. Veatch, Ph.D., is Professor of Medical Ethics and the Director of the Joseph and Rose Kennedy Institute of Ethics, Georgetown University, Washington, D.C.

1

Introduction and Overview: Ethics, Historical Case Studies, and the Research Enterprise

Harold Y. Vanderpool

Why is so much attention now being given to the ethics of research involving human subjects?[1] What is the nature and content of this ethics? What roles does ethics play or should it play in the conducting of biomedical research?

These questions are unanswerable apart from understanding the purposes and ever-increasing power of biomedical research itself. Research involving human beings has expanded exponentially over the last 60 years as nations, national and international institutions, and groups of researchers have linked their destinies and hopes to medical advances. The nature and influence of this expansion will be explored under the subheading, "The Reach of Research," below.

Studies by historians, sociologists, political scientists, and multi-disciplinary scholars have explored how, when, and by whom this research was and is being conducted. Those who deal with the ethics of clinical research should be acquainted with a number of these important, factually oriented studies, many of which are referenced in this book. Ethical judgments about the rightness or wrongness of a research protocol or some aspect of that protocol are null and void apart from a precise understanding of the research in question.

ETHICS

While necessarily relying upon its sister disciplines in the humanities and the social sciences, ethics focuses not on what individuals and groups do and how they behave, but on, what they *ought* to do and how they *ought* to behave. Ethics asks about what is right or good or virtuous; it seeks to identify and characterize moral arguments, and to investigate whether and the extent to which these arguments, or the decisions they are intended to justify, are rationally warranted.[2]

Ethics provides the means to identify and critically assess the explicit and implicit reasons for conducting research with human subjects. It also enables us to make judgments about the morality of researcher-subject relationships within the many settings in which research occurs. Ethical scrutiny provides hindsight, assists in oversight, and offers foresight.

How can ethics fulfill these roles? An inventory of the "ingredients" of ethics shows how and why ethics functions as a means for critically assessing both the rationales for human conduct and the morality of human relationships.

Ethics or ethical analysis begins with a straight-forward, jargon-free question: What actions are right or wrong, good or bad, praiseworthy or blameworthy? To ask about "actions" brings into play actors, personal interactions, and relationships. This question immediately calls forth another: By what criteria do we decide whether some action or personal interaction is right or wrong, good or bad?

Regardless of their levels of training or areas of specialization, all who "do ethics" or make ethically discerning decisions can agree on the following criteria: judgments about the morality of actions and relationships are predicated upon logical arguments, accurate facts, and coherent reasons. As we examine difficult issues, we discover that we often cannot arrive at uncontested or conclusively convincing answers, but we can be sure that we are not indulging in serious ethical inquiry if we are not seeking to arrive at answers that are the most convincing and acceptable among alternative possibilities.[3]

The salient features of ethics as a human enterprise arise from this search for coherent and defensible answers. First, ethics is a rational enterprise that endures as a centuries-long search for time-tested arguments and principles that are coherent and applicable.[4] Second, ethical reasoning rests on common and shared experiences and insights, on the facts insofar as they can be ascertained, and on ordinary logical inference. With effort and experience, most persons can become skilled in ethical analysis. Third, as critical and disciplined inquiry, ethics commissions us to make *judgments* predicated upon thoughtful analysis and deliberation. This contrasts with making assertions or voicing opinions, regardless of the frequency or certitude with which they are asserted or voiced.[5]

What the poet Wallace Stevens says of modern poetry is true for ethics:

> It has to be living, to learn the speech of the place.
> It has to face the men of the time and to meet
> The women of the time. It has to think about war
> And it has to find what will suffice.[6]

The criteria and salient features of ethics alert us to common misperceptions about ethics. Ethics should not be equated with regulations and bureaucratic rules, even though ethics informs and shapes many such rules.[7] The interesting and important ways ethics informs regulations of human-subject research will be further explored in this chapter and in the introductions and chapters that follow.

Nor should ethics be equated with all value statements and judgments, even though these judgments characteristically assess things as good or bad, right or wrong. This is true because we hold to many types of values that have little or nothing to do with ethics. For example, on the basis of prudential or practical values, we assess wrenches, cars, or human work as good, not so good, or terrible. In like fashion, we commonly make strong and, at times, highly contested judgments about aesthetic, economic, or religious matters. Ethical values are a subset within the universe of human values and valuing, even though ethical values interact in complex and multifaceted ways with other values.[8]

Ethical values and judgments pertain to the following three areas:[9]

1. Judgments about that which is ultimately good, that is, good with respect to the purposes and ends of human action;[10]
2. Judgments of human character--judgments that assign praise or blame to persons and their actions in light of their virtues of character or lack of such;[11]
3. Judgments about moral obligations--what we ought or ought not to do, how we should or should not treat others.

Concerning moral obligations, consequentialists determine the rightness or wrongness of actions according to their outcomes. Actions are judged to be right or obligatory if they will, or probably will, bring into being that which is regarded as ultimately good--human happiness, mutual respect, harmony and peace, and so on. Holding to a version of consequentialism, utilitarians regard happiness as the ultimate human good, and thus equate right or obligatory moral actions with actions that will likely produce the greatest balance of happiness over displeasure or suffering.[12] Nonconsequentialists and nonutilitarians deny that rationally calculated outcomes or consequences serve as the ultimate criterion or standard of morality. Nonutilitarians include deontologists and casuists. Deontologists equate morality with basic rules and principles of action--the principle of respecting the autonomy of others, the duty to tell the truth, certain principles of justice, and so on. Regarded as obligatory in and of themselves, these duties generate principles of procedure,[13] for example, the principle of never using persons as a means toward an end, but rather, respecting persons as end-choosing or self-choosing agents.[14] Some deontologists view these principles as multiple and interacting norms that must be played off against one another before the morality of specific acts can be determined.[15] Critical of those who equate ethics with theory-based rules of procedure and universal ethical principles, casuists accent practical moral reasoning and decision making about particular, morally troubling situations.[16]

These brief points indicate how ethics serves as a disciplined, reasoned way to identify, criticize, discover, and defend arguments and rationales that justify how humans should relate to and behave toward one another. Additional features about the nature and functions of moral inquiry will be discussed in the pages and chapters that follow. These features will be examined when they offer essential and useful ways to understand and critically assess the morality of clinical research involving human subjects.

CASE STUDIES IN THE CHECKERED HISTORY OF RESEARCH ETHICS

Discussions over the morality of deliberate medical experiments on human beings extend from Greek and Roman antiquity, to the writings of Moses Maimonides (1135-1204) and Francis Bacon (1214-1294), to debates over smallpox innoculations in the 18th century, to numerous controversies over reported abuses of human subjects after 1870, to a host of 20th century developments.[17] While many case studies of the ethics of research involving human subjects could be drawn from this long history, the brief case-sketches that follow represent notable chapters over the course of the last 60 years. Comprising the darkest and brightest periods in the history of human experimentation, these episodes continue to serve as positive and negative standards for evaluating research ethics and regulation.

Concerning ethics, episodes in the history of research with human subjects serve as cases, as heuristic devices, for thinking about the nature and function of ethics as applied to research. By using them as case examples, readers individually and in study groups can identify ethical principles that will more likely protect or permit--unwittingly or by intention--abuses of human subjects. This can be done by reflecting on the interplay between (1) types of experiments, (2) the reasons or rationales for these experiments, and (3) the ethical assumptions underlying these reasons and rationales.

The phrase "ethical assumptions" may be confusing. For example, since the sketches below include experiments conducted under Nazi supervision, should not some of them be viewed as grievously *unethical?* This question points to a distinction between two subdivisions of moral inquiry. The first is called descriptive ethics--the *nonjudgmental* task of describing and charting the many assumptions and modes of reasoning used as justifications or rationales for human behavior.[18] This involves exploring "ethical assumptions" in the social scientific sense of discovering their types and variety. Ethicists have shown that social practices and policies are never devoid of assumptions and rationales that function as moral justifications.[19] For good or ill, these systems of value shape how humans deal with war, commerce, family relationships, medical care, and biomedical research.

In addition to descriptive ethics, ethical inquiry includes normative ethics, the task of identifying and rationally justifying the grounds for determining which courses of action are right or wrong, ethical or unethical.[20] The foregoing discussion under the subheading "Ethics" dealt with some of the salient features of normative ethics. Ethical norms and theories of moral obligation function (1) as personal guides, (2) as grounds for assessing or judging others' actions, and (3) as vantage points for criticizing assumptions and modes of moral reasoning identified via descriptive ethics.[21]

The following episodes challenge us to think both descriptively and normatively. Descriptively: What assumptions and modes of reasoning served as rationales for these experiments? And what assumptions and forms of reasoning are *we* using to assess the morality of these experiments? Normatively: What ethical assumptions and modes of reasoning should we be using to assess past (and present) actions as right or wrong?

NAZI EXPERIMENTATION

During World War II, National Socialist (Nazi) German investigators experimented on unwilling and unsuspecting civilians and political prisoners for the purposes of advancing the state's goals of national and racial superiority and, more immediately, to enable Germany's fighting forces to cope with disease, injury, and life-threatening battle conditions.[22] The ideological justifications of Nazi physician-experimentalists included contributing to scientific progress--particularly, the science/pseudoscience of advancing human evolution by destroying those deemed genetically inferior and worthless.[23] The career of the infamous Dr. Sigmund Rascher exemplifies how some Nazis used their work to gain political favor and secure appointments within academic medicine.[24] Extensive, willfully harmful experiments included subjecting concentration camp internees to extreme hypothermia, high altitude decompression, mutilative wounds, typhus and other infections, toxic substances, experimental drugs, massive bleeding, and vivisections, all often ending in death.[25] Most, if not all, of these experiments were without scientific merit.[26] They were conducted in spite of and in opposition to laudable and visionary ethical guidelines on medical experimentation promulgated by the German Minister of the Interior in 1931.[27]

U.S. WORLD WAR II RESEARCH

During the Second World War medical research was planned, coordinated, and extensively funded at the federal level for the first time in U.S. history. To increase combat effectiveness while the nation was mobilized for war, this research centered on the medical problems of America's troops--dysentery, malaria, gas warfare, wounds, and wartime climatic conditions.[28] Research subjects included nonconsenting orphaned children in their teens and retarded and mentally ill persons and ward patients, as well as consenting and informed prisoners and conscientious objectors. This research was predicated upon the rationale that,

All citizens were--or were supposed to be--contributing to the war effort. . . . Some people were ordered to face bullets and storm a hill; others were told to take an injection and test a vaccine. No one ever said that war was fair, or that it should be fairer for the incompetent than the competent.[29]

Usually healthy when they volunteered or were obligingly used, most of those experimented upon endured moderate or serious sickness, and some died.[30] Unaware, nonconsenting, and deceived servicemen also suffered moderate to severe short-term and long-term injuries from mustard gas experiments in gas chambers and field tests.[31] While a number of these experiments failed to uncover useful cures, this research produced an effective influenza vaccine, developed highly effective and valuable synthetic antimalarial drugs, and discovered ways to suspend penicillin in beeswax and peanut oil so as to make it less costly and more widely used.

THE NUREMBERG TRIAL AND CODE

In its concluding decision on the war crimes of Nazi physicians and scientists, the Nuremberg Military Tribunal set forth 10 ethical principles regarding human experimentation. Replicated as free-standing principles, they are now known as the *Nuremberg Code*. Declared to be "basic principles [that] must be observed in order to satisfy moral, ethical and legal concepts," these principles stipulate that the "voluntary consent of the human subject is absolutely essential"; and that experiments must "yield fruitful results for the good of society," must "protect the experimental subject against even remote possibilities of injury, disability, or death," must "be conducted only by scientifically qualified persons," and should be terminated when there is "probable cause to believe" that "a continuation of the experiment" will likely result in harm.[32] Beyond previous codes of research ethics, the *Nuremberg Code's* consent requirements were remarkably specific--the necessity of free choice without "any element of force, fraud, deceit, duress, over-reaching, or other ulterior form of constraint or coercion"; sufficient knowledge "to make an understanding and enlightened decision" in light of "the nature, duration, and purpose of the experiment" supplied by the person "who initiates, directs or engages in the experiment"; and the right to withdraw when the experiment's continuation seems "to be impossible" physically or mentally. Although this code influenced the formation of many professional and governmental codes thereafter,[33] it has been viewed as politically naive and unduly restrictive with respect to research involving children and other populations of patients.[34] The *Nuremberg Code* nevertheless continues to be regarded by some as the gold standard for all research with competent adults, a standard that "can guide us in eliminating all unconsented-to research on competent persons throughout the world."[35]

TWO DECADES OF NONFEDERALLY REGULATED RESEARCH

Believing that the Nazi atrocities were a world apart from the work they were doing, biomedical researchers in the U.S. between 1946 and 1966 resisted ethical and regulatory oversight as intrusive to their relationships with patients-subjects and as adequately handled at the discretion of investigators.[36] Surveys of the practices and thinking of research institutions in 1960 and 1962 revealed that this trust in the conscience of investigators resulted in sporadic internal regulation and oversight.[37] Through an article published by the *New England Journal of Medicine* in 1966, Henry K. Beecher undercut the moral complacency and hands-off policies of many American physician-researchers. Beecher's exposé included 22 examples of unethical research conducted between 1948 and 1965.[38] His examples dealt with research by well-known, highly funded investigators who worked in leading medical schools and government institutions and published their findings in prestigious medical journals. Beecher showed how the research experiments he reviewed "risked the health or the life of their subjects" often without their knowledge or consent. Examples 16 and 17 became famous, widely debated cases--the injecting of live cancer cells under the skin of unsuspecting patients at the Jewish Chronic Disease Hospital in Brooklyn, New York, and the infecting of retarded children in the Willowbrook State School on Staten Island with a mild strain of infectious hepatitis.[39] The impact of Beecher's article was all the more confounding because it probed the actions and assumptions of recognized cultural benefactors, those who in a few years' time had discovered "an array of antibiotics. . . a cure for tuberculosis; a variety of drugs for treating cardiac abnormalities; a new understanding of hepatitis."[40] A disturbing number of these advances relied on research that disregarded basic principles of research ethics as set forth by the World Medical Association's *Declaration of Helsinki*, Appendix B of this book.

TUSKEGEE, 1932-1972

Yet another exposé occurred before the present-day world of research ethics and regulation was born. In July 1972, the headlines of a story by Jean Heller revealed, "Syphilis Victims in U.S. Study Went Untreated for 40 Years."[41] News stories and an *ad hoc* government panel commissioned to investigate what happened decried the way the U.S. Public Health Service had conducted a study it initiated in 1932. The study charted the many, at times devastating, effects of untreated syphilis on some 400 black men in the county seat of Tuskegee, Alabama. Finding "no evidence that informed consent was gained from the human participants in this study," the *ad hoc* panel declared that this experiment was "ethically unjustified" at its inception in 1932, not to speak of the subjects' being kept unaware and uninformed for another 40 years. Compounding its moral problems, "penicillin therapy should have been made available to the participants . . . not later than 1953," when penicillin became generally available. In a separate memo, one of the panelists, Jay Katz, recalled the Nuremberg Military Tribunal, whose decision rendered the harms and violations of the Tuskegee Syphilis Study "intolerable in this country or anywhere in the civilized world."[42] In the face of criticisms about the study's scientific reliability and questionable therapeutic value, its scientific defenders maintained that it contributed to a first-hand knowledge of the pathological sequelae of advanced syphilis and was useful in the development of new serologic tests. In December 1974 the U.S. government agreed to pay a $10 million out-of-court settlement to subjects-plaintiffs and their survivors. In addition, the U.S. Department of Health and Human Services (DHHS) has been making yearly payments to cover the medical, nursing care, and other expenses of the research subjects, their spouses, and their progeny--payments that exceeded $1.8 million in 1994.[43]

FEDERAL REFORM, 1973-1981
Contemporary research ethics and regulation in the U.S. evolved step by step in response to the exposés between 1966 and 1972 as well as to other controversies in medical ethics and momentous changes in civil rights and the law.[44] In response to the turmoil over Beecher's article, the Food and Drug Administration (FDA) (1966) and the National Institutes of Health (NIH) (1971) developed internal policy guidelines. These were codified as federal *regulations* by the U.S. Department of Health, Education, and Welfare in 1974.[45] In response to the recommendations of a congressionally created National Commission for the Protection of Human Subjects of Biomedical and Behavioral Research (1974 - 1978), these regulations were revised in 1981 then, in turn, formulated as "Common Federal Policy" for additional federal agencies in 1991.[46] The institutions and dynamics of present day biomedical research regulations were thus assembled:

- Peer review by local review committees, commonly called IRBs (institutional review boards) in the U.S.;[47]
- Assurance of compliance contracts between local institutions and federal agencies;[48]
- Detailed federal and local regulations;[49]
- Officially sanctioned ethical principles set forth as guides for the resolution of ethical problems;[50]
- Updated instructions with respect to interpreting and following all of the above.[51]

In spite of ongoing criticisms over the ethical flaws, bureaucratic complexities, and time-consuming costs of these developments, they have been effective, perhaps greatly effective, in reducing harmful injuries to research subjects.[52] Meanwhile, this research resulted in dramatically increased knowledge about the nature of human disease and disability, and it has generated a vast array of new diagnostic and therapeutic modalities.[53]

AFTER 1981

Following the revisions of the U.S. federal regulations in 1981, a decade of calm ensued, during which time many persons naively assumed that the ethics of research involving human subjects had become settled and noncontroversial. Beginning in 1992, this calm was shattered by new revelations about abusive and denigrating mustard gas experiments during World War II, alarming radiation experiments on unaware subjects thereafter, and nightmarish harms to persons in an NIH drug trial.[54] The 1990s have also given rise to a host of new problems and concerns, such as initiatives favoring the inclusion of far greater numbers of women and minorities in biomedical research. These initiatives led to the recent adoption of sweeping guidelines by the NIH, The Inclusion of Women and Minorities as Subjects in Clinical Research. These guidelines apply to all NIH-sponsored research, and are reproduced in this volume's Appendix E.

Each of the chapters in this collection identifies and discusses the many, ever-continuing, and changing concerns over the ethics and regulations of research involving human subjects at the present time. Altogether, they comprise not one, but numerous case studies on the nature and import of research ethics. An overview of the topics in these chapters is given in the last subheading of this chapter, entitled "This Book's Imperatives."

THE REACH OF RESEARCH

Thousands of researchers and administrators, hundreds of thousands of research subjects, billions of dollars, reputations, profits, and promise: these are the markings of contemporary biomedical research involving humans. Although the full-scale reach of this research is not known, my research confirms the following profiles.

Presently, the DHHS awards approximately $5.5 billion per year for research involving human subjects.[55] Its ethics-oversight branch, the Office for Protection from Research Risks (OPRR), has multiple project-assurance contracts with 420 institutions in North America, including the 127 U.S. medical schools. A survey of several major medical centers reveals that, on average, each center's IRB has between 1,300 and 1,600 research projects/protocols under active and/or continuing review.[56] These include projects subject to both expedited review and full IRB review.[57] Each medical school surveyed reviews 350 to 540 new research protocols per year, which call for the recruitment of between 10,000 and 20,000 subjects for the institution's biomedical research.[58] It is likely that the 25 U.S. medical schools that are receiving the highest levels of extramural grant funding from the NIH are recruiting some 250,000 research subjects each year. In 1993 the NIH granted the U.S.'s 127 medical schools $3.9 billion for extramural research for some 15,240 protocols, not all of which is for clinical research involving human subjects.[59]

Notably, Henry K. Beecher predicated the "urgency" of his 1966 exposé on the remarkable growth of federally funded biomedical research and on a growing emphasis on research in medical schools and university hospitals "increasingly dominated by investigators."[60] Beecher indicated that NIH funding had risen to $436 million in 1965. That year the NIH funded between 1,500 and 2,000 research projects.[61] To begin to grasp the extent of biomedical research in the U.S. at the present time, one should note that, allowing for inflation, the NIH now grants the equivalent of its entire 1965 budget to its top 22 grant-receiving medical centers.[62] Medical schools, however, comprise only 30 percent of the institutions that now have multiple project-assurance agreements with the OPRR. In addition, the OPRR has single-project-assurance contracts with at least 1,000 other groups and institutions.

The FDA is responsible for regulating a somewhat separate solar system of research involving human subjects. Paul Goebel, chief of the Institutional Review Branch of the FDA, reports that the FDA is responsible for the oversight of 1,200 IRBs, many of which are also regulated by the NIH through multiple project-assurance agreements. In addition, the FDA exercises exclusive oversight over another approximately 5,000 IRBs that focus on intraocular-lens research. The FDA's database of 1,200 IRBs includes hospitals, geographically based nonprofit committees, and a number of free-standing, for-profit IRBs.[63] This last group contracts with various researchers, many of whom work for and with pharmaceutical, medical device, and biotech companies.

Goebel comments that "most of the research in the U.S. is conducted under the purview of the FDA, not the OPRR," because "most studies are funded by drug companies that fall outside of the OPRR's auspices."[64] He estimates that *industry*-sponsored research with human subjects is more than twice that of universities, and this research likely involves at least 1 million subjects each year.[65]

For-profit IRB companies that operate under FDA oversight include eight to 10 companies that focus solely on approving or disapproving research protocols according to the regulatory guidelines of the DHHS and FDA.[66] One of these companies employs 18 full-time staff members and reviews an estimated 3,500 research projects per year throughout the world.[67]

Altogether, funding for biomedical research from federal, state, local, philanthropic, and industry sources had reached the amazing sum of $22.5 billion by 1990.[68]

Behind these statistics are increasingly powerful and symbiotic linkages between researchers, academia, industry, and the government, linkages that comprise a medical-industrial, research-industrial complex.[69] As Beecher indicated 30 years ago, the academic careers and fame of physician-investigators are inextricably linked to their publications as well as to their expertise in securing grant support. In turn, the financial stability and reputations of researchers' medical institutions are rooted in their abilities to develop notable programs of research, to attract top-notch investigators, and, increasingly, to develop commercial, technology-transfer ventures with industry.[70] Complementing these, the long-term needs of pharmaceutical, drug-device, and biotech industries are based on "the five Ps" of medical centers: patients, prestige, patents, publications, and personnel.[71] To complete the circle, the U.S. government and the governments of other developed nations, view innovative medical technology and a strong biomedical industry as essential to favorable balances of trade, economic competitiveness, and the ability to assure a "fuller life" for citizens.[72]

The ethics of research involving human subjects is the standard-bearer of an awesome responsibility: how to respect and protect human subjects of research within the framework of these powerful, pro-research initiatives. This responsibility can and should be borne not only by ethicists but by all who seek to examine and apply ethical reasoning to research with human subjects--professionals and nonprofessionals alike. To be relevant and responsible, research ethics must be informed by and appreciative of the ethically justifiable purposes and ends of the institutions and individuals who are expanding the reach of research. The ethics of research must negotiate between the moral interests of protecting and showing respect for the human subjects of research and those of enabling researchers to continue humankind's historic battle against the forces of death, disability, and disease.

THIS BOOK'S IMPERATIVES

The foregoing discussions of ethics, episodes in the checkered history of research ethics, and the reach of research account for this book's contents. For the sake of clarity and comprehension, its chapters are arranged into four parts, each of which is introduced by a "road map" essay that identifies overarching issues, places its chapters in the context of current regulation and debate, and flags notable issues discussed by each author.

The chapters in Part I serve the following three purposes. First, the chapters by Albert R. Jonsen, Robert M. Veatch, and Terrence F. Ackerman display the continuing debate over whether the benefits of biomedical research should be balanced with, or curtailed by, the principles of respecting and protecting the human subjects of research. As major voices in the debate, these authors identify the basic principles of research ethics, illustrate how they should be applied, and differ over how they should be interpreted and prioritized. Second, Carol Levine indicates how and why the principle of justice has achieved new focus and influence over the last 15 years. Her chapter acquaints readers with some of the recent and dramatic changes in research ethics--in particular, research pertaining to AIDS and women's health. It also forecasts momentous changes adopted in 1994 for all NIH-funded projects regarding the inclusion of women and minorities in research.[73] Third, Charles R. McCarthy charts future challenges that will be faced by IRB members and administrators, as well as those who assume responsibility for reforming the regulations and ethics of research. The agenda of issues identified by McCarthy is extended by Fletcher and Miller in Chapter 7.

The essays in Part II focus on critical issues of conflict of interest that infest the just-sketched world and reach of research involving human subjects. The chapter by John C. Fletcher and Franklin G. Miller tackles what the stance of the federal government ought to be vis-à-vis controlling, supporting, or forbidding controversial areas of biomedical research. Their chapter critically examines the brief but turbulent career of "public bioethics," that is, bioethics analysis and policy formation at the federal level. They do this for the purpose of defining and shaping federal policy. Stuart E. Lind charts and analyzes the many ways financial issues and incentives influence clinical investigation. Beyond finger pointing on the one hand and defensiveness on the other, Lind challenges readers to reflect on and constructively deal with ethical issues of sponsorship, coercion, and the profit motive in research with human subjects. John La Puma discusses a largely uncharted but emerging and significant topic in the ethics of research with human subjects--physicians' involvements in post-marketing investigation. La Puma wrestles with the critical connections between the biomedical industry's marketing techniques, the laudable goal of assessing the efficacy of new drugs, and physicians' conflicts of interest.

Part III explores issues surrounding a controversy that became public in the late 1980s--the fear that adhering to Western research ethics in developing countries constituted "medical-ethical imperialism."[74] How should research with human subjects be conducted in developing countries? Should the construction and ranking of underlying ethical principles of this research be different from that of the operative principles of the U.S., Canada, and Western Europe? Exploring these issues provides insights regarding the nature and character of ethical inquiry, offers perspectives on how U.S. regulations should be interpreted and applied in non-Western settings, and assists IRB members in their review of Western-sponsored research conducted abroad.[75]

Similar to the chapters in Part I, the essays in Part III display ongoing ethical debates and examine present and developing regulations. Involved for years as a speaker and consultant in the development of national and international guidelines for research ethics, Robert J. Levine critically examines the adequacy and authority of the three historic codes of research ethics--the *Nuremberg Code*, the *Declaration of Helsinki*, and the *International Ethical Guidelines for Biomedical Research on Human Subjects* developed by the Council for International Organizations of Medical Sciences (CIOMS), each of which is printed in this book's appendices. Levine argues that the *Nuremberg Code* and the *Helsinki Declaration* are far less adequate than CIOMS's *International Ethical Guidelines*--particularly in transcultural research. He believes that damage, confusion, and consternation are caused by those who continue to appeal to the *Nuremberg Code* and the *Helsinki Declaration* as ultimate sources of ethical guidance.

Nicholas A. Christakis (U.S.A.) and Carel B. IJsselmuiden (South Africa) and Ruth R. Faden (U.S.A.) join the debate initiated by Levine: should ethical principles articulated in the West, including informed consent and its underlying principle of respect for persons' autonomy, be understood as universally required in cross-cultural biomedical research, or should it be subject to multiple (or culturally plural) interpretations and applications? The issues in this debate have long intrigued philosophers and ethicists, but they have only recently achieved urgency in the ethics of human-subject research. Because it explores the time-bound nature, limits, and conceptual problems of Western research ethics, this debate may have important implications for the future shape of research ethics in the West.

Part IV deals with four critical, cutting-edge areas of human research, each one the subject of controversy, ongoing deliberation, and, at times, entire conferences. Benjamin Freedman addresses ethical issues in cancer research. He shows how cancer trials presage ethically infused problems in other clinical arenas, and he raises challenging and innovative issues over the need to expand IRBs' ethical responsibilities. Instead of their present, narrowly defined functions, IRBs should be dealing with no less than a "superset" of ethical issues inherent to clinical trials from their design stage through their application in medical practice.

William G. Bartholome identifies the ethical blind spots in the current U.S. federal regulations involving research with children and makes his own contributions to the ethics of pediatric research. Based upon his mastery of and participation in explorations of pediatric research since the 1970s, Bartholome critically evaluates the contemporary literature, illustrates how core ethical principles apply to controversial protocols, and forecasts future challenges.

Constance M. Pechura profiles the science, regulations, and ethical issues regarding three hotly contested areas of research--on fetal tissue, on fetuses, and on embryos. With great clarity, she describes the interplay between scientific and technological advancements, ethical debates, and political pressures. Pechura's essay presents an agenda of philosophical and ethical issues for future analysis.

Part IV ends with Eric T. Juengst's chapter on a policy agenda for genome research. His discussion deals with 10 ethical questions that neither current rules nor practices completely address, including how to investigate the inheritance patterns of extended families, how to deal with the social and psychological risks of genetic studies, and when and how to disclose the interim results of such studies.

Altogether, these authors deal with "Critical Issues in Specialized Areas," the title of Part IV. Readers should nevertheless note that this final section does not encompass all the issues and areas that are discussed elsewhere in this volume--research pertaining to women's health, AIDS, post-marketing studies, and so on. The challenges are extensive and continuing.

NOTES

1. As its title indicates, this book explores the ethics of research *involving*, not *on*, human subjects. Though constantly used past and present, the preposition "on" connotes a position over others, whereas "involving" refers to the many levels of researcher-subject interaction. I thank Robert J. Levine for bringing this wording to my attention, and for his critical and helpful review of this chapter.

2. A.J. Dyck, *On Human Care: An Introduction to Ethics* (Nashville: Abingdon, 1977), 22.

3. H.Y. Vanderpool, "The Ethics of Clinical Experimentation with Anticancer Drugs," in *Cancer Treatment and Research in Humanistic Perspective*, ed. S.C. Gross and S. Garb (New York: Springer, 1985), 16-46, esp. 27-31.

4. A readable and useful discussion of ethical theories and principles vis-à-vis their applications in bioethics is found in T.L. Beauchamp and

J.F. Childress, *Principles of Biomedical Ethics,* 4th ed. (New York: Oxford University Press, 1994), 3-119.

5. As a form of reasoned discourse, ethical inquiry is suspended when persons assert that the rightness or wrongness of an action in question is based on some authority--for example, the authority of self, of a family member, a famous person, or a hallowed book or tradition. Such sources may indeed be, and at times are, wellsprings of moral guidance and insight, but their contributions must be identified and shown to be relevant and convincing before they can carry moral weight.

6. W. Stevens, "Of Modern Poetry," in *The Palm at the End of the Mind,* ed. H. Stevens (New York: Vintage Books, 1972), 174-75.

7. See the humorous and informative article by Andrew Taylor, Jr., who indicates how ethics is not what it is often taken to be, that is, the work of bureaucrats who "have wrapped medical (and animal) ethics with rules and regulations endowing that area of human activity with a rapacious capacity to gobble time and generate reams of paper work." A. Taylor, "Don't Confuse Me with Ethics: I Already Know What's Right," *Journal of Nuclear Medicine* 33 (1992): 296-303.

8. For example, ethical values are often compatible with and/or in conflict with other types of values. H.Y. Vanderpool, "Values, Valuing, and Ethics," in *The Values and Ethics of Medicine,* ed. H.Y. Vanderpool *et al.* (Galveston, Tex.: The University of Texas Medical Branch, 1994), 1-10.

9. For this outline I am indebted to the discussion of G.C. Graber, A.D. Beasley, and J.A. Eaddy in *Ethical Analysis of Clinical Medicine* (Baltimore: Urban Schwarzenberg, 1985), 99-102.

10. This is another point at which ethics intersects with nonmoral values, because these values are often viewed as the ultimate ends for human action. Consider, for example, the hedonistic value of happiness and/or pleasure, or (for Friedrich Nietzsche) the creative power of the human spirit, or (for Judaism, Christianity, and Islam) faithfulness to God and the holiness of life. See, for example, W. K. Frankena's discussion, "Intrinsic Value and the Good Life," in *Ethics* (Engelwood Cliffs, N.J.: Prentice-Hall, 1973), 79-94.

11. A succinct and clear discussion of virtue or character ethical theories is found in Beauchamp and Childress, *Principles of Biomedical Ethics,* 62-69.

12. This point of view is maintained by only one school of utilitarians. See Frankena, *Ethics,* 34-60; and Beauchamp and Childress, *Principles of Biomedical Ethics,* 47-55.

13. These principles often represent summations of extensive philosophical/moral inquiry. Since the principles or rules themselves are

viewed as determinates of moral obligation or duty, this approach to ethics is technically termed deontological--from the Greek word *deon* (that which is needful or obligatory).

14. Frankena, *Ethics*, 12-33; Beauchamp and Childress, *Principles of Biomedical Ethics*, 56-62; Dyck, *On Human Care*, 54-73, 92-113; and Vanderpool, "Ethics of Clinical Experimentation," 27-31.

15. Drawing upon the work of W.D. Ross, whose thinking is further discussed by Albert R. Jonsen in Chapter 3 of this book, each of these principles is viewed as *prima facie* (at first view) obligatory, as "an obligation that must be fulfilled unless it conflicts on a particular occasion with an equal or stronger [*prima facie*] obligation." Beauchamp and Childress, *Principles of Biomedical Ethics*, 28-40, at 33 (emphasis added). Robert M. Veatch's analysis in this book's Chapter 2 also exemplifies that of a nonconsequentialist who holds to multiple and interacting deontological principles (see especially Veatch's note 10). See also Vanderpool, "Ethics of Clinical Experimentation," 28-29.

16. A.R. Jonsen and S. Toulmin, *The Abuse of Casuistry* (Berkeley, Calif.: University of California Press, 1988), 1-19, 333-43; Beauchamp and Childress, *Principles of Biomedical Ethics*, 92-100; and Jonsen in Chapter 3 of this book.

17. G.H. Brieger, "Human Experimentation: History," *Encyclopedia of Bioethics*, (New York: Macmillan, 1978), 684-92; D.J. Rothman, "Research, Human: Historical Aspects," *Encyclopedia of Bioethics*, revised ed. (New York: Simon & Schuster Macmillan, 1995), 2248-58; and S.E. Lederer, *Subjected to Science: Human Experimentation in America before the Second World War* (Baltimore: Johns Hopkins University, 1995).

The term "experimentation" is ambiguous in that it can refer both to present-day controlled research (including randomized clinical trials) and to testing or trying something new or tentatively (which typified most past medical research and important degrees of patient care at present). To seek to avoid confusion, the terms "experiment" and "experimentation" will be used to refer to research involving human subjects in the past, while the terms "research," "biomedical research," and "clinical trials" will be used for contemporary controlled biomedical research. See the discussion in R. J. Levine, *Ethics and Regulation of Clinical Research*, 2d ed. (Baltimore: Urban and Schwarzenberg, 1986), 8-10.

18. Dictionaries commonly refer to this meaning of "ethics" as the second or third way the term is used. For example, in *Webster's New Collegiate Dictionary* (Springfield, Mass.: G. and C. Merriam, 1981), the second definition of ethics is rendered as "a set of moral principles or values" and "a theory or system of values." The first of the "three kinds

of thinking that relate to morality" listed by Frankena is that of "descriptive empirical inquiry," the goal of which is "to describe or explain the phenomena of morality." Frankena, *Ethics*, 5. Although descriptive ethics dwells on the taxonomy of moral assumptions and modes of reasoning within human culture, it is unavoidably "judgmental" in the weak sense of being value laden or value infested. This is true for all forms of human discourse, including scientific and medical thinking and writing. Provocative discussions of the many values inherent to concepts of health and disease are found in A.L. Caplan, H.T. Engelhardt, Jr., and J.J. McCartney, eds., *Concepts of Health and Disease* (Reading, Mass.: Addison-Wesley, 1981).

19. As soon as politicians and policy makers--including those who overtly appeal only to science and the social sciences--argue why some course of action ought or ought not to be undertaken, moral assumptions and modes of reasoning are brought into play. This appears to be true even for those who expressly discount the influence of moral reasoning. See Dyck, *On Human Care*, 18-23; and H.Y. Vanderpool, "B.F. Skinner on Ethics and the Control of Retarded Persons," *Linacre Quarterly* 45 (1978): 135-51.

20. This task accords with the first and most common definition of "ethic" in many dictionaries: "the discipline dealing with what is good and bad and with moral duty and obligation," (*Webster's*) or "a principle of right or good conduct," in *The American Heritage Dictionary*, 2d college ed. (Boston: Houghton Mifflin, 1982), 467.

21. Frankena, *Ethics*, 12-60.

22. As previously indicated, one area of ethical inquiry explores judgments about that which is ultimately good with respect to the purposes and ends of human action. This ultimate good was and is identified with the hedonistic value of happiness and/or pleasure by many utilitarians. In contrast, Aristotle associated this end (for Aristotle a means-end) with *arete*, the excellence encompassing human virtue (wisdom, courage, temperance, and justice) and intelligence within human communities--which Aristotle believed would result in happiness. The national, racial, and evolutionary ends of the Nazi party constituted a form of consequentialist nation-state tribalism, which is commonly but wrongly equated with utilitarianism. Consequentialists identify right or obligatory moral actions with outcomes or consequences, but they differ greatly with respect to what ultimate end(s) or goal(s) they have in mind. For discussions of the good and good ends, see A.K. Bierman, *Life and Morals: An Introduction to Ethics* (New York: Harcourt Brace Jovanovich, 1980), 380-414; and Frankena, *Ethics*, 79-94. The tradition of associating the Nazi experiments with utilitarianism likely stems from the influential article by Leo Alexander, "Medical Science Under

Dictatorship," *New England Journal of Medicine* 241 (1949): 39-47, esp. 39, 45. For the charge that Nazi physicians "grounded their actions on utilitarian principles," see, for example, F. Rosner *et al.*, "The Ethics of Using Scientific Data Obtained by Immoral Means," *New York State Journal of Medicine* 91 (1991): 54-59, at 55.

23. I. Van Der Sluis, "The Movement for Euthanasia, 1875-1975," *Janus*, 66 (1979): 131-72; and R.J. Lifton, *The Nazi Doctors* (New York: Basic Books, 1986).

24. Currying the favor of Heinrich Himmler, the Reichsfuhrer of the SS (*Schutzstaffel*, or Defense Echelon), and others, Rascher attracted the attention of high officials in the Nazi party. Accused of financial irregularities, the murder of an assistant, and scientific fraud, Rascher was executed, presumably on Himmler's orders. R.L. Berger, "Nazi Science–The Dachau Hypothermia Experiments," *New England Journal of Medicine* 322 (1990): 1435-40, esp. 1438-39.

25. For the text of the charges against Nazi physicians that details these experiments, see Telford Taylor, "Opening Statement of the Prosecution, December 9, 1949," in *The Nazi Doctors and the Nuremberg Code*, ed. G.J. Annas and M.A. Grodin (New York: Oxford University Press, 1992), 67-93. See also Eva Mozes-Kor, "The Mengele Twins and Human Experimentation: A Personal Account," in *Nazi Doctors and the Nuremberg Code*, ed. Annas and Grodin, 53-59; and Rosner *et al.*, "Ethics of Using Scientific Data," 54-59. Similarly brutal experiments were performed by Japanese doctors and scientists during World War II. In exchange for their scientific data and in the name of national security, U.S. authorities did not seek to prosecute these experimenters. See the summary discussions of A.M. Capron, "Human Experimentation," in *Medical Ethics*, ed. R.M. Veatch (Boston: Jones and Bartlett, 1989), 137-38; and P. M. McNeill, *The Ethics and Politics of Human Experimentation* (Melbourne, Vic., Australia: Cambridge University Press, 1993), 24-26; and the recent comprehensive study by S.H. Harris, *Factories of Death: Japanese Biological Warfare 1932-45 and the American Cover-Up* (London: Routledge, 1994).

26. Berger, "Nazi Science," 1435-40.

27. M.A. Grodin, "Historical Origins of the Nuremberg Code" in *Nazi Doctors and the Nuremberg Code*, ed. Annas and Grodin, 121-44. The 1931 regulations specified that "experimentation shall be prohibited in all cases where consent has not been given," that prior experiments on animals must serve to clarify and confirm the validity of human research, that experiments "shall be prohibited if it in any way endangers" the lives of children or young persons, and that no trials should include dying persons. *Ibid.*, 130-31 (which gives the full text of these regulations).

28. This episode in the history of human experimentation has been uncovered by D.J. Rothman, "Ethics and Human Experimentation: Henry Beecher Revisited," *New England Journal of Medicine* 317 (1987): 1195-99; and D.J. Rothman, *Strangers at the Bedside* (New York: Basic Books, 1991), 30-50.

29. Rothman, *Strangers at the Bedside*, 49-50.

30. Rothman indicates that six out of 238 subjects in a sulfonamide treatment protocol died apparently because of kidney damage. He adds that "there is no indication that the subjects or their relatives had any idea that they were part of an experiment." *Ibid.*, 35.

31. C.M. Pechura and D.P. Rall, eds., *Veterans at Risk: The Health Effects of Mustard Gas and Lewisite* (Washington, D.C.: National Academy Press, 1993). Similar experiments were conducted by Australian doctors and physiologists on Aborigines and armed-service personnel. McNeill, *Ethics and Politics*, 29.

32. See the full text of the code in this book's Appendix A. Notably, these principles were included in the 1931 ethical guidelines of the Reich Minister of the Interior (see note 27 above).

33. For example, it influenced the *Declaration of Helsinki* of 1964, and in modified form it was adopted by the Joint Chiefs of Staff of the U.S. Army, Navy, and Air Force in 1953, as indicated by J.R. Taylor and W. Johnson, "Summary of the Department of the Army Report" (1975), in *Veterans at Risk*, ed. Pechura and Rall, 379-438. The complete text of this U.S. armed services code, which was designated "Top Secret," is given in Annas and Grodin, *Nazi Doctors and the Nuremberg Code*, 343-45. In Chapter 10 of the present volume, Robert J. Levine further discusses the influence of the *Nuremberg Code*.

34. In his thoughtful overview of the ethics and regulation of human experimentation, A.M. Capron remarks, "The Nuremberg code in some ways amounted to a retreat from the German regulations [of 1931] which had emphasized institutional and not merely individual responsibility." Capron, "Human Experimentation," 135-72, at 146. See also the discussion of Fletcher and Miller in Chapter 7 at note 10 in the present volume. In the present book's Chapter 10, Levine argues that the *Nuremberg Code* should be viewed as flawed and time-bound. An outstanding discussion of the ways informed consent was defined, altered, and applied to biomedical research after Nuremberg is found in R.R. Faden and T.L. Beauchamp, *A History and Theory of Informed Consent* (New York: Oxford University Press, 1986), 151-232.

35. G.J. Annas and M.A. Grodin, "Where Do We Go from Here?" in *Nazi Doctors and the Nuremberg Code*, 314. Jay Katz concludes his assessment of this code by saying that it is "a remarkable document that stands alone in its unequivocal declaration of the rights, perhaps even

inalienable rights, of subjects to consent to participation in research."
J. Katz, "The Consent Principle of the Nuremberg Code: Its Significance
Then and Now," in *Nazi Doctors and the Nuremberg Code*, 227-39, at 235.
See also J. Katz, "Human Experimentation and Human Rights," *Saint
Louis University Law Journal* 38 (1993): 21-25.

36. Rothman, *Strangers at Bedside*, 51-69. In his 1959 review of the
history and ethics of research, Henry K. Beecher spoke of the crippling
effect of the *Nuremberg Code's* consent requirements on various types of
research and in favor of his view against setting down "many rules" in
the conducting of research. H.K. Beecher, "Experimentation on Man,"
Journal of the American Medical Association 169 (1959): 461-78.

37. The 1962 survey indicated that only nine of 52 reporting institutions (out of 86 departments of medicine contacted) had a documented
procedure for approving research involving human subjects, 16 of 52
had developed consent forms for research subjects, and 22 had review
committees that performed advisory functions. See the discussion of
W.J. Curran, "Governmental Regulations of the Use of Human Subjects
in Medical Research: The Approach of Two Federal Agencies," in *Experimentation with Human Subjects*, ed. P.A. Freund (New York:
George Braziller, 1969), 402-54, at 407. Later surveys in 1970 uncovered
"inadequate ethical concern" among many American investigators, 28
percent of whom, for example, would willingly approve of very high-
risk, low-benefit research. Peer review of protocols was found to be
weak and permissive in one-third of the institutions polled, and "the
poorer patients in hospitals" were bearing undue burdens of risky
research. B. Barber, "The Ethics of Experimentation with Human
Subjects," *Scientific American* 234 (1976): 25-31.

38. H.K. Beecher, "Ethics and Clinical Research," *New England
Journal of Medicine* 274 (1966): 1354-60. For a discussion of Beecher's
career and publications respecting the ethics of research, see Rothman,
Strangers at Bedside, 70-84.

39. Faden and Beauchamp, *History and Theory*, 161-64; and Levine,
Ethics and Regulation, 70-71. Lederer indicates that by the 1930s many
American physician-researchers had achieved celebrity status and the
public's confidence. Lederer, *Subjected to Science*, 126-38.

40. Rothman, *Strangers at Bedside*, 79.

41. J. Heller, "Syphilis Victims in U.S. Study Went Untreated for
40 Years," *New York Times*, 26 July 1972, 1, 8. Heller was alerted to this
study by an Associated Press colleague, Edith Lederer. Lederer had been
contacted and informed by Peter Buxtun, who, beginning in 1966 as an
employee in the Public Health Service, had been lobbying for the
study's termination on ethical grounds. See the superb historical narra-
tive by J. H. Jones, *Bad Blood* (New York: Free Press, 1993), esp. 188-205.

42. An abbreviated version of the *Final Report of the Tuskegee Syphilis Study Ad Hoc Advisory Panel* (Washington, D.C.: U.S. Public Health Service, 1973), is found in *Ethics in Medicine,* ed. S.J. Reiser, A.J. Dyck, and W.J. Curran (Cambridge, Mass.: MIT Press, 1972), 316-21. See also Faden and Beauchamp, *History and Theory,* 165-67.

43. The court settlement is discussed in Jones, *Bad Blood,* 212-19. The yearly costs are from unpublished remarks by Gary B. Ellis, Director of the Office for the Protection from Research Risks, at an annual conference sponsored by Public Responsibility in Medicine and Research (PRIM & R), 31 October 1994, Boston, Mass.

44. See Faden and Beauchamp, *History and Theory,* 81-234. Rothman's historical account deals with the interplay among the medical-ethics controversies over heart transplantation; congressional hearings on the ethical, legal, and social implications of biomedical advances; the recurring scandals over the Tuskegee Syphilis Study; as well as uncovered scandals over unethical contraceptive research in Tennessee and San Antonio, Texas. Rothman, *Strangers at Bedside,* 168-89.

45. The FDA called for Institutional Review Committees and informed consent in 1971. For developments in the U.S. between 1961 and 1983, see the discussion of Fletcher and Miller in Chapter 7 of the present volume, 158-66. Rothman discusses FDA and NIH responses to Beecher in *Strangers at the Bedside,* 87-100. The completed federal regulations were presented on 30 May 1974 by the Department of Health, Education, and Welfare (now called the Department of Health and Human Services) and were listed as Title 45, *Code of Federal Regulations (CFR),* part 46.

46. The 1991 regulations are duplicated in this book's Appendix D. They were printed in the *Federal Register* on 18 June 1991 under the titles of 16 U.S. departments, including, as revised, under Title 46 *CFR,* part 46, of the Department of Health and Human Services. These regulations include Subparts B ("Activities Involving Fetuses, Pregnant Women, and Human In Vitro Fertilization"), C ("Involving Prisoners as Subjects"), D ("Protection for Children"), and a final section on "Expedited Review Procedures." Henceforth, I will refer to the National Commission for the Protection of Human Subjects of Biomedical and Behavior Research by the abbreviated title of the National Commission.

47. On the local level, IRBs are called by many names--research ethics committees, local review committees, human investigation committees, and so on. Each local IRB is entrusted with the power to approve, revise, and/or disapprove all human-subject research protocols. Each IRB is responsible for "balancing . . . society's interests in protecting the rights of subjects and in developing knowledge that can benefit the subjects of society as a whole." The National Commission

for the Protection of Human Subjects of Biomedical and Behavioral Research, *Institutional Review Boards: Report and Recommendations* (Washington, D.C.: DHEW Publication No. (OS) 78-0008, 1978), 1. IRB members are to work closely with investigators and in keeping with current federal regulations. See Levine, *Ethics and Regulation*, 321-63, at 325. For a history of the development and use of these committees, see R.J. Levine, "Research Ethics Committees," *Encyclopedia of Bioethics*, revised ed. (New York: Simon & Schuster Macmillan, 1995), 2266-69; and the discussion of Franklin and Miller in this book's Chapter 7, note 10.

48. These agreements require that each institution has a local IRB that must be sure that each research proposal accords with federal regulations. "In effect, having set the standards for approval of projects (including minimal requirements for diversity of IRB membership), the government delegates the execution of its rules to research institutions based on their assurance that they will comply." Capron, "Human Experimentation," 147. Universities, medical centers, and many research institutes secure compliance-with-regulation contracts through the Office for the Protection from Research Risks (OPRR), the regulatory division within the U.S. Department of Health and Human Services. Hospitals and clinics that conduct human research for drug and medical-device companies must either have their own IRBs or utilize the services of for-profit IRB companies. FDA regulations require drug and medical-device sponsors of research to make commitments about the nature of such IRB review. Capron outlines the steps that must be taken to satisfy these assurance contracts. *Ibid.*, 147-48. Levine briefly discusses and contrasts the differing styles of oversight by the FDA and OPRR in *Ethics and Regulation*, 357-59. Perspectives on the functions of the OPRR and the contributions of IRBs are offered by Charles R. McCarthy, "Experience with Boards and Commissions Concerned with Research Ethics in the United States," in *Research Ethics*, ed. K. Berg and K. Tranoy (New York: Alan R. Liss, 1983), 111-22.

49. For current U.S. federal regulations, see note 46 above and Appendix D. The vignette given here on the emergence and character of U.S. regulations is both similar to and different from that of other nations. H. Sass, "Comparative Models and Goals for the Regulation of Human Research"; A. Shapira, "Public Control Over Biomedical Experiments Involving Human Beings: An Israeli Perspective," in *The Use of Human Beings in Research*, ed. S.F. Spiker *et al.* (Boston: Kluwer Academic, 1988), 47-89, 103-19; and P. Riis, "Experiences with Committees and Councils for Research Ethics in Scandinavia," in *Research Ethics*, 123-29.

50. Notably, the National Commission for the Protection of Human Subjects of Biomedical and Behavioral Research, "Belmont Report: Ethical Principles and Guidelines for Research Involving Human Subjects," *Federal Register*, 44 (19 April 1979): 23192-97, which is printed as Appendix C of this book.

51. Guidebooks on understanding and applying federally mandated U.S. policies for biomedical and behavioral research were first produced in the early 1980s. The most recent guide deals with the jurisdiction and administration of IRBs, compares regulations of the FDA and the Department of Health and Human Services, provides an extensive discussion of the ethical dimensions of IRB review, and discusses issues pertinent to special classes of research subjects--women, children, cognitively impaired persons, prisoners, and so on. The Office for the Protection of Research Risks *et al.*, *Protecting Human Research Subjects: Institutional Review Board Guidebook* (Washington, D.C.: U.S. Government Printing Office, 1993). The most thorough-going scholarly discussion of the interplay between these regulations and the work of the National (1974-1978) and the President's (1980-1983) Commissions, as well as the extensive medical ethics literature through 1985, is R.J. Levine, *Ethics and Regulation*.

52. This raises complex questions about the degrees and frequency of injuries to research subjects over time. Upon surveying the literature on injuries to research subjects from the mid-1970s through the early 1980s, R.J. Levine concludes that "the role of research subject is not particularly hazardous in general." Levine nevertheless registers a menu of worries over the various physical, psychological, and social risks and harms inherent to this research. R.J. Levine, *Ethics and Regulation*, 39-54, at 40. Published discussions of harmful experiments that continue to occur remind us that a *reduction* of injuries caused by research still means that hazards and injuries continue. J. Katz, "Human Experimentation and Human Rights," 41-51; B. Freedman, "Multicenter Trials and Subject Eligibility: Should Local IRBs Play a Role?" *IRB: A Review of Human Subjects Research* 16 (January-April 1994): 3; M.K. Cho, "Are Clinical Trials of Cell Transplantation for Duchenne Muscular Dystrophy Ethical?" *IRB: A Review of Human Subjects Research* 16 (January-April 1994): 12-15; and note 54 below.

53. T.E. Malone, "The Moral Imperative for Biomedical Research," in *Biomedical Research: Collaboration and Conflict of Interest*, ed. R.J. Porter and T.E. Malone (Baltimore, Md.: Johns Hopkins University, 1992), 3-32.

54. Addressing the widely held belief that problems in research ethics had been resolved, A.M. Capron commented prophetically in 1989, "today the subject is often naively viewed as one of settled ethical

principles . . . and multifaceted procedures. History suggests that such claims must be viewed skeptically: the principles may be less conclusive and the guidelines less protective than they appear." Capron, "Human Experimentation," 128. As Fletcher and Miller indicate in Chapter 7, pp. 160-66 of the present volume, turmoil continued during the 1980s over research on fetal tissue, human fertilization, genetics, and factors related to human behavior. The mustard gas experiments were brought to light in 1993 by a study conducted by the Institute of Medicine on behalf of the Department of Veterans Affairs. Pechura and Rall, *Veterans at Risk.* An *ad hoc* Advisory Committee on Human Radiation Experiments between 1946 and 1974 was formed by an executive order by President William Clinton in January 1994. The committee's reports indicate that these experiments were far more frequent and widespread than government officials had reported or admitted. The 1993 NIH drug trial on fialuridine (FIAU) resulted in neurological damage, severe toxicity, and liver failure on the part of seven research subjects, two of whom were probably saved from death by liver transplants. In the face of media alarm and investigations by the NIH and FDA, the National Academy of Science's Institute of Medicine (IOM) conducted a review of this and previous FIAU trials. While the IOM Committee found "nothing to suggest that the investigators were negligent," or that, given previous trials on the drug, the tragedy was preventable, it set forth a number of recommendations that would likely control for, but not "absolutely prevent" the recurrence of similar tragedies. Institute of Medicine, *Review of the Fialuridine (FIAU) Clinical Trials* (Washington, D.C.: National Academy Press, 1995), 151. Benjamin Freedman discusses several grim examples of unethical research and the ethical pros and cons of using information derived by immoral means in "Research, Unethical," *Encyclopedia of Bioethics* revised ed. (New York: Simon & Schuster Macmillan, 1995), 2258-60.

55. Gary Ellis, Director of the OPPR, telephone conversation with author, 2 September 1994. Combined with the funding supplied by other branches of the U.S. government--the Alcohol, Drug Abuse, and Mental Health Administration and the Departments of Defense, Energy, and Veterans Affairs--some $9.5 billion was being used to support biomedical research and development in 1989. An excellent survey of this support is provided by A.K. Dustira, "The Funding of Basic and Clinical Biomedical Research," in *Biomedical Research*, 33-56.

56. This author's survey yielded the following figures: Johns Hopkins, 1,500; the University of Alabama, 2,500; the University of California at San Diego, 2,000; the University of Michigan, 2,000; the University of Pennsylvania, 3,000; the University of Texas, Southwestern (Dallas), 1,600; the University of Washington (Seattle), 3,000; and

Vanderbilt University, 3,100. Like so much of the data on the funding and extent of biomedical research involving human subjects, these figures are not precise in their numbers and meaning. These high numbers likely include newly reviewed protocols, those subject to expedited review (see note 57 below), and research projects that are subject to continuing review (annual reapprovals). The discrepancies between these figures likely indicate that some of these institutions were reporting only their number of biomedical research projects subject to either expedited or full IRB review (as was the case with Southwestern in Dallas), while others were including behavioral and epidemiological studies that dealt with medical issues. Having recently completed an in-house survey of its research programs, the University of Washington reported that its 3,000 figure included all its epidemiological and behavioral research projects, but that its "biomedical" research included approximately 1,400 research projects: 1,000 the subject of full committee review and 400 for expedited review. Southwestern estimated that of its 1,600 active protocols, less than 320 were subject to expedited review.

57. Expedited review is allowable for protocols that involve no more than "minimal risk" to research subjects or for protocols that were previously approved, but that need minor changes. Such review is expedited in that only one or more experienced reviewers designated by the IRB chairperson (not the full IRB) can review and approve the protocol in question. "Minimal risk means that the probability and magnitude of harm or discomfort anticipated in the research are not greater . . . than those ordinarily encountered in daily life or during the performance of routine physical or psychological examinations or tests." See the 1991 federal rules and regulations (45 CFR, part 46, secs. 102 (i) and 111) in Appendix D of this book. Expedited review was first authorized by the DHHS in 1981.

58. These data are tentative. Executive administrators of IRBs readily state that they "have a good handle" on their total number of protocols but not on the number of research subjects that are being recruited. The University of Washington estimates that its biomedical research probably involves between 15,000 to 20,000 research subjects (a small portion of the approximately 300,000 subject-participants in its combined biomedical, behavioral, and epidemiological research). Other institutions estimate that some 10,000 subjects are being recruited for their biomedical research on a yearly basis.

59. These figures are from NIH's 1993 ranking of extramural awards to medical schools. While they are categorized as "research" funds, they do not indicate the amounts that are targeted for basic research, animal research, or clinical research involving human subjects.

60. Beecher, "Ethics and Clinical Research," 1354.

61. Rothman, *Strangers at Bedside*, 53, 59.

62. Although a separate study would need to be done in regard to the effects of inflation on biomedical research, a rough measure of these effects can be derived from consumer price indexes and estimates of the effect of inflation on the purchasing power of the dollar. These measures indicate that inflation caused the price of goods and services to increase 4.6 times between 1965 and 1993. To be equivalent with present-day purchasing power, the NIH's 1965 budget of $436 million would thus need to be $2 billion in 1993. In 1993, the NIH granted $2.04 billion in extramural research funding (a figure that excludes the NIH's training and fellowship grants) to 22 top-funded U.S. medical schools for some 3,098 research projects. These inflation figures are drawn from the *Statistical Abstract of the United States* (Washington, D.C.: U.S. Government Printing Office, 1994), 466-68.

63. An analysis and overview of one of these committees is provided in S.S. Herman, "A Noninstitutional Review Board Comes of Age," *IRB: A Review of Human Subjects Research* 11 (March-April 1989): 1-6.

64. Paul Goebel, telephone conversation with author, 28 September 1994. It is nevertheless clear that many studies funded by drug companies remain under the OPRR's purview insofar as they occur in institutions that receive federal support and maintain project assurance agreements with the NIH. Goebel added that at the present time more than 1,000 investigational new drugs (INDs)--many with more than one research protocol--are being researched under the sponsorship of drug companies and the oversight of the FDA.

65. As indicated by this figure, and the equally conjectural estimate of 250,000 research subjects for the top 25 U.S. medical schools above, there is little data on the number of research subjects recruited each year, on their socio-economic status, on the levels of risks they face, or on the number of subjects recruited for respective medical specialties.

66. See the 1992 in-house "Guides" of Independent Review Consulting (IRC) Inc., San Anselmo, Calif. For 14 years beginning in the 1970s, IRC's president, Erica Heath, administrated the IRB at the University of California at San Francisco. Heath believes that the OPRR "does a shoddy job" in its review and oversight of university-based IRBs. She has published examples of consent forms "that really honored subject autonomy" and confidentiality. E. Heath, "Improving Confidentiality in Pharmacoeconomic Studies," *Arena Newsletter* 7 (July 1994), 6-7.

67. This company, Western IRB, mostly works for U.S. firms, but each year it conducts protocol reviews in Great Britain, continental Europe, Canada, South America, and India. The company's CEO, Dave Boston, says that Western IRB "keeps its review boards separate from its business" and charges the same fee regardless of whether the protocol in

question is approved or disapproved. D. Boston, telephone conversation with author, 20 September 1994.

68. Dustira, "Funding of Basic and Clinical Biomedical Research," 34-46.

69. These phrases are used by Thomas E. Malone and Jay Katz, respectively. Malone says that medicine and industry are following "in the footsteps of the military, the nuclear, and the space establishments to become part of a medical industrial complex in which the researchers, the health care providers, and the manufacturers who supply them will be closely linked." Malone, "Moral Imperative," 30; and Katz, "Human Experimentation and Human Rights," 38. Concerns over the newly emerging "medical-industrial complex" were registered 15 years ago by Arnold S. Relman, "The New Medical-Industrial Complex," *New England Journal of Medicine* 303 (1980): 963-70.

70. P.G. Waugaman and R.J. Porter, "Mechanisms of Interaction between Industry and the Academic Medical Center," in *Biomedical Research*, 93-118.

71. T. Cooper and M. Novitch, "The Research Needs of Industry: Working with Academia and with the Federal Government," in *Biomedical Research*, 187-98, at 191.

72. C.C. Vaughan *et al.*, "The Contribution of Biomedical Science and Technology to U.S. Economic Competitiveness," in *Biomedical Research*, 57-76.

73. See Appendix E of this book for the 28 March 1994 NIH *Guidelines on the Inclusion of Women and Minorities as Subjects in Clinical Research*.

74. C.B. IJsselmuiden and R.R. Faden, "Research and Informed Consent in Africa--Another Look," *New England Journal of Medicine* 326 (1992): 830-33.

75. The most recent IRB guidebook asks, "Why must foreign sites abide by DHHS regulations?" It answers that this must be done "to ensure that all DHHS-supported or -conducted research involving human subjects provides subjects with protections that are at least equivalent to those afforded by DHHS regulations . . . those required by 45 *CFR* 46." Later this guidebook stipulates that although IRBs in America should be responsive to "local laws" and "population differences," IRBs dealing with "another," presumably non-American geographical or cultural setting, "may not take into account pertinent local factors." OPPR *et al.*, *Protecting Human Research Subjects*, 2-8, 2-11. The apparent discrepancy between researchers having to follow U.S.-equivalent protections of human subjects in non-U.S. settings and their being allowed to adjust Western ethics to the mores of minority populations within their own countries is far from resolved.

PART I

Current Debate Over Research Ethics and Regulations

Introduction to Part I

Harold Y. Vanderpool

Why does debate continue over the ethics and regulation of research involving human subjects? Whatever the controversy, what roles should ethical reasoning play in the decisions of institutional review boards (IRBs)?

IRBs AND ETHICAL REASONING

To begin with the roles of ethical reasoning, consider the position of *The Belmont Report*, which was published in the *Federal Register* in 1979 for the express purpose of setting forth "ethical principles that should serve as "guidelines" for IRBs' decisions.[1] *The Belmont Report* asserts that the rules and regulations governing research

often are inadequate to cover complex situations; at times they come into conflict, and they are frequently difficult to interpret or apply. Broader ethical principles will provide a basis on which specific rules may be formulated, criticized and interpreted.[2]

The import of these points is great for all who conduct clinical trials or are responsible for their regulatory oversight. Researchers and IRB members are mistaken if they merely attempt to conform in cookbook fashion to the letter of ethical codes and regulatory guidelines. Conformity alone is impossible because at times the rules of codes and guidelines conflict with each other, and they escape easy application.[3] While the range of decisions by IRB members and investigators are *delimited* by codes and regulations, decisions about their meaning and application constantly call for ethical reflection and discretion.

The Belmont Report itself is an interpretive exposition of research ethics at the federal level. Its framers viewed it as assisting researchers, subjects, and reviewers to understand the "ethical issues inherent in research" for "the resolution of ethical problems" arising from that research. Inescapably, all researchers and IRB members bring *their own* interpretive points of view into play as they prepare for, carry out, or oversee research involving human subjects. Ethical awareness expands, challenges, and shapes these points of view.

WHAT REASONING, WHAT PRINCIPLES?

Debate continues over the ethics and regulations of research with human subjects because of disagreements over the meaning and priority of basic ethical principles inherent to research. *The Belmont Report* identifies the following "three basic ethical principles": respect for persons, beneficence, and justice. Respect for persons means "that individuals should be treated as autonomous agents" and "that persons with diminished autonomy are entitled to protection." Beneficence is defined as "an obligation" encompassing two rules--do no harm, and maximize possible benefits and minimize possible harms.[4] Justice pertains to "who ought to receive the benefits of research and bear its burdens." In turn, each of these principles is especially pertinent to three respective applications: respect of persons applies to securing the informed consent of the subjects of research; beneficence especially applies to systematic and comprehensive harm-benefit analysis; and justice pertains to "fair procedures and outcomes in the selection of research subjects."[5]

Notably, *The Belmont Report* does not indicate how its three ethical principles (not to speak of additional principles within these three) should be weighted or prioritized. According to Albert R. Jonsen, a member of the National Commission that composed the report and the author of this Part's Chapter 3, IRBs are charged with weighing these principles and deciding how they should be applied.[6] Willingly or unwillingly, IRB members are expected to deliberate philosophically and ethically. This deliberation includes, but is not exhausted by, the principles articulated in *The Belmont Report.*[7]

Here matters become very interesting--and controversial. Should the three, free-standing principles of *The Belmont Report* be interpreted as more or less weighty depending upon the *particular circumstances* of the research in question? This is argued in Jonsen's provocative and crafted essay. Or should the work of the National Commission--work that included *The Belmont Report*--be viewed as giving birth to a new approach to research ethics--an approach predicated on the assumption that clinical research is "an obligation that society must undertake on behalf of its members"? Terrence F. Ackerman argues this perspective in Chapter 4.[8] Or should Belmont and the work of the National Commission be viewed as giving "absolute priority" to respect for persons' autonomy over the general good of society? Robert M. Veatch argues this viewpoint in Chapter 2.[9]

Yet far more is at stake in these authors' essays than disagreements over interpreting *The Belmont Report*. Veatch represents those who hold that respecting persons as autonomous, self-choosing agents should never be superseded or undermined by probable benefits to society.[10] This view stresses that persons should neither be morally *wronged* nor *harmed*.[11] Wrongs to persons include deception, not keeping promises, and touching or making a bodily intervention without express permission.[12] The notion of moral wrongs in research involving human subjects deserves more attention and analysis than it has yet received. Should wrongs (like harms) be morally ordered as, for example, grievous, regrettable, or excusable (under various circumstances)? Other than the individual who is wronged, who can determine a wrong's severity?

Jonsen and Ackerman represent "balancers," who view the principle of benefitting others via innovative biomedical research as outweighing autonomy in specific and circumscribed situations.[13] This position is implicit in federal regulations that detail what all informed consent should include *and* allow consent to be waived under stipulated circumstances.[14] Rooted in his extensive experience, Jonsen's intriguing exploration of the respective weights of moral principles in specific circumstances displays the cogency of casuistry, an approach to ethical decision making that has increasingly influenced bioethicists over the last 20 years.[15] Ackerman marshals arguments in favor of requiring persons to be involved in beneficial and harm-removing research "at modest cost to their own interests."[16] When is it moral to conscript unwitting or reluctant research subjects in society's battles against disease and disability? By drawing us inside these highly charged debates, these chapters enhance our understanding of research ethics and regulations and sharpen our decision-making abilities.

Beyond these controversies over how the ethical principles of *The Belmont Report* should be understood and applied, a national and international debate has recently emerged over the standing of *Belmont's* three basic principles themselves. Are the principles of respect for persons, beneficence, and justice "quintessential" and universally applicable, or are they culturally bound and limited?[17] Due to its import, this debate is placed in a separate part of this book--Part III. This part begins with an essay by Robert J. Levine, who questions the universal validity of the ethical and regulatory principles of the *Nuremberg Code* and the *Declaration of Helsinki* due to their errors and time-bound objectives.

THE PURVIEW OF IRBs

More effective decision making results from an enhanced understanding of research ethics for several reasons--the ability to identify otherwise unnoticed ethical problems, the ability to argue one's position well, the ability to formulate solutions with greater confidence, and so on. These abilities are valuable for researchers, administrators, and IRB members alike.

But what is the purview of IRBs, whose functions include educating their respective research-conducting communities? In Chapter 13, Benjamin Freedman briefly describes the "normal" and limited ethical concerns of many, if not most IRBs--the "tweaking" of consent forms, and so on. Based on extensive research on clinical trials, Freedman indicates why the ethical issues of research should be expanded to "a superset, rather than a subset" of scientific and clinical issues arising from "the design, management, interpretation, and application of clinical trials."[18]

Because Freedman's analysis focuses on cancer research, his chapter is placed in Part IV of this book. As indicated, however, his discussion is conceptually and ethically innovative. By challenging not the principles of research ethics, but the extent to which they should be applied, Freedman raises critical questions regarding IRB members' responsibilities.

JUSTICE

The principle of justice surfaces in two places in the 1991 U.S. federal regulations. Concerning a just selection of research subjects, these regulations state that selection must be "equitable" and that IRB members "should be particularly cognizant of the special problems of research involving vulnerable populations."[19] Concerning IRB membership, the regulations seek to assure fairness in protocol review by means of a "diversity of the [IRBs'] members." This includes diversity with respect to race, gender, and cultural background; the inclusion of one or more members who know firsthand about the needs of vulnerable subject populations; and at least one IRB member who is not affiliated with the IRB's institution.[20]

The Belmont Report discusses subject selection criteria much more extensively than these federal regulations. While *Belmont* mentions that justice pertains to both the benefits and burdens of research, it dwells on the burdens--the unjust treatment of disadvantaged black men in the Tuskegee syphilis study; a warning about recruiting easily available and manipulated welfare patients, racial and ethnic minorities, and persons confined in institutions; and the injustice of recruiting persons in research protocols who, later on, will probably not be "the beneficiaries of subsequent applications of the research" in question. In Chapter 4 Carol Levine charts how the principle of justly apportioning the *benefits* of research became pervasive and powerful in the 1990s. She describes how and why justice now centers on the *inclusion* of under-represented groups of research subjects--as evident in the regulations that were adopted in March 1994 by the National Institutes of Health (NIH). These regulations are required for all NIH-funded projects and are given in this volume's Appendix E.

Levine's challenging discussion rests on the thesis that in the late 1970s and early 1980s women and minorities were significantly excluded from research in order to avoid repeating historical abuses of research subjects. This contrasts with the thesis that these persons were excluded because of gender bias and racial discrimination.[21] Levine's analysis raises important questions over how a rationally just system of research resource allocation might be designed. What weights ought to be given to life-threatening conditions on the one hand and life-flourishing initiatives on the other? How should research allocation priorities be determined with respect to such factors as age, ethnicity, or the social contributions of those who stand to benefit?

ETHICS AND REGULATION

The relationships between ethics and regulations are not as simple as they might seem. As noted in Chapter 1, one of the three major areas of ethical inquiry deals with judgments of moral obligation--what humans ought or ought not to do, how we should or should not treat others.[22] Similar to judgments of moral obligation, regulations also proscribe and prescribe behavior. As apparent from the foregoing discussion of *The Belmont Report*, the ethical principle of respect for persons, for example, was "packaged" and applied as procedural guidelines regarding informed consent.

Yet ethical judgments differ from regulations in important ways. First, the rational and experiential "oughts" of ethics become "musts" in regulations that are backed by the force and penalties of law. Second, regulations of research involving human subjects include more than "packaging" the *ethics* of research into procedural, behavioral guidelines for researchers. After the oughts or purposes of ethics are stated as regulatory procedures, additional regulations are formulated for the purposes of their being followed and enforced.[23]

Third, no easy, one-to-one relationship exists between general principles of ethics and their being transposed into specific rules of regulatory procedure. Even as all moral rights or wrongs cannot and should not be stated as regulations,[24] so also adherence to existing regulations does not automatically mean that even weighty moral principles are being honored. Some of the back-and-forth relationships between ethics and regulations are exemplified in the essays by Carol Levine (Chapter 5), Charles R. McCarthy (Chapter 6), and John C. Fletcher and Franklin G. Miller (Chapter 7).

Consider, for example, how the U.S. federal regulations of 1983 and 1991 state very briefly that the selection of subjects should be "equitable," but then give no procedural directives on how to apportion the burdens and benefits of research more fairly via egalitarian selection and recruitment of subjects.[25] Carol Levine shows how, in response to a broad-based movement for greater access to the benefits of research, new regulations to ensure just allocation of resources were put in place by federal grant-sponsoring agencies. Beginning in 1990, these agencies drew up explicit procedural requirements regarding the recruitment of greater numbers of women, minorities, and AIDS patients into ongoing and newly established research initiatives. Having surfaced as a broad based social-ethical concern in the early 1990s, the principle of justly apportioning the benefits of research was transposed into particular and required procedures well before the new, more sweeping guidelines were adopted by the National Institutes of Health (NIH) in March of 1994.[26]

NIH's 1994 *Guidelines on the Inclusion of Women and Minorities as Subjects in Clinical Research* (reproduced in Appendix E of this book) now require measures that exceed those previously adopted. They require that women and members of minorities and their subpopulations must be included in "all NIH-supported biomedical and behavioral research projects involving human subjects, unless a clear and compelling rationale and justification establishes . . . that inclusion is inappropriate with respect to the health of the subjects or the purpose of the research."[27] The inclusion of these groups must not be delimited by the costs involved and must be predicated on programs and outreach efforts designed to actively include these groups in clinical studies. For all NIH-funded projects, IRBs are now charged with the task of upholding these new mandates without compromising former regulations--for example, the requirement of making sure that the incentives and rewards associated with recruitment initiatives avoid coercion or undue influence.

In Chapter 6 Charles R. McCarthy raises other important issues of ethics and regulation. Forecasting future changes and challenges, he wonders whether IRBs will be able to retain their present degree of self-regulation in the face of congressional probes of reported instances of IRBs' noncompliance. McCarthy also identifies several issues that are not addressed in the 1991 *Code of Federal Regulations* or *The Belmont Report*--for example, how to improve the spotty records of National Data and Safety Monitoring Committees and how to rectify the lack of regulatory procedures over compensating harmed and injured research subjects. McCarthy asks how these and newly emerging issues can be dealt with when the present *Code of Federal Regulations* cannot be changed without the approval of all 16 federal agencies.

The essays in this section and those that follow illustrate how, once reformed, the ethics and regulations of human subjects' research are ever reforming. Although complaints will continue to be made over the ethical complexities and bureaucratic constraints of research involving human subjects, this research has expanded exponentially since the 1970s. The symbiosis between ethics and regulation established at the federal level in the U.S. after 1974 seems to have *justified*, not just curtailed, new and expanding research initiatives. By being responsive to changing social sensitivities, ethical ferment and regulatory adjustments appear to ease the public's anxiety and increase the public's trust in the ever-expanding reach of clinical research.

NOTES

1. This report merits the category of "required reading." The latest version of the guidebook, published by the Office of the Protection from Research Risks (OPRR), is entitled *Protecting Human Research Subjects: Institutional Review Board Guidebook* (Washington, D.C.: U. S. Government Printing Office, 1993). The OPRR is the division within the U.S. Department of Health and Human Services (DHHS) that is responsible for assuring that researchers and their institutions comply with federal regulations regarding human subjects research. Its guidebook designates *The Belmont Report* as its "seminal policy statement on the protection of human subjects of research," which contains principles that "are now accepted as the three quintessential requirements for the ethical conduct of research involving human subjects," *xv-xxi*. Existing U.S. federal regulations, however, barely mention ethics. In discussing "Assurances of Compliance," the regulations say that each institution needs "a statement of principles" governing its IRB. "This may include an appropriate existing code, declaration, or statement of ethical principles" (45 *Code of Federal Regulations (CFR)* Part 46.103.b.l.). The

current U.S. *Code of Federal Regulations* is reprinted in Appendix D of this book. Under the subject of IRB membership, the regulations stipulate that "the IRB shall be able to ascertain the acceptability of proposed research in terms of institutional commitments and regulations, applicable law, and standards of professional conduct and practice" (45 *CFR* 46.107.a).

2. That *The Belmont Report* is to be used by IRBs is clear both implicitly (from its title and its appearance in the *Federal Register)* and explicitly. Under section C (Applications), part 2 ("Assessment of Risks and Benefits") the report discusses procedures that will make "communication between review board members and investigators less subject to misinterpretation"; and it discusses how to determine whether "an investigator's estimates of the probability of harm or benefits are reasonable."

3. Several areas of conflict are discussed in chapters that follow. Consider, for example, how the "basic elements of informed consent" in 45 *CFR* 46. 116a conflict with the various ways consent can be waived in 116d.

4. Other expositions and authors maintain that this definition of beneficence should be distinguished as two principles—beneficence (providing benefits and balancing benefits against risks and harms) and nonmaleficence (the norm of avoiding the causation of harm). The "four-principles approach" of Beauchamp and Childress thus includes respect for autonomy, nonmaleficence, beneficence, and justice. T.L. Beauchamp and J.F. Childress, *Principles of Biomedical Ethics*, 4th ed. (New York: Oxford University Press, 1994), 37-38.

5. These quotations are taken from all the major, admirably brief, sections of *The Belmont Report*.

6. A. Jonsen, Chapter 3, p. 64 of this book.

7. See the discussion on "doing ethics" in Chapter 1. Other ethical principles and/or dimension of research involving human subjects include privacy, confidentiality, promise-keeping, and the virtues of character and disposition of researchers as moral agents. See the discussion of J.F. Childress, "The Normative Principles of Medical Ethics," in *Medical Ethics*, ed. R.M. Veatch (Boston: Jones and Bartlett), 28-48, esp. 36-37; and (on virtue), A. Jonsen, Chapter 3, pp. 68, 80-81 of this book.

8. T. Ackerman, Chapter 4, p. 91 of this book. Ackerman carefully delimits the extent to which this social obligation should affect the individual.

9. R. Veatch, Chapter 2, pp. 51-53 of this book.

10. For Veatch, respect for persons is a deontological, duty-based moral principle that can be counterbalanced only by some other nonconsequentialist duty. For a discussion of deontology versus utilitarianism (or some other version of consequentialism), see Chapter 1, p.

4 of this book. Other autonomists include Hans Jonas, Jay Katz, and George Annas. See H. Jonas, "Philosophical Reflections on Experimenting with Human Subjects," in *Experimentation with Human Subjects*, ed. P. Freund (New York: George Braziller, 1969), 1-31; J. Katz, "The Regulation of Human Experimentation in the United States--A Personal Odyssey," *IRB: A Review of Human Subjects Research* 9 (January/February 1987): 1-6; J. Katz, "Human Experimentation and Human Rights," *Saint Louis University Law Journal* 38 (1993): 7-54; and G. J. Annas and M. A. Grodin, *The Nazi Doctors and the Nuremberg Code*, ed. Annas and Grodin (New York: Oxford University Press, 1992), 3-11, 307-14. These writers share a common aversion to past justifications of abuses of research subjects in the name of a society's well-being.

11. R. Veatch, Chapter 2, pp. 47-49 of this book. Some investigators and IRB members assume that their primary moral duty involves protecting research subjects from risks of harm--as connoted by the name of the Department of Health and Human Service's (DHHS's) ethics oversight agency, the Office for Protection from Research Risks (OPRR). This assumption is indebted in part to certain of the federal regulations themselves, wherein expedited review is allowed for research that "involves no more than minimal risk" (45 *CFR* 46.110); and the requirement of obtaining informed consent can be waived (in part) because the experiment in question "involves no more than minimal risk to the subjects" (45 *CFR* 46.116.d). Against the view that "What's the harm?" is the fundamental question for research ethics, Parker and Lidz comment in their analysis of coercion that "it is deception, misinformation, and unknowing or unwilling participation contrary to participants' interests . . . against which IRBs should seek to protect study participants." L. S. Parker and C. W. Lidz, "Familial Coercion to Participate in Genetic Family Studies: Is There Cause for IRB Intervention?" *IRB: A Review of Human Subjects Research* (January-April 1994): 6-12, 9.

12. R.J. Levine discusses how laws of negligence penalize offenders if that negligence results in harm, whereas laws of battery make it "wrong *a priori* to touch, treat, or do research upon a person without consent. Whether or not *harm* befalls the persons is irrelevant; it is the 'unconsented-to touching' that is *wrong*." R. J. Levine, *Ethics and Regulation of Clinical Research*, 2d ed. (Baltimore: Urban & Schwarzenberg, 1986), 97 (emphasis added). Compared to data about how often persons are harmed in research involving human subjects (see this book's Chapter 1, notes 52 and 54), data on wrongs is extremely sketchy--in part because of difficulties of observing and verifying such wrongs.

13. The rhetoric of "balancing" has been used ever since the U.S. Congress began to debate the need to regulate medical research involving human subjects. For example, on the Senate floor in October 1962,

Senator Jacob Javits of New York affirmed, "I am for experimentation . . . but we must hold the balance between . . . the right of the individual to know how his life is being disposed of . . . and the virtues of experimentation." Quotation from R. R. Faden and T. L. Beauchamp, *A History and Theory of Informed Consent* (New York: Oxford University Press, 1986), 203.

14. The detailed elements of informed consent are listed in 45 *CFR* 46.116.a. In addition to the examples provided by Jonsen in Chapter 2, patients-subjects who are brought to emergency rooms with severe head injuries illustrate circumstances in which informed consent has to be waived if research on new therapies is conducted. E. D. Prentice *et al.* "An Update on the PEG-SOD Study Involving Incompetent Subjects: FDA Permits and Exception to Informed Consent Requirements," *IRB: A Review of Human Subjects Research* 16 (January-April 1994): 16-18.

15. For a discussion of casuistry and Jonsen's theoretical perspective, see Chapter 1 above at note 16. For changing perspectives in medical ethics, compare the approaches voiced by Tom L. Beauchamp and James F. Childress in the first edition of their influential book, *Principles of Biomedical Ethics* with their latest, 4th edition. T.L. Beauchamp and J.F. Childress, *Principles of Biomedical Ethics* (New York: Oxford University, 1979), 3-55; and *Principles of Biomedical Ethics*, 1994, 17-119. In their 4th edition, Beauchamp and Childress discuss and critique their former "deductivist, covering-precept" model of ethical reasoning that deduces moral judgments "from a preexisting theoretical structure of normative concepts." They then opt for "coherentism," an approach that "is neither top-down nor bottom-up," 14-28, quotations from 14 and 20.

16. Ackerman, Chapter 4, pp. 96-98, 101 of this book. Arguments based on implicit social contracts in favor of a duty to participate in research have been advanced by Arthur L. Caplan, "Is There an Obligation to Participate in Biomedical Research?" in *The Use of Human Beings in Research*, ed. S. F. Spiker *et al.* (Boston: Kluwer Academic Publishers, 1988), 229-48.

17. See note 1 above for the OPRR's position on the "three quintessential" ethical requirements contained in *The Belmont Report.*

18. B. Freedman, Chapter 13, pp. 323-28, 335-36 (quotes from 336) of this book.

19. 45 *CFR* 46.111.a.3 in Appendix D of this book.

20. 45 *CFR* 46.197.a, b, and d.

21. The gender and racial bias thesis is argued by Rebecca Dresser, "Wanted: Single, White Male for Medical Research," *Hastings Center Report* 22 (January-February 1992): 24-29.

22. See Chapter 1, pp. 3-4 of this book.

23. Federal regulations of research thus include behavioral guidelines for *researchers,* as well as guidelines for IRB *reviewers* that include requirements for IRB reporting and compliance. For the interplay between these regulatory functions, see Chapter 1, pp. 10-11 of this book.

The abuses of Nazi experimenters indicate how the existence of regulations and laws governing researchers are ineffective without a framework of mandated and ongoing oversight at the local and federal levels.

24. With respect to the regulations of research with human subjects, the relationships between the many parties involved and the numerous circumstances that arise are so varied and complex that a mountain of regulations laden with countless "ifs" and "thens" could not address them all. See the discussion and examples of when ethical norms should not be enforced as law in Beauchamp and Childress, *Principles of Biomedical Ethics,* 1979, 11-12.

25. The revised 1991 regulations briefly expand upon those of 1983 by adding that IRBs "should be particularly cognizant of the special problems of research involving vulnerable populations, such as children, prisoners, pregnant women, mentally disabled persons, or economically or educationally disadvantaged persons" (45 *CFR* 46.111.a.3). This addition continues the emphasis on protecting vulnerable populations from the burdens and risks of research. Nothing is mentioned about allocating the benefits of research more equitably. Both sets of regulations assume that vulnerable populations of patients will be protected from bearing undue burdens by regulations that govern protocol design, the consent process, and the composition of IRBs.

26. Required procedures concerning the inclusion of women and minorities in study populations were set forth, for example, in *NIH Guide for Grants and Contracts* 20 (N. 32, 23 August 1991): 1-3. Before the new inclusionary guidelines were adopted by the NIH in March 1994, the 1993 OPPR *Guidebook* stipulated that the in-house procedural requirements of the NIH and other agencies must be followed by IRBs. The guidebook legitimated this change of rules under the single "equitable" clause of the *Code of Federal Regulations, Institutional Review Board Guidebook,* 3-23 to 3-26 and 6-11 to 6-17.

27. *NIH Guidelines on the Inclusion of Women and Minorities as Subjects in Clinical Research,* III.A. in Appendix E of this book. Critical questions over a preceding version of these guidelines are raised by Marcia Angell, "Caring for Women's Health--What is the Problem?" *New England Journal of Medicine* 329 (July 1993): 271-72.

2

From Nuremberg
Through the 1990s:
The Priority of Autonomy

Robert M. Veatch

It may turn out that the period from Nuremberg to the 1990s will be seen as the high-water mark for the principle of autonomy in clinical research. I am going to suggest that if that is so, it will pose significant moral risks to society in general and to the research enterprise in particular.

The core of the old Hippocratic ethic is that whatever the clinician does should be done for the benefit of the individual patient. Many lovers of the Hippocratic Oath probably do not realize that, taken seriously, the oath prohibits all research with human subjects, at least research designed to produce generalizable knowledge. Thus the centuries of medical ethics prior to the middle of the present century--centuries that were in the Hippocratic tradition--were essentially without a commitment to autonomy or self-determination. Clinical research is not undertaken for the benefit of the individual. Innovative therapy may be, but not full-blown research that focuses on production of socially useful knowledge.[1]

From the time of Claude Bernard in the 19th century, we have been headed for this crisis. Bernard realized the crucial importance of doing systematic research.[2] He may not have realized that it was in direct conflict with Hippocratic clinical ethics.

NUREMBERG AND AUTONOMY

All this came to a head at Nuremberg. Nuremberg made it clear that some members of the medical profession had abandoned the Hippocratic commitment. These members believed that they could benefit society by compromising some subjects--for the good of the *Volk*. True, they had a bizarre notion of who was a member of their society, but theirs was essentially a logic of subordinating the individual to the interests of the larger group.

In 1946 at Nuremberg the world had a stark choice between two plausible options, neither of which allowed for serious infringements of the interests of others for the good of the *Volk*. It could have returned to pure Hippocratism, making all clinicians single-mindedly loyal to their individual patients. Logically, this would have made all clinical research--that is, all research designed to gain generalizable knowledge--unethical. Or it could have come up with a new ethic that would permit "use" of subjects without violating their integrity as members of the moral community.

We made the second choice. The second principle of the *Nuremberg Code* said, "The experiment should be such as to yield fruitful results for the good of society. . . ."[3] Taken by itself, this second principle, of course, opens the door to a full-blown utilitarianism. The individual could be sacrificed for the good of the social cause.

But the research enterprise was rescued by the introduction of a whole new idea, self-determination or autonomy. The first article of Nuremberg, the one given first prominence, is that "the voluntary consent of the human subject is absolutely essential."[4] The moral principle of autonomy (and its subsidiary consent doctrine) thus saved medical research from a retreat to Hippocratic individualism.

AUTONOMY AND BALANCING THEORIES

Nevertheless, single-minded respect for autonomy comes at an awful price, or at least so say autonomy's critics. If autonomy is the highest moral priority, investigators are put to awful trouble. There are enormous costs in trying to inform subjects in order to comply with moral, legal, and administrative requirements. Sometimes there is no real reason to believe that patients would be hurt if we just assumed that patients could be used for research and we finessed the consent process that respect for autonomy requires. Given the data on the low number of reported harms to research subjects, there are very strong reasons in terms of social costs why autonomy should be compromised.

AUTONOMY AND BENEFICENCE

Aren't there times when autonomy just has to give way to social benefits? I don't think so. Consider the following case that I encountered some years back while serving on an IRB in New York. An investigator wanted to do some biochemical studies on normal human tissue. Not wanting to take the tissue from normal volunteers, he asked the IRB for approval of a study that would secure placental tissue from the delivery room. This tissue is usually discarded, but it would have served the investigator's purposes well. Surely no one would have objected to putting it to a good use.

The IRB easily agreed that the study offered benefits equal to the risks. That was easy; there were no risks. But then the committee turned to the question of consent. The investigator proposed that no consent be obtained. The IRB members were divided. The majority thought that getting consent was a silly waste of time. A minority thought that the women should be asked, that asking them would show respect for them as persons. Some women might have felt that they would want to know about the use of their tissue even if there were no risk involved. Still, the majority of the IRB members (including females) thought that consent would serve no purpose. The women were in no danger. The placentas would have been otherwise discarded.

I took this case to a class I was teaching at Vassar College. Since it had only recently been converted to a coeducational institution, the students were mostly female. About one-third agreed with the IRB. Two-thirds would have wanted to be asked. They said that they would feel violated if they were not asked. They wanted to be respected as persons.

There were two good reasons to respect the women's autonomy and ask them to agree to the use of their tissues. First, there was a utilitarian reason. A significant number of them might have been mad if they had found out that they had not been asked: mad at the researcher, researchers in general, the hospital, and at the research enterprise. Not only this investigator, but researchers in general, could have suffered from a bad public outcry against researchers perceived as unethical or uncaring. From the utilitarian perspective, informing subjects and securing their consent may turn out to be a wise investment of time. It just would not be a good investment of the good will that still exists toward research to spend it on short cuts that could be perceived as abusive.

Second, and more fundamental, it just would not be a decent way to treat a human being. It would treat them as a means to someone else's ends without their approval. It would leave them feeling violated. Treating persons as means and not ends violates the fundamental Kantian imperative. From the perspective of a formalist or deontologist, there are behaviors that are morally wrong even if they do not do harm to people. Failing to show them respect as persons by using them as means to another's end without their consent is the epitome of such a wrong.

AUTONOMY IS FEASIBLE

Part of the complaint of researchers against the priority for autonomy is that they feel that respecting autonomy makes research impossible. I think that this is almost always just plain false. Consider the case of the research with the placentas. One could have gotten consent during prenatal visits. They only would have needed a few to agree. Even the more militant Vassar students said that they would have agreed if asked.

Blank-check or uninformed consents. In many research projects a "blank-check" or "uninformed" consent upon admission would make research easier. For example, for use of medical records for research, many would probably agree to a blanket authorization. The use of body wastes also probably would qualify. Patient/subjects need not consent to a specific protocol or to the use of specific information.

Is such a blank-check consent adequate to respect autonomy? Under the reasonable-person standard, the investigator must tell the subject what he or she would reasonably want to know in order to consent. In some cases, some people may only want to know that their records may be used for some research. In those cases autonomy would be adequately respected. Researchers would have told them all they wanted to know to make an informed choice. Autonomy would be respected.

Misinformed blank-check consents. But what of the cases in which such blank-check consents would leave patients misinformed? What of cases in which it would leave them failing to grasp the true nature of the use of their information or wastes? One of the elements of an informed consent is the purpose of the study. Why is this included? Obviously not to protect subjects from risk. In some cases, such as the placenta study, there is none. Rather it is to permit subjects to refuse to be part of a project that is offensive to them.

Consider, for example, a proposed psychiatric study of adolescent females who refused to abort their first pregnancy. The apparent goal of the study was to better understand the psychological make-up of the refusers in order to intervene to help them overcome their resistance to abortion. It is clear that the record search would have done no harm to these young women; they would never again be first-time abortion refusers and could not be affected by the search of their records (provided confidentiality from outside disclosure would be adequately maintained). Still, they clearly could have had strong objections to the purpose of the study. They also might have objected to the breach of confidentiality that would arise when the researchers themselves--strangers to these unwitting subjects--would see highly sensitive, personal psychiatric information. When patients are asked to sign a blank-check consent for research use of records, how can they be protected from the rare instance when they would strongly object to participating in the study, not because of the risks, but because of their objection to the purpose of the study or to the invasion of privacy?

Using IRBs to test the reasonable-person hypothesis. I would propose as a solution to this problem a provision that if any investigator wants to rely on blanket consents for the use of medical records or bodily wastes or for clandestine observation of patients, the IRB must be informed and must approve. The investigator would be claiming that merely telling the patient of the general possibility of such research would adequately inform the patient, would tell the patient all that the reasonable patient would want to know. If the investigator were to rely on such blanket consents without violating the patient's autonomy, he or she would have to be able to support the hypothesis that the patient would not want to be told anything about the study other than the general fact that some research use might be made of the patient. The IRB would have to be asked to verify that such a hypothesis was plausible. When it did, then the research could proceed without violating the autonomy of the patients.

A problem with IRB judgments about consent. When an IRB is asked to evaluate the adequacy of a consent, it must guess what patients would want to be told. But the IRB's guess of what subjects need in order to have their autonomy respected may not be right. If the IRB had been evaluating consents for those Vassar students, the IRB would have guessed wrong.

There is no basis for assuming that a male-dominated group of professional researchers would guess correctly about what a group of female subjects with different ages, education, and value systems would want to know in order for their autonomy to be respected. If the reasonable-person standard is the correct one for evaluating consents in an era of autonomy, and I believe that it is, then the judgment of the investigator, of a consensus of investigators, or of the IRB about what subjects would want to be told can never be certain.[5] This is one of the serious flaws with a balancing strategy that relies on wisdom or *phronesis* (or what can sometimes better be called biased intuitions or a gut feeling) supported in one way or another by both Albert Jonsen and Terrence Ackerman in this book. There is no way to assure consistency or objectivity if IRBs or investigators are urged to balance off competing claims. Any person asked to trade off competing moral principles will necessarily be influenced by deeply held, poorly understood biases.

A better approach would be to ask a group of potential subjects whether they would want to be told of the proposed research. Some colleagues and I did precisely that in a study designed to test the feasibility of empirically documenting what groups of subjects would want to be told in order to make their consent truly informed.[6] An IRB was trying to guess whether or not those who donated to a blood bank would want to be told that their blood was going to be used for research. Finally, we drew a sample of blood donors and asked them; 52 percent said that they would want to be asked.[7]

Ruth Faden has done something similar.[8] She and her colleagues wanted to figure out which side effects of Dilantin patients in a seizure clinic would want to be told about. They particularly wanted to compare what patients wanted to be told with what the clinicians believed they should be told. They found that the patients' views were very different from those of the physicians in the clinic. In general, patients wanted to be told of many more side effects than clinicians believed necessary to disclose. They particularly wanted to know about certain cosmetic effects (such as increased hair growth) even though they acknowledged that being informed would not dissuade them from agreeing to the medication.

If one wants to respect autonomy and is clever in the way research is designed, respecting autonomy is almost always feasible. It can be done without enormous inconvenience. Failing to do so runs a terrible risk to the research enterprise. More importantly, it runs the risk of failing to treat patients as autonomous agents who are partners in the research enterprise. Social benefits, by themselves, never can justify such a violation.

JUSTICE AND THE LIMITS OF AUTONOMY

Does this mean that there is never any basis for overriding autonomy? I don't think so. Both Ackerman and Jonsen make the fundamental mistake of assuming that, if autonomy is to be overridden, it is to be by the principle of general beneficence, by the social good served by the knowledge to be gained.[9] They grasp the fact that there are cases in which it is terribly implausible to give autonomy absolute priority, and they jump to the erroneous conclusion that the interests of others in society (what Mill called the harm principle) provide the basis for limiting autonomy. That, I am convinced, is a serious mistake.

OTHER WAYS OF OVERRIDING AUTONOMY

Social benefit is not the only moral principle that can conflict with autonomy. There are other moral duties that are part of the general duty to show respect for persons. They include the principles of truth telling, fidelity to promises, and avoidance of killing. They are as fundamental as autonomy. They are not based on producing benefits and avoiding harms. I therefore refer to them as principles that are not consequence maximizing. Sometimes I simply call them deontological duties.[10] Occasionally a duty based on one of these principles can come into conflict with autonomy. This is quite rare in research medicine, but when they do conflict, autonomy does not always win out over these principles related to respect for persons, even if it does always win out over producing social benefits.

JUSTICE AS OVERRIDING AUTONOMY

The principle of justice also can be viewed as a duty separate from merely producing social benefits. Justice requires distributing benefits fairly. Nonutilitarian theories of justice hold that there is some pattern of distribution of goods that is inherently morally right, even if it does not maximize aggregate net benefits. In an egalitarian world, that can mean arranging social practices so that they benefit the least well off. Even if such an arrangement fails to benefit society as a whole as much as some other practice would, defenders of an egalitarian principle of justice would say that the distribution is right, at least *prima facie*.

If justice is a moral principle independent of social beneficence, then it is possible that sometimes justice can legitimately restrain autonomy even if social beneficence cannot. Thus, in theory there may be cases in clinical research in which the desperate medical needs of the least well-off could justify compromising autonomy. Probably that won't happen often, but it can.

For instance, suppose there were an epidemic leading to terribly traumatic death in small children believed to be spread by adult carriers who themselves suffered no symptoms. If record searches of possibly infected adults, against their consent, were deemed necessary to study the epidemiology of the disease, autonomy might be seen as losing out, not because of the great good to be done, but because of the fact that a group who were among the worst-off had claims of justice against the relatively well-off suspected carriers. It is not necessarily the amount of good expected, but the relative well-being of the ones whose autonomy is violated and the ones to benefit, that justifies compromising autonomy.

It is crucial to realize that although Jonsen and Ackerman appeal to *The Belmont Report* and the work of the National Commission to support their appeal for balancing strategies, there is no evidence that the commissioners actually supported balancing. Both *The Belmont Report* and the federal regulations list principles that must be satisfied. The most reasonable reading of that requirement is that they all must be satisfied before research is ethically acceptable. Hence, the report on children permits only minimal risk or minor increase over minimal risk if specified conditions are met.[11] The fact that only limited risk is tolerable, regardless of the potential benefit, supports the view that the

National Commission was not willing to go the full way to balance beneficence and respect for subjects as Jonsen and Ackerman suggest.[12] If they were, they would logically permit larger and larger risks to children for larger and larger social gains. Likewise, the requirement of assent of children and permission of parents that is a condition of such research would make no sense if society were willing to balance social benefit against respect for the rights of nonconsenting subjects; it would make good sense if respect for persons were lexically ranked above general beneficence.

Some might question how authorization of research on nonconsenting subjects based on parental permission is consistent with an absolute priority of respect for persons over general beneficence. First, the fact that there is any such limit on research that could serve the general welfare significantly is itself telling. Second, it is a mistake to assume that respect for the rights of children completely prohibits parental decisions to authorize minimal risks to the child for the good of others. Parents are expected to teach their children charity; requiring a small child to contribute a portion of an allowance to charity is either not contrary to the child's long-term interest at all or, if it is, it is consistent with the parental responsibility to train the child in social responsibility. That is surely not the same as permitting the parent to sacrifice the child for the greater social good. The National Commission's recommendations on children make sense only if respect for the individual is given an absolute priority over the social good.

Even the provision for exceptions by a National Ethical Advisory Board supports this claim. Note that it is not just any social good that can justify nonconsenting research; it is limited to problems affecting the health and welfare of children. Moreover, it must be necessary to prevent or alleviate a *serious* problem. That I take to be an implicit appeal to compromise the integrity of a child only when others have a claim of justice, not when they have claims grounded in general beneficence. Consider two cases that could involve recruitment of children in ways requiring approval from the National Board. In one, very large numbers of people could benefit modestly while in another a small number of children could have a "serious problem alleviated." It is possible that the total amount of good could turn out to be exactly the same in the two cases. Yet the National Commission recommends board authorization only in the second case, a result incompatible with balancing approaches that would, in principle, permit general beneficence to outweigh the rights of the minority if only the aggregate good were great enough. Jonsen and Ackerman cannot explain why the second case is different from the first; a theory that permits justice to compete with autonomy but gives autonomy an absolute priority over beneficence does provide an explanation.

PRACTICAL LIMITS ON JUSTICE-BASED CONSTRAINTS

While it may be true that in theory the principle of justice could constrain autonomy, it is critical to emphasize how unusual those circumstances would be. Rigid requirements would have to be met if justice were to override autonomy. In effect this is a decision to sacrifice bodily integrity, privacy, and self-determination for the benefit of the least well-off. This flies in the face of some of America's most cherished values. It should be done very carefully.

The closest analogy I can think of is with military conscription. Conscription deprives citizens of liberty and autonomy at some risk to bodily integrity for the good of society. I believe that this is only justified in the name of justice, not simply aggregate social utility.

Additional criteria must be met if conscription is to be ethical. Whether the conscription is into the military or into the medical-research enterprise, there must be public due process. An act of Congress is necessary to legitimate military conscription. It should also be necessary to authorize compromises with the autonomy of research subjects.

To be ethical, there would have to be substantive as well as procedural fairness in the policy. The policy would have to satisfy the criterion of publicity; that is, the policy would have to be announced publicly so that all would know about it and have the right to challenge it. (That, in effect, is what the proposal to submit special cases before a public national board would accomplish.) Moreover, everyone who could be used in the study would have to be equally exposed to the risk of being conscripted. There would have to be a public-appeal process. Finally, conscription of subjects would have to be the least invasive way to accomplish the end sought.

I think it is extremely unlikely that *any* compromises with the autonomy of research subjects would be able to satisfy these criteria. Until they do, priority must be given to the autonomy of potential subjects to decline to be part of some investigator's personal ambitions.

A FINAL TEST CASE: AUTONOMY AND THE RIGHT OF ACCESS TO EXPERIMENTAL TREATMENTS

As a final test of this slightly qualified lexical priority of autonomy in research with human subjects, consider the cases of people who are increasingly demanding the right of access to experimental treatments before those treatments have completed their clinical trial process and met FDA requirements for general use.

AUTONOMY AS A LIBERTY RIGHT

AIDS has taught us that autonomous, rational people may perceive that it is in their interest to gain access to experimental chemotherapeutic agents such as AZT and ddI. This is also true of desperately ill cancer patients. Moreover, the same case can be made for access to experimental treatments for less dramatic, less terminal conditions. Men and women want to take aspirin to attempt to prevent myocardial infarction. They do so based on preliminary evidence or even rumor.

It is crucial to realize that their views are not irrational. In some cases it makes sense to want to try an untested drug when one decides that, compared with the alternative, the potential benefits justify the risks involved.

All randomized clinical trials must be justified ethically by a sincerely held belief that the risks and benefits of two treatment options are more or less equal. We must be at or near what I for many years have called the "indifference point."[13] Others have called this the point of "equipoise."[14]

Estimating the risks and benefits is inherently a subjective process. Some people may calculate the risks and benefits of the options in an atypical manner. They may have a rational but subjective preference to be in one of the different groups (or arms) of a randomized clinical trial, even while the investigators and the IRB are honestly indifferent. If their preference is for the standard treatment, right now they have an automatic right of access. If their preference is for the experimental treatment, right now they have no such right of access.

Does a priority for autonomy give them a right of access to experimental agents, not only over-the-counter agents such as aspirin, but also restricted drugs controlled by investigational new drug (IND) research?

AUTONOMY IS A LIBERTY RIGHT

Autonomy is a liberty right. It gives people the right to be left alone, to be protected from unconsented touching. It is the right to be free from conscription into research without consent. It does not give one an entitlement to controlled investigational agents. Thus, if an individual can gain access to it--say, if it is available as an over-the-counter preparation--he or she has the right to use it in a way not proved beneficial.

Still, if it is rational for some people to have preferences for experimental agents even while investigators remain at their indifference points, it might be in such a person's interest to get access to not only over-the-counter drugs, but to experimental agents as well.

It sometimes is a decent and noble thing for investigators to help such patients pursue their interests. Hence, we now have policies permitting compassionate-use exemptions, treatment INDs, and parallel-track uses. If investigators were willing to cooperate with subjects who had rational, subjective preferences for IND agents, then their own autonomy as well as that of the subjects would support their providing the agents to them.

But do they ever have a moral duty to cooperate in helping to provide access to such investigational agents? At first, it would seem that they have the moral right, but not the duty, to cooperate. To grant any more would violate the autonomy of the investigator. The researcher as well as the subject would have rights grounded in autonomy.

But what is the implication of the claim that justice can sometimes override autonomy (even if general societal benefit cannot)? An egalitarian view of justice holds that the worst-off patients have claims of justice that sometimes override autonomy. Many of the patients we are talking about easily qualify as among the worst-off members of society: AIDS patients or metastatic cancer patients, for example. In principle, I believe that these patients have an entitlement-right claim to access to experimental agents. That claim is *prima facie*; it can be overridden by other considerations. Still, morally they have a legitimate and rationally defensible claim to the experimental agents. If they are plausibly among the least well-off, they have claims of justice that may override the autonomy of the investigators. In such cases, I believe that the priority of autonomy would disappear. The investigators would have a moral duty to help the least well-off gain access to experimental treatments when they had a rational, if subjective, belief that the treatment would be in their interest. It is what we owe to the least well-off among us. Then, and only then, would autonomy give way, not in favor of maximizing aggregate social benefits, but in favor of a *prima facie* principle of justice.

CONCLUSION

Autonomy has been a key principle in the transition from the pure patient-centered paternalism of the Hippocratic era to one in which human subjects can be used as a means to social ends. Autonomy commands a priority that cannot be surrendered to mere social beneficence. If autonomy is to be given the priority that it deserves, the autonomy of investigators, as well as that of patients, must be respected. Autonomy stands between us and a moral abyss. I have tried to show what a very cautious compromise of autonomy might look like, one grounded not in social beneficence but in justice. Until we develop such a guarded alternative to autonomy and know precisely how we will protect ourselves from the dangers of naked utilitarianism, I am not willing to compromise on giving autonomy an absolute priority.

NOTES

1. For the distinction between research and innovative therapy, see R.J. Levine, "The Boundaries Between Biomedical or Behavioral Research and the Accepted and Routine Practice of Medicine," in *The Belmont Report: Ethical Principles and Guidelines for the Protection of Human Subjects of Research,* by the National Commission for the Protection of Human Subjects of Biomedical and Behavioral Research (Washington, D.C.: U.S. Government Printing Office, 1978), Appendix I, 1-1 - 1-44.

2. C. Bernard, *An Introduction to the Study of Experimental Medicine,* trans. H.C. Greene (New York: Dover, 1957).

3. *The Nuremberg Code,* Appendix A of this book.

4. *Ibid.*

5. President's Commission for the Study of Ethical Problems in Medicine and Biomedical and Behavioral Research, *Making Health Care Decisions: A Report on the Ethical and Legal Implications of Informed Consent in the Patient-Practitioner Relationship,* vol. 1 (Washington, D.C.: U.S. Government Printing Office, 1982), 27.

6. R. Winer *et al.,* "Informed Consent: The Use of Lay Surrogates to Determine How Much Information Should Be Transmitted," in *The Patient as Partner -- A Theory of Human-Experimentation Ethics,* ed. R.M. Veatch (Bloomington, Ind.: Indiana University Press, 1987).

7. *Ibid.,* 168.

8. R.R. Faden *et al.,* "Disclosure of Information to Patients in Medical Care," *Medical Care* 19 (19 July 1981): 718-33.

9. Jonsen, Chapter 3 of this volume; and Ackerman, Chapter 4, pp. 93-99.

10. In calling them deontological, I realize that some rule utilitarians also support these principles on the grounds that adhering to them maximizes consequences better than any other set of rules does. Thus not all who subscribe to these principles can be labeled deontologists. I have developed my view of these nonconsequentialist principles in R.M. Veatch, *A Theory of Medical Ethics* (New York: Basic Books, 1981), borrowing generously from the classic, W.D. Ross, *The Right and the Good* (Oxford: Oxford University Press, 1939).

11. National Commission for the Protection of Human Subjects of Biomedical and Behavioral Research, *Research Involving Children: Report and Recommendations* (Washington, D.C.: U.S. Government Printing Office, 1977).

12. Jonsen, in Chapter 3 of this book; and Ackerman, in Chapter 4 of this book.

13. Veatch, *The Patient as Partner,* 210-11.

14. B. Freedman, "Equipoise and the Ethics of Clinical Research," *New England Journal of Medicine* 317 (1987): 141-45; N. Johnson, R.J. Lilford and W. Brazier, "At What Level of Collective Equipoise Does a Clinical Trial Become Ethical?" *Journal of Medical Ethics* 17 (March 1991): 30-34.

3

The Weight and Weighing of Ethical Principles

Albert R. Jonsen

This essay is about the metaphor in the common expressions, "What is the weight of this moral principle? How do we balance this principle against that one?" In this metaphor, principles are like pineapples or prize fighters. Each one of them is a material object with mass and dimensions; each one weighs in at so many kilos or pounds and, when put on a scale and measured against other objects, tips the balance or is tipped. What is the moral meaning behind the metaphor? How has that moral meaning functioned in deliberations about the ethics of research involving human subjects?

A passage written by the doyen in the field of law and ethics of human experimentation, Professor Jay Katz, exemplifies marvelously the use of the metaphor. In his essay, "The Nuremberg Code Consent Principle: Then and Now," Professor Katz reflected,

Had the [Nuremberg] Tribunal been aware of the tensions that have always existed between the claims of science and individual inviolability . . . it might have suggested that a balancing of these competing quests is necessary. . . . Even if the Tribunal had been aware of this problem, I hope it would not have modified its first principle, "The voluntary consent of the human subject is absolutely essential." It is this assertion that constitutes the significance of the Nuremberg Code then and now. Only when that principle is firmly put into practice can one address the claims of science and the wishes of society to benefit from science. Only then can one avoid the dangers that accompany *a balancing of one principle against the other that assigns equal weight to both;* for only if one gives primacy to consent can one exercise the requisite caution in situations where one may wish to make an exception to this principle, but only for clear and sufficient reasons.[1] (Italic added.)

From this passage, the words "only then can one avoid the dangers that accompany a balancing of one principle against the other that assigns equal weight to both" provide the text for this essay about moral metaphors. I preface the essay with my confession of belief in Professor Katz's creed, lest it appear that, in making distinctions, I depart from its strong central affirmation: the voluntary consent of the subject is the absolutely essential feature of the code and of the ethics of research with human subjects.

First, then, some clarification of the metaphor itself. We know weight and weighing from experience: we pick up a heavy box of books; we step on a bathroom scale; we toss some items out of a suitcase to lighten the load. Seldom do we have recourse to physics for a scientific explanation of that experience. When we do, we learn that weight is the force on a body due to gravity and that $W = M(mass)g(gravity)$. Moving rapidly from physics to the history of science, we learn that the word "gravity" was first used in 17th-century English to describe, not the force field of a celestial body as it did after Newton, but rather "heaviness"--as distinct from "lightness." Moving from the history of science to linguistics, we realize that in its original Latin, *gravitas* means both "the heaviness of a material body or object" and "the seriousness of a subject or the social importance of a person." Thus, Caesar could write of *gravitas armarum*, or "heavy weapons," and Cicero of *gravitas sententiarum*, or "serious opinions." Why the link between physical and moral heaviness?

A sentence from the great Jesuit mathematician Clavius, who wrote in pre-Copernican days, suggests the reason for the link. "The earth," he said, "insofar as it is the greatest weight [*gravitas*], tends naturally to the natural point which is the center of the universe."[2] The gravity of a person, an event, comes from the fact that it tends to center itself, to become the point around which other persons, events, or opinions circle. It becomes, as Milton wrote of "some beauty . . . the cynosure of neighboring eyes," the focus of attention and admiration.

MORAL PHILOSOPHY AND BIOETHICS

Now this rapid voyage through physics, linguistics, and poetry brings us to philosophy and to moral philosophy in particular. The scholarly tradition of moral philosophy has not been particularly concerned about weighing and balancing, since it has, from Plato down to Rawls, been absorbed in the task of finding a single architectonic principle with the power of pulling into ordered lines all possible moral rules or maxims, like satellites orbiting an intellectual center. Weighing and balancing are, in the classical systems, less important than ordering and inferring. Even Rawls, who invoked the metaphor in his famous "reflective equilibrium," considered that an advantage of his other technique of "lexical ordering" was that it "avoids having to balance principles at all; those earlier in the ordering have an absolute weight with respect to later ones and hold without exception." Utilitarianism, he noted, "is a single-principle conception with one ultimate standard; the adjustment of weights is, in theory, settled by reference to the principle of utility."[3] Rationally impressive theory, deep but elegantly simple, is the elusive goal of modern moral philosophy. That elegant simplicity is, in Spinoza's phrase, an *ethica modo geometrica*, "theory is moral geometry." We all know that, while tables and chairs, buildings, and ballistic missiles have weight, their geometry has none.

Contemporary bioethics is a child of that classical tradition, but, having been born in the 1960s, it is a conflicted flower child: it cannot but speak in the language of principle and theory that it inherited, but it liberates itself from that inheritance by chanting four principles and paying equal reverence to at least three distinct types of ethical theory: deontology, consequentialism, and contractarianism. It has, until quite recently, blithely ignored the consequent confusion and incoherence. Look at most of the textbooks of bioethics--they open with chapters explaining in neutral terms the dominant ethical theories and principles, never making it clear whether the reader should select one or use all.

In their deservedly popular text, *Principles of Biomedical Ethics,* Beauchamp and Childress have moved further. After expounding the types of ethical theory, they proposed what they call a "composite theory," which "permits each basic principle to have weight without assigning a priority weighing or ranking.

Which principle overrides in a case of conflict will depend on the particular context, which always has unique features."[4] They have noted that Baruch Brody's "pluralistic theory" has much in common with their "composite theory."[5] They then recalled W.D. Ross's proposal about *prima facie* duties, in which "the overriding duty is found by locating 'the greatest balance of right over wrong in the circumstances of conflict between those principles,'"[6] and they agreed in part with his "metaphor of weights moving on a scale." Yet, even with this departure from the rigid adherence to a single theory and a univocal principle, we are left with some mystery. What does it mean to say, as Beauchamp and Childress did, "What principle overrides . . . will depend on the particular context, which always has unique features"? How do the unique features of a particular context provide weight to a principle or tip the balance toward one rather than the other?

PRINCIPLES, PROBLEMS AND PRACTICES

These important questions are open to interminable debate at the speculative level. If the debate must issue in some concrete recommendations for action, however, speculation must attend to the exigencies of practical reasoning and, in so doing, may learn something. This was the case, I submit, when Congress established the National Commission for Protection of Human Subjects of Biomedical and Behavioral Research in 1974. During the previous decade, medical science had been the beneficiary of growing public support and funding. Then the revelation of several episodes in which the rights and welfare of human subjects of research had been abused began to tarnish the moral probity of the research enterprise. Congress, pressured from various sides, set up a body to recommend ways to protect the rights and welfare of subjects in the light of general ethical principles that should govern the conduct of research. This was the first public body charged with the task of relating ethics to public policy. As such, it had to bring speculative moral philosophy into the real world of moral commitments and moral conflict. It had to turn abstract principles into practical resolutions.

Congress specified the tasks of the National Commission: it was to study several particular problems, such as research with the human fetus, with children, with the mentally infirm, and with prisoners; it was also charged with developing general ethical principles relevant to research with human subjects. For the purpose of this essay, I will discuss the way in which the National Commission responded to the mandate to "identify the requirements for informed consent to participation in biomedical and behavior research by children . . . or their legal representatives."[7] The National Commission's report, *Research Involving Children,* was issued in September 1977, and its recommendations were issued as regulations in the *Federal Register* on 8 March 1983.[8] As a member of that Commission, I can agree with Leonard Glanz's comment that these "were among the most difficult for the policymakers to draft and adopt."[9] One reason for the difficulty lay in the formulation of the congressional mandate, "to identify the requirements for informed consent . . . by children . . . or their legal representatives."

It has often been noted that the first principle of the *Nuremberg Code,* "voluntary consent . . . is absolutely essential," was shaped in response to the moral abominations of the Nazi concentration-camp experiments. The victims of this deadly exploitation were as far from volunteers as humans could be. Persons in captivity were the center of attention. It has also been noted that so primary and absolute a principle unequivocally excludes from research children or others who are mentally incompetent. This exclusion was eliminated by the *Declaration of Helsinki,* 1964, which admits the consent of legal guardians for such subjects.[10]

The National Commission had to wrestle with two issues that went beyond the principles enunciated in the *Nuremberg Code* and the *Declaration of Helsinki*: Is it ever the case that a child's consent should be sought and respected? What should be the conditions of a valid consent by a legal representative? These were difficult enough, but then a further problem loomed, one that the congressional mandate had not foreseen, but which the commissioners felt they must address. What would be the ethical course if the nation encountered a danger to children's health that had to be met by research that posed significant danger to the children who would be its subjects? Could legal guardians, held to protect the best interest of their charges, consent to such research? We knew that such situations had existed in the not-distant past: would the epidemics of poliomyelitis have been beaten back by vaccines without such dangerous experimentation? We could not, in 1972, have foreseen the AIDs epidemic that would begin to threaten the lives of children a decade later.

At the same time that the National Commission was working on the *Children's Report*, it was developing what became known as *The Belmont Report,* a document that would state the general ethical principles governing research with human subjects. The *Nuremberg Code* and the *Declaration of Helsinki* were both statements of principles; the commission hoped to propose even more basic moral foundations for the practice of human research. At the same time, it recognized that basic moral foundations had to be linked with specific practices that could be incorporated in the activities of research. After considerable debate and wide consultation, the commission enunciated three basic ethical principles that should govern all research with human subjects, namely, respect for autonomy, beneficence, and justice. It associated these three general principles with the practices of informed consent, risk-benefit assessment, and fair-selection processes. These three practices would incorporate the three principles into the actual conduct of research in the clinical setting. The report did not suggest any directions for weighing or balancing these principles should conflict arise between them, nor did it provide clues about whether the practices were ever open to exception or limitation. It did not give detailed recipes about how particular "tough cases" should be resolved. Recognizing, however, that these questions would arise, the commission endorsed the policy of establishing institutional review boards (IRBs) in each research institution. These review boards would be charged with the interpretation and application of the principles and practices in every case in which an investigator wished to use a human person as a research subject. *The Belmont Report* was issued in 1978.[11]

ABSOLUTE PRINCIPLES

The basic ethical principles of *Belmont* certainly looked like W.D. Ross's *prima facie* principles, although those words appear nowhere in the document. The old Oxford don must have smiled in his philosophical heaven to see these latter-day Americans adopt his ethical theses. The commissioners, most of whom had never read a word by Professor Ross, were thinking like him, and they eventually found themselves faced with the same problems that he had left unsolved in his books: How does one determine actual duty when several *prima facie* rules conflict? The *Children's Report* pushed that problem from the speculative to the practical and required an answer that could be translated into public policy.

When the National Commission undertook the *Children's Report*, it encountered a strong wall: the powerful interdiction of theologian Paul Ramsey against any research that does not directly benefit the individual child subject.[12] Ramsey himself had argued this position before the commission, but, despite his powerful logic and persuasive rhetoric, he had not prevailed. The commission had also listened to Jesuit theologian Richard McCormick and, in the end, inclined to his thesis that nontherapeutic research could be permitted when there can be a reasonable presumption that the child would consent.[13] But, having accepted this position, the commissioners realized that they had to go beyond a statement of principle. They were in the position of "the reasonable person," in the language of the common law, or the "ideal observer," in moral philosophy: they had to decide on such matters as the degrees of risk that a "reasonable child" would accept, the significance and the likelihood of anticipated benefit to the child, and the importance of the results of the research to other children and to the society itself. Only so could we make sense of the phrase "reasonable presumption." Thus, the recommendations of the *Children's Report* are studded with terms like "minimal risk," "minor increase over minimal," "more than minimal risk," "experiences reasonably commensurate," and "significant benefit." The commission realized that these terms required definition. At the same time they realized that, as a recent article on the subject put it, "The term(s) cannot be defined without specifying a context: minimal risk to what end, from whose point of view and under which situation . . . 'minimal risk' is relational, context-dependant."[14] The commissioners had been transmogrified into a covey of casuists, debating, not the principles of things, but the "who, what, when, where, why and how much" of particular situations.

The fifth and sixth recommendations of the *Children's Report* inspired great debate. The fifth recommendation stated that "research in which more than minimal risk to children is presented by an intervention that does not hold out the prospect of direct benefit for the individual subject may be conducted," and it then stated five conditions for approval of such research. The sixth recommendation stated that any research that could not be approved under the conditions of recommendation five could be considered by a National Ethical Advisory Board if it presented the "opportunity to understand, prevent or alleviate a serious problem affecting the health and welfare of children." These two recommendations shattered the unanimity of the commission. Over the four years of the commission's life, almost all recommendations had issued from the consensus of the commissioners. Now, two commissioners dissented from Recommendation Five, and three different opinions, concurred in by various commissioners, were issued. In the end, however, a commission dedicated to the principle of respect for autonomy and to the rule of informed, voluntary consent, had concluded that it was not inconceivable that a nonconsenting subject could be subjected to research that was of no direct benefit or, more precisely, that legitimate surrogates could assent to procedures that might not be in the best interest of their charges.

How could we show our faces before Dr. Katz, who, as we noted above, has said that the first principle of Nuremberg should be taken literally, that it is absolutely essential? Not only had we stretched it to include proxy voluntary consent, but we had envisioned the possibility that such consent might be given when the interests of the subject would not be protected and promoted. Yet, remember that Dr. Katz went on to say, "Only if one gives primacy to consent can one exercise the requisite caution in situations where one may wish to make an exception to the principle, but only for clear and sufficient reasons."

What does the term "absolute" mean if exceptions can be entertained? Once again, a bit of etymology may help us understand. Absolute derives from the Latin *absolvere*, which, in the past-perfect participle, is *absoluta*, meaning, "separated, cut free from." A principle or rule is absolute when considered apart from circumstances. Thus, it does not mean "without exception" but rather "considered in itself." In this sense, "absolutely necessary" says nothing about the weight of the principle; it merely says, "in principle necessary." Considerations about weight must come from elsewhere. Let us explore in hopes of finding the source of moral weight.

HOW MORAL PRINCIPLES ACQUIRE WEIGHT

In the opening pages of this essay, Father Clavius, a pre-Copernican astronomer, was quoted as saying that the earth has gravity because it falls to the center of the universe. Similarly, a moral principle is "weighty" when it falls to the center of consideration within the universe of moral considerations relevant to the problem under consideration. Its weight is its importance or significance in deliberation about the issue. That "weight" derives from several related sources. First, it comes from the way in which a society in a particular cultural tradition cultivates certain ideas and values, enacting and reinforcing them in its intellectual, social, and religious life. Second, it comes from the critical examinations to which such central ideas are subjected by what passes for philosophy in the society. Each of these sources is extremely complex; social and intellectual history, as well as current sociology and philosophy, are required to clarify them. There is a third source of weight in ethical decision making, rather different than these two, which I will explain after reviewing the first and second sources.

The first source of moral weight is the intellectual, social, and cultural traditions of a community. Certain moral notions accumulate weight as a tradition rolls through time. Take as a recent example Robert Bellah's work on the idea of "individualism" in American culture, reported in his book, *Habits of the Heart*. Bellah wrote, "American cultural traditions define personality, achievement, and the purpose of human life in ways that leave the individual suspended in glorious, but terrifying, isolation."[15] This is the modern precipitate from a long "historical conversation," which includes "biblical and republican strands." Our current American emphasis on "respect for autonomy" as an ethical principle is inexplicable outside of that tradition. The tradition of political and moral liberalism, as it becomes mainstream within a culture, has pushed to the margins of the culture—the population margins and the intellectual margins—other principles that are incompatible or fit clumsily at best. For example, religious zealotry, which demands that all conform to an orthodoxy, is intellectually and politically incompatible with liberalism and respect for autonomy. Thus, but not without strife, it is pushed to the margins and, not without strife, it may be kept there. It has little or no weight in deliberations about moral and social issues within the dominant culture, although it may flourish within minority communities.

Thus, in our culture, respect for persons is a principle that has considerable weight. It outweighs the marginalized principles that I mentioned above. It also outweighs other principles that are commonly accepted as worthy but have "lost weight" by attrition of the social conditions in which they flourished. For example, it would be commonly accepted that "family loyalty" or "respect for elders" were good things; however, given significant changes in the sociology and economics of the family in our culture, these good things are much less weighty as ethical notions than they were in earlier times. Clearly, the principle of autonomy outweighs a panoply of other moral notions that may serve major purposes in other cultures but are only minor functions in our own. Punctilious etiquette toward persons of various social classes, rigorous conventions of honor, and elaborate linguistic formulas are important morally in other societies, but not in ours. Thus, in this sense it is not difficult to find some principles that have more weight than others within a social tradition.

The weight that comes from cultural tradition may be encapsulated in various views of moral character and moral roles that are fostered in those traditions. In a society that promotes the belligerent defense of homeland, courage is a prized virtue; in one that promotes individual autonomy, the virtues of enterprise and ingenuity are encouraged. Thus, principles that are weighty in a cultural tradition derive further weight at the level of personal character. This is also true, I believe, of social roles within societies, where a certain moral character will typify a certain role: the honest politician, the competent lawyer, the compassionate doctor, the solicitous minister, and so forth. The general principles of a moral tradition take on a more personal face. In a moral debate, persons who cultivate those characters and enact those roles may weigh the appropriate principles more heavily. Thus, we often note that physicians prefer beneficence over autonomy.

These anthropological observations do not get us very far, however. It is not the balancing of central against marginal principles or significant against trivial ones that causes moral perplexity. It is the balancing of central and significant ones against each other. It is possible to demonstrate that individualism, with its consequent ethical principle of respect for persons, is central in American culture. However, it is also possible to demonstrate that beneficence, the duty to help others, has played a consistent place in Western culture and American life. Similarly, justice and fairness are central and significant notions. The problem of balancing arises when autonomy must be balanced against beneficence and beneficence against justice. These notions all have, in the abstract, equivalent gravity or, put less surely, it is difficult to show by theoretical argument how one should prevail over the other.

In the first instance, then, the weight of any principle derives from the gravity that pulls it into the center of any cultural and critical deliberations about a moral issue. The pull comes from the collective attraction that an idea exerts on a social community existing within a moral tradition and from the moral character endorsed in that tradition. If that community's history or social complexion fosters a certain idea, it will, when issues summon it, appear in the public discussion; if the idea is absent or marginal, it will be invisible or silent. Thus, "holy war" and "ethnic cleansing" do not appear as weighty moral notions in certain cultures, while they have powerful attraction in others. Note how in recent times books and articles published in the United States struggle to explain the history and sociology of those "foreign" cultures where these ideas are weighty. Much more needs to be said about the problems that arise if one accepts this explanation of the first source of moral weight. What about relativism? What about societies in which invidious principles (such as, in our view, "holy war" and "ethnic cleansing") prevail? What about societies in which critical reflection repudiates central cultural concepts? How do competing, critical, innovative moral notions force their way into a moral tradition? It is impossible to pursue these questions here. I will be bold enough to assert my thesis in the belief that these problems can be addressed in a reasonable fashion.

A second way in which a moral principle puts on weight comes from the critical reflection of what passes for philosophy within the culture. I say, "what passes for" not out of disdain, but in recognition that in some cultures there is a formal intellectual enterprise that is called philosophy; while in others, intellectual life runs in other courses but there is, nonetheless, a recognized cultural wisdom that articulates ideals and announces priorities for social and personal life. Whenever this happens, respected thinkers select certain principles, ideals, and virtues for special attention. These principles are drawn from those available in the cultural tradition; the philosophers promote them to the center of the system of reflective thought that they construct. Their gravity becomes apparent when other ideas are drawn into their orbit and circle around them as implications. Thus, the notion of the individual as autonomous subject enthralled the thinkers of the Enlightenment and gradually attained a central place in the thought of leading philosophers such as Hobbes, Locke, Rousseau, and Kant. The philosophical reflections of British liberalism and American pragmatism have elaborated and refined the ideas. The principle of respect for persons becomes a familiar, indeed indispensable, notion among those who read and write in the Western philosophical traditions; those who ignore it do so at peril of exclusion from the philosophical society, and those who criticize it must fight an uphill battle.

This sort of weight, however, is somewhat illusory. A system of moral philosophy is not a morality. Although some such systems attain great prominence in a culture and exercise a powerful influence on common ideas of morality—take Confucianism in China—they are generally rather peripheral to the moral life of a people. Thus, while those who read and write philosophy may give great weight to a principle because it has made a system of thought coherent and convincing, that principle may not be as weighty in the lives of those who live the morality of the culture. Even if they do acknowledge its importance, they may not give it the preeminence or the priority accorded to it within the system of thought. For example, in recent years we have seen the principle of autonomy fall to the center of bioethics. It is congenial to American moral tradition; it is central to much of Western moral philosophy. However, we are beginning to hear protests from those who speak with other voices within the dominant moral tradition and who are in the process of elaborating alternative moral philosophies. Similarly, John Rawl's *Theory of Justice*, an unquestionably prominent work in moral philosophy, argues for the centrality of a principle of compensatory justice. The authority of the author and the elegance of the argument make the notion weighty; yet it carries little weight outside the scholarly community. A weighty tome does not a weighty argument make.

PRINCIPLES AND CIRCUMSTANCES

Weighty principles, then, acquire their gravity from tradition and character, as well as from systems of moral reflection. There is, I suggest, a third way in which the metaphor of weight might be employed. In this third way, it refers not so much to principles as to the ultimate moral decision. A moral decision follows consideration of various features of a situation, including both principles and circumstances. In this third view it is the considerations, rather than the principles themselves, that are weighty. The importance of any principle in the first instance does not of itself establish its priority in relation to any other principle. Many moral principles coexist within a moral tradition; many of them seem of equivalent importance and, on their faces, do not announce their superiority over their competitors. When the circumstances surrounding a moral problem are specified in some detail, however, a sense of priority begins to emerge and begs to be investigated more closely. It is simple enough to say that the truth must be told and to assert that the innocent should not be harmed. Both are weighty principles within our moral tradition. However, consider the story that St. Augustine and Immanuel Kant both told, and that simplicity dissolves into moral perplexity: an innocent man is hiding in your home from the agents of a tyrant who is bent on arresting him, and those agents ask you whether he is there. Which of the two weighty principles should prevail? Arguments can be made on both sides: Augustine and Kant argued for the priority of truth telling. Thousands of brave persons who protected heretics from Inquisitors and Jews from Nazis preferred the principle of protecting the innocent. I suggest that it is not the weight of the principle itself that tips the balance; it is the accumulated weight of the variety of circumstances that cluster around the principles in question that does so. When we hear the story, we want to know more. Precisely who is this person and of what does his innocence consist? What is the nature of the tyranny and why do they seek him? What is the likelihood that he will be found regardless of what you say? What are the consequences to you and your family if exposed? Are there alternatives to disclosure? (Admittedly, the example limps because, in critical situations, such prudential reflection is often impossible and may even be repugnant; still, the example is a historical one over which many good minds have puzzled.)

The circumstances of the case are themselves weighty: some circumstances are lightweight and count for little in our evaluation; others are heavyweight and demand attention. Indeed, we might seriously consider changing the terms of the metaphor: the principles are the scales on which the burdens of circumstances are placed. Principles do weigh on a final decision; however, the scales dip, not under the principles' weight, but under the accumulated circumstances that pull on one or the other principle.

This may seem odd. The circumstances of cases, the "who, what, when, where, why, how, and how much," are factual descriptions. How do they give moral weight to the principles? Are they not what many philosophers have called the "nonmoral" features of a moral problem? Are they not simply "facts" that lie on one side of "Hume's hurdle," over which the ethicists must leap to get from fact to value? I have always thought this a peculiarly narrow view of moral situations. I would rather say that the circumstances function as "morally appreciated" features of a situation. While they are not themselves derivations of moral principle, they are evaluated in relation to principles and values. Thus, in the *Children's Report* one can find an attempt to evaluate what might constitute a minor increase over minimal risk by a comparison with the ordinary experiences of children either in sickness or health. The assumption is that we can appreciate in general ways what "the good life" is for a child and appreciate the extent to which some research intervention departs from that.

St. Thomas Aquinas, in his voluminous treatise on human action, asked whether the theologian should take note of the circumstances of human acts. He answered, rather surprisingly, "The theologian considers human acts according as they are found good or evil, better or worse; and this diversity depends on circumstances."[16] This answer surprises readers who assume that St. Thomas, patron of Roman Catholic theologians, must have been firmly committed to absolute principles and certainly would have repudiated the relativism that this statement suggests. Yet, it would not surprise readers who know that the medieval saint was a dedicated follower of Aristotle, who wrote, "Matters of practical conduct have nothing invariable about them . . . they require human beings to consider what is appropriate to specific circumstances and to the specific occasion."[17] Aquinas, apparently unfazed by the perils of situationism and relativism, went on to assert that circumstances can contribute to the greater or lesser seriousness of a moral fault (a point that few would quibble with) or even change the "species" of the moral act itself (a more contentious claim). He gave an example appropriate to his time: theft is a species of moral act (based on the principle, do not appropriate for oneself the property of another); the time and place of a theft are circumstances that would not usually make a theft anything but a theft. If the place of the theft were a church and the object stolen a sacred object, however, the moral species would become sacrilege, the profanation of a holy place--a much more heinous sin than theft.[18] Similarly, in an example given not by Aquinas but by many of his followers, the moral theologians of the 17th and 18th centuries, an underpaid servant who takes food for his family from the larder of his master does not commit theft. In these cases, circumstances of place, of wealth and poverty, and of servitude supplement the principles and make us look upon them in certain ways. The principle of protection of property weighs much more heavily when the property is sacred (in Aquinas' culture) and becomes lighter when the property of another is needed to sustain life. In each case, the circumstances are "morally appreciated."

By "morally appreciated circumstances" I mean the way in which certain facts are associated with certain goals and perspectives that can themselves be subject to moral evaluation. For example, I register so many pounds on my bathroom scale. That avoirdupois can be considered overweight in relation to many perspectives: the statistical norm for my height and age in a relevant population, the cultural standards for fashionable appearance, the risks associated with cardiovascular morbidity and mortality, the ability to maneuver at sports, and so on. Each of these perspectives can be morally evaluated; goals that I set in relation to them can be assessed in light of those values. The actual fact of how many pounds I weigh can be "morally appreciated" in view of those goals and perspectives. In their light, I can evaluate whether my concern about my weight arises from vanity, from responsibility for my health, from enjoyment of tennis, or from thrift about purchasing new shirts and trousers. The actual number of pounds may differ in moral relevance depending on this evaluation.

Turn from the minor moral matter of my avoirdupois to the more serious issue of research with children. The circumstantial observations such as "minor," "minimal over minor," "risks commensurate," and so on, that I use in the moral appreciation of my avoirdupois are used as well as in the moral appreciation of research proposals regarding children. They lend weight to the principles in the situation. In addition, the circumstances under consideration in any case are of quite different sorts and may seem incommensurable or imponderable: the classical problem of apples and oranges. In any particular case we may be forced to evaluate a health risk, a personal preference, the protection of a person against harm, a financial cost, or a scientific question. These do not sort into the same basket. Thus, we must view the case as a whole and assess how the various weights accumulate. So, we find ourselves pondering "small risks," "significant costs," "minimal harms," "doubtful competence," and so forth, not singly but cumulatively. We must often do our weighing in scales that have more than two pans. We find ourselves saying, "Well, all things considered, I believe this is the right thing to do."

Up to this point, we have been pondering the metaphor of weighing in moral discourse. While I have not researched the origins of the metaphor, I surmise that it might have been imported from the cognate field of jurisprudence. There, the idea of weighing the pleas of various parties in a scale has contributed not only to the language of law, but even to its most prominent icon, blindfolded Justice holding a balance. This ancient image has been updated. As William Winslade wrote, "The symbol of the scales of justice is closely tied, in recent American legal thinking, to the idea that adjudication consists in a balancing of interests . . . after all the relevant interests are placed on the scales, the judge is supposed to rule in favor of the interests which have more weight."[19] The metaphor of balance works best in ethics when the various considerations relevant to moral choice are viewed as, in some sense, quantities. Thus, the metaphor is easily adapted to classical utilitarianism, in which pleasures and pains are assumed to have quantitative properties. The 18th-century English philosopher and jurist Jeremy Bentham wrote, "Sum up all the values of all the pleasures on the one side and those of all the pains on the other. The balance, if it be on the side of pleasure, will give the good tendency of the act upon the whole. . . ."[20] Whether the consideration be "interests" in American jurisprudence or "pleasures and pains" in classical utilitarianism, the content loaded onto the balance is assumed to be relatively homogeneous and to differ only in such relatively quantifiable characteristics as "intensity," "duration," and "extent." When moral philosophies emphasize principles, these principles can also be given weight in the sense explained above, namely, from the moral traditions, moral character, and systematic moral reflection within a culture. When facing any particular moral dilemma in real life, however, the principles and the values are embedded in a complex of circumstances. These circumstances are of such diverse sorts that it is almost impossible to find common features to weigh against each other.

FIT AS MORAL METAPHOR

Since this essay is about moral metaphors, it might be appropriate to examine another metaphor long used by moral philosophers. The metaphor of "fit" has very ancient roots in Western moral thought. It was a central notion in the moral doctrines of the Sophists and the Stoics; it was the key to Aristotle's concept of practical judgment (the word *epikeia*, often poorly translated as "equity," literally means "the fitting"); and it has come down to recent times in the writings of such authors as Ross and Bradley and as the major theme of H. Richard Niebuhr's ethics of responsibility. We echo this ancient idea even in common language when we say that this or that act was "suitable" or "fitting." Fit implies a context, structure, or design--made up of diverse elements--into which some feature of moral discourse, either a principle or a judgment, is set. When so set, it is seen to be of the right measure, size, and shape, making a harmonious pattern. This old moral metaphor has been used in many ways: for the Sophists, moral choice fit the situation of time and place; for the Stoics, moral behavior fit the harmonious movement of the universe; for Aristotle, modifications of law suited the intent of the original legislator. This metaphor appeared in St. Thomas Aquinas's discussion of the place of circumstances in moral judgment. He wrote, "Acts are proportionate to their end by a certain commensurateness that comes from the due circumstances."[21]

I venture the suggestion that the metaphor of fit is more illuminating than the metaphor of weight when it comes to understanding how circumstances influence moral judgment. Moral judgment is a patterned whole into which principles, values, circumstances, and consequences must be fitted. The particular judgment itself must be fitted into a larger set of judgments about the moral suitability of behavior and practices. I wish to suggest that the metaphor of fittingness allows for a more coherent understanding of the idea of "moral appreciation" of "the nonmoral facts" that make up the circumstances of a case. It is difficult to "appreciate" weighing and balancing (although the loss of a few pounds may be a cause for joy and a plump hog may make a farmer rejoice). Appreciation is an aesthetic concept: we appreciate a painting, a landscape, a symphony, or a good play--whether drama or a throw from shortstop to second base to first base. This sort of aesthetic appreciation arises, in part, from the harmonious fitting together of various elements that may be, in themselves, heterogeneous.

A moral judgment about a case is, I think, similar. Principles, values, circumstances, and consequences must be seen as a whole. The judgment about them comprises them all together: we do not, in Platonic fashion, turn our eyes from a vision of moral principle down to the nonmoral facts of a case; instead, we sweep facts, values, consequences, and principles into a single vision. The English moral philosopher Francis Hutcheson, often given credit for inventing the "ideal observer" theory of moral judgment, wrote, "When we say one is obliged to an action, we mean . . . that every spectator, or he himself upon reflection, must approve his action, and disapprove his omitting it, if he considers fully all its circumstances."[22] Apart from the merits of the ideal observer theory (which in the hands of its later proponents curiously ignores how "all its circumstances" fit into moral judgment), the sentence properly expresses the content of moral judgment. Hutcheson's words echo, at five centuries distance, the words of Aquinas quoted above about an act's "commensurateness which results from the due circumstances."

THE NATIONAL COMMISSION

A return to the deliberations of the National Commission will provide two instances that illustrate this idea. First, in the *Children's Report*, the maxim "do no harm," while not explicitly cited, is all pervasive. Since children generally cannot give consent (a circumstance), the principle of respect for autonomy is of less weight than the principle of nonmaleficence. However, the maxim "do no harm" must be refined in the context of research. It is necessary to clarify what constitutes harm and how research might do harm. Although much of that clarification was tacit and implicit, the commission's conclusions bear witness to the realization that there are harms of many sorts and many degrees, that most research maneuvers do not do harm but pose risks of harm, and that these are of many sorts and degrees. A harm such as deliberate death or maiming, such as took place in the Nazi research, is unquestionably unethical; how should the harm that comes from a needlestick to draw blood be judged? Is it more harmful or risky if the child is healthy and normal than if the child is a leukemia patient for whom needlesticks are routine? Is a change of daily activities for research observation a harm or risk of harm? Would it be so if the change involved placing the child for a day in the care of strangers rather than familiar caretakers? Should it be considered a harm to be assigned by a random process to a treatment regimen that turns out, at the conclusion of the study, to be the less effective treatment that was tested? These and many other variations on the theme of harm and risk are essential to any reasonable judgment that the maxim "do no harm" is being honored or violated. It is the total picture in the instant case that allows such a judgment to be made. The moral weight of "do no harm" is manifested only amidst the greater and lesser, the probables and the possibles of quite particular circumstances.

In a second example, the National Commission's *Report on the Fetus as Research Subject* reported a debate among the commissioners. All commissioners agreed that only minimal risk should be tolerated when the subject of research cannot give consent. They agreed that this maxim should hold whether a fetus is going to be aborted or not. However, they disagreed over what might constitute minimal risk to a fetus whose existence is about to be ended by abortion. "Some members hold that no procedures should be applied to a fetus-to-be-aborted that would not be applied to a fetus-going-to-term. . . . Others argue that, while a woman's decision for abortion does not change the status of the fetus *per se*, it does make a significant difference in one respect--namely, in the risk of harm to the fetus."[23] The latter position is exemplified by a study seeking to learn whether a certain drug crosses the placenta: when the drug is administered prior to abortion, harms such as ototoxicity or nephrotoxicity, which might appear in a infant carried to term, will not affect a fetus that will be aborted within hours of the administration of the drug. Thus, the timing and the intent of the mother, both circumstances, determine whether the maxims, "do no harm" and "treat fetuses as research subjects equally," are applicable. Here, the weight of "do no harm" is determined by the circumstances of time and place and maternal intent.

These examples illustrate how the principles and maxims that are invoked in any case of moral perplexity are "sized" by being "fitted" into contexts and patterns of circumstances. Any principle or maxim, true enough in itself, becomes relevant and important (or irrelevant and less important) within such a factual pattern. If one final shift of metaphor might be permitted, the principles and maxims "come into focus" against a background of circumstances. Change the background, either by addition or removal of some fact or by a heightening or shading of the circumstances, and one or another maxim will appear more vividly and centrally. Seeing these patterns constitutes an essential part of moral judgment.

Any trained moral philosopher knows the epistemological conundrums that trail such assertions. In particular, the description of moral judgment as analogous to aesthetic judgment raises eyebrows. Apart from memories of Kierkegaard and Nietzsche, the problem of subjectivism immediately appears. One need not be a moral philosopher to recognize that, if ethics is like artistic appreciation, then *de gustibus non est disputandum* (there is no disputing about tastes). Finally, the inevitable and somewhat unwelcome companion of ethical aestheticism is ethical intuitionism, a highly problematic (though not entirely discredited) metaethical theory. I shall not confront these problems here. Instead, I will return to the history of the National Commission and propose that one way of avoiding the epistemological problem of subjectivism is to put a group of reasonably intelligible persons together to argue about an ethical problem and to demand of them a resolution, as Congress did demand from the National Commission.

The commission sought to give guidance on how we might recognize conditions in which great dangers might threaten large numbers of children and to evaluate how likely it would be that such dangers might be alleviated by certain investigations. In such situations, regardless of what course is chosen, some benefits may be foregone and some harm may be done. The commission stated, "Rather than attempt to resolve the dilemma in the abstract . . . the ethical argument should be made, not over a hypothetical case, but over an actual situation, in which the real issues and the likely costs of any solution can be more clearly discerned," and it thus left such problems to the deliberations of a National Advisory Board. Note that it did not leave such discernment to the local IRBs that were otherwise given considerable discretion in interpreting the other principles. It reserved the interpretation of this principle alone to a highly visible and highly accountable national body. This reservation represented the "requisite caution in situations where one may wish to make an exception to the principle, but only for clear and sufficient reasons," of which Professor Katz spoke. The situation cannot be envisioned in advance, because the weight, the seriousness of the particular circumstances, needs concrete specification.

One can have a principle that is absolute, in the sense of very weighty; that is never out of sight; that guides and controls all deliberations about an issue, but to which an exception can be made, in Dr. Katz's words, "for clear and sufficient reasons." But those clear and convincing reasons can be perceived only in the particular situation, not in abstraction from it. The concept of balancing principles is, as he says, "dangerous" if, deceived by the metaphor, we believe we can weigh two absolute and weighty principles, such as the importance of scientific advance relative to the importance of personal autonomy, on some metaphysical scale. Rather, the weighty principle of autonomy dominates all our deliberations about the ethics of human research because both our cultural heritage and our critical reflection refuse to sacrifice individuals to the common welfare. Yet, we can appreciate situations in which quite specific harms to many may force us to contemplate exposing some to risks so that all might be saved. Exceptions are painful and specific, and the reasons that justify them never ought to be generalized nor routinized.

Take, for example, the tragic epidemic that struck my home, Seattle, in January 1993. Within about three days, 400 persons, mostly children, were struck with devastating illness caused by Escherichia coli 015:H7 in undercooked, contaminated hamburger meat purchased at many Jack-in-the-Box restaurant outlets. Two children died and many were close to death; many who recovered will have chronic gastrointestinal and renal problems. Initially, it could not be estimated how many of the thousands of children who ate at those outlets, and perhaps others, had ingested the pathogen and would become ill. Suppose that a pharmaceutical company had a powerful antimicrobial ready for testing with critically ill adults. Suppose that it was already known that the drug had rare but potentially serious side effects and that someone suggested that this be given prophylactically to all children who had eaten at fast food places over the previous week. Should this more-than-minor risk for some children who would not otherwise have been infected be permitted? This is the kind of concrete problem that must be assessed in the situation, in order to discern whether clear and sufficient reasons warrant a specific exception to an absolute principle.

Assessment in the situation requires that a group of concerned persons must gather together all of the relevant information. That group would first act as if they were epidemiologists, searching for the causes; evaluating the seriousness of the crisis, its extent, and the likelihood that it might spread; and examining the data about the investigational drug. The group then would have to go on to act as a group of "ethicists," aware of the principles and maxims such as protection of the innocent, respect for autonomy, avoidance of harm, concern for the public welfare, and so forth. Each of these principles could be proposed and defined. A moment would come, however, when the group as epidemiologists and the group as ethicists would have to become one. It would have to answer the question: Can any risk of harm to an individual be permitted in order to avoid some risk of harm to the population? The maxims about avoiding harm and about protecting the public would move into focus as answers would be suggested to the questions: "How much harm? How likely? How certain? How otherwise avoidable?"

When the group entered this debate, it would merge the assessment of factual circumstances and the assertion of philosophical principle into prudent judgment. The weighing and balancing of principles does not depend on any moral equivalent of the laws of physics. It is done by practical moral judgment, discretion, prudence or, in Aristotle's idiom, *phronesis*. Despite the recent resurgence of interest in this notion, many philosophers consider it exasperatingly vague. Indeed, it does frustrate those who are searching for the architectonic principle of morality. But, vague as it is, moral judgment is truly moral only if exercised by persons who are, as Aristotle insisted, imbued with justice, friendship, and magnanimity. In more contemporary language, these are people who both hold firmly to clear principles about justice, human dignity, and welfare and have the discretion to differentiate between the serious, the ordinary, and the trivial in the situations of human living. We know that there are a few such persons--precious few--in our world. Thus, we hope that in the deliberations of fairly appointed committees and commissions, which are publicly visible and accountable, we may find something resembling the *phronesis* that alone can render reasonable and prudent decisions about particular moral perplexities.

NOTES

1. J. Katz, "The Nuremberg Code Consent Principle: Then and Now," in *The Nazi Doctors and the Nuremberg Code*, eds. G. Annas and M.A. Grodin (New York: Oxford University Press, 1991), 236-37, emphasis added.

2. C. Clavius, "In Sphaeram" (1591), quoted in P. Redondi, *Galileo Heretic* (Princeton, N.J.: Princeton University Press, 1987), 38.

3. J. Rawls, *Theory of Justice* (Cambridge: Harvard University Press, 1971), 43, 41.

4. T.L. Beauchamp and J.F. Childress, *Principles of Biomedical Ethics* (New York: Oxford University Press, 1989), 51.

5. B. Brody, *Life and Death Decision Making* (New York: Oxford University Press, 1988).

6. W.D. Ross, *The Right and the Good* (Oxford: Oxford University Press, 1930), Ch. 2.

7. U.S. Public Law 93-348, 1974.

8. National Commission for the Protection of Human Subjects of Biomedical and Behavioral Research, *Research Involving Children*

(Washington, D.C.: U.S. Government Printing Office, 1977); 48 *Federal Register* (1983), 9818.

9. L. Glanz, "The Influence of the Nuremberg Code on U.S. Statutes," in *Nazi Doctors*, 192.

10. S. Perley *et al.*, "The Nuremberg Code: An International Overview," in *Nazi Doctors*, 149-73. The *Declaration of Helsinki* is in Appendix B of this book.

11. DHHS, *The Belmont Report: Ethical Principles and Guidelines for Protection of Human Subjects of Research*, DHEW Publication 0578-0012 (Washington, D.C.: U.S. Government Printing Office, 1979), Appendix C of this book.

12. P. Ramsey, "The Enforcement of Morals: Nontherapeutic Research in Children," *Hastings Center Report* 8 (1978): 7-9.

13. R. McCormick, "Proxy Consent in the Experimentation Situation," *Perspectives in Biology and Medicine* 18 (Autumn 1974): 2-20.

14. B. Freedman, A. Fuks, and C. Weijer, "In Loco Parentis: Minimal Risk as an Ethical Threshold for Research upon Children," *Hastings Center Report* 23 (March-April 1993): 13-19.

15. R. Bellah *et al.*, *Habits of the Heart: Individualism and Commitment in American Life* (New York: Harper and Row, 1986), 6.

16. Thomas Aquinas, "Summa Theologiae" I-II, q.7, a.2, in *The Basic Writings of Saint Thomas Aquinas*, ed. A.C. Pegis (New York: Random House, 1945), 241.

17. Aristotle, "The Nicomachean Ethics" II, ii, 3, 1104a, in *The Basic Works of Aristotle*, ed. R. McKeon (New York: Random House, 1941), 953.

18. Aquinas, "Summa Theologiae" I-II, q.18, aa.10-11, *Basic Writings*, 330-33.

19. W.J. Winslade, "Adjudication and the Balancing Metaphor," *Proceedings of the World Congress for Legal and Social Philosophy* (Brussels: 1971), 403-7.

20. J. Bentham, "The Principles of Morals" IV, 5, in *British Moralists*, ed. L.A. Selby-Bigge (New York: Dover Press, 1965).

21. Aquinas, "Summa Theologiae" I-II, q.7, a.2, *Basic Writings*, 241.

22. F. Hutchinson, "An Essay on the Nature and Conduct of the Passions," I, *British Moralists*, 408.

23. National Commission for the Protection of Human Subjects of Biomedical and Behavioral Research, "Research Involving the Fetus," in *Ethics in Medicine*, ed. S.J. Reiser, A.J. Dyke, and W.J. Curran (Cambridge, Mass.: MIT Press, 1977), 471.

4

Choosing Between Nuremberg and the National Commission: The Balancing of Moral Principles in Clinical Research

Terrence F. Ackerman

Careful review of codes, commentaries, and regulations suggests a basic dichotomy in the conceptual frameworks for assessing the moral permissibility of clinical-research activities. In one approach, the fulfillment of duties to subjects--respect for their autonomy, protection of their welfare, and fair treatment vis-à-vis others--should absolutely constrain promotion of the general welfare through the conduct of clinical research. Developing ethical guidelines for clinical research involves specifying the content of duties to subjects and the manner in which research must conform to these requirements. In the other approach, promotion of the general welfare through clinical research and the fulfillment of subject-related duties represent competing moral demands that must be balanced against one another. Developing research ethics involves both specifying the content of these competing moral demands and formulating the criteria according to which they should be weighted in order to arrive at norms for the conduct of clinical research.

The development of these alternative conceptual frameworks can be traced in the decades following the Second World War. The first approach is evident in the requirements of the *Nuremberg Code* and the various versions of the *Declaration of Helsinki*, which emphasized the full satisfaction of duties to subjects. In contrast, the reports of the National Commission for the Protection of Human Subjects of Biomedical and Behavioral Research and the subsequent federal regulations distilled from them adopt the stance that duties to subjects and pursuit of the general welfare must be balanced against one another in arriving at guidelines for clinical research.

This exploration of these alternative approaches will include formulating their basic tenets, clarifying the background assumptions that underlie each, illustrating their articulation and application in the literature of research ethics, and examining how the methods of research ethics differ for these respective positions. Assessment of their comparative adequacy as conceptual bases for research ethics will focus on two key issues: whether there are duties incumbent on society to promote the general welfare through the conduct of clinical research, and whether there are duties incumbent on individuals to accept minor compromises of their moral interests when necessary for the execution of clinical-research activities. The results of this analysis suggest that a version of the balancing approach is the most defensible conceptual framework for the development of research ethics.

THE ABSOLUTE PRIORITY OF DUTIES TO SUBJECTS

Between the end of World War II and the establishment of the National Commission for the Protection of Human Subjects of Biomedical and Behavioral Research, codes and commentaries on research ethics focused on articulating norms of behavior for protecting the moral interests of human subjects. Although the philosophical presuppositions of these codes and commentaries were rarely expounded, their treatment of the moral parameters for clinical research and the circumstances of their articulation are suggestive of a basic moral framework and its guiding assumptions. This basic moral framework assigns absolute priority to the fulfillment of subject-related duties. Perhaps the clearest interpretation of "absolute priority" is the notion--developed later by Rawls--of the "lexical ordering" of moral principles.[1] According to the lexical-ordering strategy, the requirements of duties assigned higher priority must be fully satisfied before the requirements of duties possessing lesser priority can be met. Applied to clinical research, this means that pursuit of the general welfare through research interventions must be constrained by full satisfaction of duties to subjects. As generally accepted since the time of The Belmont Report, these duties cluster around three categories of subjects' interests: exercising autonomous choice, protecting and promoting personal welfare, and securing fair treatment vis-à-vis others.[2]

The conceptual framework that assigns absolute priority to the fulfillment of subject-related duties is best considered a schema under which a variety of individual moral positions might be arrayed. These individual positions are differentiated by the specific interpretation assigned to the content of duties to subjects. For example, an important moral issue has concerned the permissibility of using nontherapeutic interventions with subjects who are unable to consent. Several views have been proffered within the framework of the absolute-priority view. Some have maintained that respect for autonomy prohibits the use of nontherapeutic interventions with subjects unable to consent.[3] Others maintain that the duty to respect autonomy is not applicable to persons incapable of exercising autonomy. Rather, the duty to protect subjects from harm is the pertinent duty. Some argue that fulfillment of this duty is compatible with the use of nontherapeutic procedures involving subjects unable to consent, provided that these procedures involve "negligible risk" or "no discernible risk."[4] Still others maintain that this duty is satisfied provided that nontherapeutic procedures do not involve an increment in risk beyond what the subject would encounter if engaged in normal daily activities outside the research context.[5] Each of these positions may fall within the absolute-priority schema, however, provided that it requires that pursuit of the general welfare in research employing nontherapeutic procedures be constrained by full satisfaction of duties to subjects as specified.

Moral commitments typifying the absolute-priority view are apparent in both the *Declaration of Helsinki* of 1975 and the *Nuremberg Code.* The *Declaration of Helsinki* asserts that "concern for the interests of the subject must always prevail over the interests of science and society."[6] This general-priority commitment is reflected in the manner in which specific moral issues are addressed in both codes. One issue is whether involvement of competent adult persons in research is ever permissible without adequately informed consent (for example, in research involving deception). The *Nuremberg Code* asserts, in its very first line, that "the voluntary consent of the human subject is absolutely essential," and the *Declaration of Helsinki* requires that "in any research on human beings, each potential subject must be adequately informed of the aims, methods, anticipated benefits and potential hazards."[7] Another issue concerns the permissibility of using nontherapeutic research procedures with subjects unable to consent. In insisting that the voluntary consent of subjects is "absolutely essential," the *Nuremberg Code* clearly precludes such research. No less emphatic is the *Declaration of Helsinki's* requirement that in research involving nontherapeutic procedures, "the subjects should be volunteers," thereby excluding persons unable to consent. A third issue concerns the conditions under which therapeutic procedures can be evaluated in clinical trials. The *Declaration of Helsinki* makes it clear that the harm/benefit ratio of treatment for subjects participating in clinical trials may not be less favorable than that available outside the trial. In "any medical study, every patient . . . should be assured of the best proven diagnostic and therapeutic methods," and their involvement is appropriate "only to the extent that medical research is justified by its potential diagnostic or therapeutic value for the patient." Thus, the informed consent of competent adults is required, subjects unable to consent may not be exposed to harm for reasons unrelated to their own welfare, and subjects may not be involved in trials of therapies if their best interests are not thereby served.

More importantly for present purposes, full satisfaction of the specific rules formulated in these codes for protecting the interests of human subjects is a necessary condition for the moral permissibility of clinical-research activities. No modification of these rules, justified by reference to the role of research activities in promoting the general welfare, are countenanced in either code.[8] Duties to subjects always constrain pursuit of the general welfare.

Underlying this approach that assigns absolute priority to the fulfillment of subject-related duties are certain key assumptions. First, although medical research is viewed as producing many significant improvements in the welfare of the members of society, its contributions are considered morally desirable, not morally mandatory. Second, it is assumed that the members of society are not morally obligated to participate as subjects in research activities or to accept modifications in rules protecting their interests for the benefit of others. Third, it follows that the function of moral rules applicable to the conduct of clinical research should primarily be to assure that the interests of subjects are not compromised.

These assumptions are often unstated or poorly articulated in commentaries using the absolute-priority framework. Perhaps only Hans Jonas, in his classic essay, "Philosophical Reflections on Experimenting with Human Subjects," has clearly formulated these framework assumptions.[9] Jonas asserted that, although "progress is by our own choosing an acknowledged interest of society, . . . the melioristic goal is in a sense gratuitous." Thus, "our descendants have a right to be left an unplundered planet; they do not have a right to new miracle cures." Moreover, he claimed that persons have no obligation to come to the aid of persons in need by participating in research. Despite the nobility of self-sacrifice, the "surrender of one's body to medical experimentation is entirely outside the enforceable 'social contract.' " Finally, he insisted that protecting human subjects is the essential function of social rules for regulating human research. The dangers of the morally tainted "reification" of human subjects intrinsic to medical research "calls for particular controls by the research community and by public authority" sufficient to mitigate potential violations of the interests of research subjects.

The absolute-priority view and its underlying assumptions reflect the tenor of the times in which they were formulated. The Nazi atrocities were a recent memory.[10] Critical assessments of the inadequacies of the protection of human subjects in more "civilized" societies were accumulating. The works of Beecher and Pappworth, and widely discussed revelations regarding the Jewish Chronic Disease Hospital Study and Tuskegee Syphilis Study gave substance to these concerns.[11] Moreover, statutory and regulatory safeguards for the protection of human subjects were only beginning to emerge, being brief in detail, narrow in scope, and informal in their procedural requirements.[12] Thus, this ethical framework for the analysis of clinical-research activities was highly pertinent to the most pressing problems posed during this era.

BALANCING SUBJECT PROTECTIONS AND RESEARCH GOALS

It was in the atmosphere of these deeply protectionistic concerns that the National Commission for the Protection of

Human Subjects of Biomedical and Behavioral Research was established. A key task assigned to the commission was to devise recommendations for enhancing the protection of vulnerable research subjects. Nevertheless, the 1983 revision of the Department of Health and Human Services regulations on the protection of human subjects, which follows closely the recommendations of the commission, suggests a clear conceptual departure from the approach assigning absolute priority to the fulfillment of subject-related duties.[13]

The weighting strategy suggested by the federal regulations is not formally articulated or consciously applied. Moreover, its particular applications are not entirely consistent with one another, nor is it applied to all the relevant regulatory issues for which it might be used. Nevertheless, this weighting strategy seems to provide a plausible interpretation of the moral commitments implicit in the federal regulatory requirements.

In contrast to the absolute-priority view, the federal regulations suggest that pursuit of the general welfare should be balanced against fulfillment of subject-related duties in formulating guidelines for research activities. This balancing strategy seems to involve some recognition of both pursuit of the general welfare and fulfillment of subject-related duties in situations where they conflict, but with greater weight assigned to satisfaction of the latter group of duties. The specific weighting strategy involves two points.[14] First, presumptive priority is assigned to duties to subjects, requiring their full satisfaction in most circumstances. Second, this presumption may be overridden if it is necessary to undertake research activities that may prevent or remove important harms to others and if there will be no more than minor compromises in protections of the interests of subjects. In developing this interpretation of the federal regulations, it is useful to consider both baseline rules for approval of research by an IRB (institutional review board) and exceptions that allow research not satisfying these conditions.

The presumptive priority assigned to full satisfaction of duties to subjects in most circumstances is clearly suggested in section 46.111, which lists basic conditions for approval of research by an IRB. This section specifies that to approve research "the IRB shall determine that all" of the requirements therein listed "are satisfied." These requirements cover each major category of subject-related duty. Duties to respect personal autonomy are reflected in requirements that "informed consent will be sought" and that adequate provisions be made "to protect the privacy of subjects and to maintain the confidentiality of data." Duties of fair treatment are represented in the requirements that "the selection of subjects [be] equitable" and that "appropriate additional safeguards [be] included" to protect subjects especially vulnerable to coercion or undue influence. Duties to protect the welfare of subjects are reflected in the requirements that "risks to subjects [be] minimized" and that "risks to subjects [be] reasonable in relation to anticipated benefits." In addition, a beneficence duty generally endorsed in the sections on special subjects is represented in the requirement that nontherapeutic procedures involving more than minimal risk may not be employed with subjects unable to consent or who are otherwise especially vulnerable.

However, other sections of the federal regulations introduce exceptions to these rules suggesting that the presumptive priority assigned to full satisfaction of subject-related duties may sometimes be overridden. It is interesting to contrast these provisions with the requirements of *Nuremberg* and *Helsinki*. First, while *Nuremberg* and *Helsinki* insist that the consent of subject or surrogate is a necessary condition for ethically acceptable research, section 46.116 of the *Code of Federal Regulations* specifies that consent requirements can be altered or waived provided that (1) the research involves no more than minimal risk to the subjects; (2) the waiver or alteration will not adversely affect the rights and welfare of the subjects; (3) the research could not practicably be carried out without the waiver or alteration; and (4) whenever appropriate, the subjects will be provided with additional pertinent information after participation.

Second, both *Nuremberg* and *Helsinki* require the consent of the subjects who will undergo nontherapeutic procedures. For the federal regulations, the baseline rule is that nontherapeutic procedures may be used with subjects who are unable to consent or who are otherwise especially vulnerable, provided that these procedures involve no more than minimal risk. Unlike the earlier codes, however, the federal regulations also embrace an exception to the baseline rule. In section 46.406, it is indicated that nontherapeutic procedures involving more than minimal risk may be used with children only if (1) the risk represents a minor increase over minimal risk; (2) the intervention presents experiences commensurate with those inherent in the life situation of the subjects; and (3) the intervention is likely to yield vitally important knowledge about the subjects' disorder or its treatment. A similar exception is suggested by the National Commission in its recommendations on research with those institutionalized as mentally infirm, although the latter recommendations were never approved for inclusion in the federal regulations.[15]

These exceptions to baseline moral rules formulated in the federal regulations suggest the broad outlines of the general conditions under which the presumptive priority in favor of full satisfaction of duties to subjects may be overridden. One condition is that it must not be practicably possible to conduct the research unless the exception to full satisfaction of duties to subjects is allowed. For example, the regulations specify that waiver or alteration of consent requirements is permissible only if "the research could not be practicably carried out" without it. Similarly, the regulations on research with children allow the use of nontherapeutic procedures involving more than minimal risk only when the research is likely to produce "vitally important knowledge" that could not otherwise be secured. A second condition for permitting exceptions is that compromise in the fulfillment of duties to subjects must be narrowly circumscribed. For example, alteration or waiver of consent is permitted only when it does not "adversely affect the rights and welfare" of subjects and the research risks are only "minimal." Likewise, use of nontherapeutic research procedures with children involving more than minimal risk is permitted only when the risk "represents a minor increase" over minimal risk. A third condition suggested by the regulatory exceptions is the requirement that the knowledge generated be useful in removing or preventing important harms. For example, the use of nontherapeutic research procedures involving more than minimal risk is permitted with children only when "vitally important" knowledge for understanding or ameliorating the subjects' disorder might be generated. Thus, a position emerges according to which the presumptive priority in favor of full satisfaction of duties to subjects may be overridden when compromises in their interests are minor and are practicably necessary for the conduct of research that may remove or prevent important harms to others.

DIFFERENT ASSUMPTIONS

Underlying this kind of view is a group of assumptions very different from those implicit in the absolute-priority view. They rarely are formally articulated, but they can be distilled as logical presuppositions of the specific guidelines for research formulated in the federal regulations and the weighting strategy embedded in them. The first assumption is that the development of generalizable knowledge through clinical research constitutes an obligation that society must undertake on behalf of its members. If the conduct of clinical research were merely desirable, then the importance of the knowledge to be gained in research could never be sufficient to compromise the full satisfaction of baseline duties to subjects. Since the federal regulations permit the presumption in favor of full satisfaction of these duties to sometimes be overridden, they must assume the existence of a moral obligation to conduct clinical research.

The second assumption is that individual members of society have a moral obligation to accept minor compromises in their interests as research subjects when it is necessary to remove or prevent important harms to others. If participation in clinical research is merely an especially praiseworthy contribution to the general welfare of society, then those who participate as subjects could not be required to accept any compromises in the full satisfaction of duties that investigators have toward them as subjects. Because the federal regulations endorse certain exceptional conditions under which some compromise in the full satisfaction of duties to subjects is allowed, however, it follows that they assume an obligation on the part of subjects to accept these conditions when necessary for the development of generalizable knowledge.

A final key assumption is that the guidelines developed for the conduct of clinical research have a dual function. One is to protect the moral interests of research subjects against serious compromise by others. The other is to facilitate the development of forms of generalizable knowledge that will provide improved means for removing and preventing harms to persons caused by disease and injury. Given their dual function, research guidelines must formulate norms that balance pursuit of the general welfare through clinical research activities against the fulfillment of baseline duties to subjects.

Current federal regulations on the conduct of IRB research with humans derive, in substantial part, from the recommendations of the National Commission for the Protection of Human Subjects. Although the commission was created with the critical charge of formulating guidelines to assure that serious abuses of human subjects would be eliminated, it was also deeply impressed by the need to encourage clinical-research activities. Indeed, it considered these activities to be so important to the welfare of members of society that it believed that there are circumstances in which some minor compromises in the fulfillment of baseline duties to human subjects are justified. In this way, the recommendations of the National Commission and the federal regulations represent a repudiation of the absolute-priority view.

The subsequent literature of research ethics has wavered between the balancing approach and the absolute-priority view. This can be seen in the manner of addressing particular questions, such as the issue of using medical records in epidemiological research without the explicit consent of subjects. Some theorists attempt to resolve these issues simply by delineating the requirements of duties to subjects. They hold that permissible research must satisfy these prior constraints. For example, Robert Veatch maintains that the requirement of respect for personal autonomy cannot be modified because of the potential contribution of research activities to the general welfare. In his view, epidemiological research involving medical records satisfies this requirement only if (1) subjects give explicit prior consent for use of their medical records in specific studies, (2) they provide prior blanket consent for use of their records in research of this general type, or (3) it can be determined that reasonable persons would not object to the use of their medical records in a specific investigation being contemplated.[16] In contrast, other theorists address this issue by asking what policy would strike a suitable balance between pursuit of research goals and protection of the moral interests of subjects. For example, Roberts and colleagues investigated the concerns of subjects who participated in a study of the prior medical histories of women with breast and bowel cancers.[17]

Prospective subjects were identified by reviewing a tumor registry without their prior consent. The authors asserted, however, that when epidemiological research addresses socially important questions and medical records must be used without prior consent for valid scientific design, then minor infringements on the rights of subjects are morally justified. Moreover, they maintained that this policy is justifiable even though a small number of subjects might object to unconsented disclosure of their medical condition to investigators.[18]

The conclusions of these interlocutors do not mesh, because different weighting strategies and framework assumptions ensure divergent conclusions. Thus, a crucial question emerges: Which is the most defensible weighting strategy for use in addressing moral issues in clinical research? This question can be resolved by determining which approach has the most defensible underlying assumptions.

ARGUMENTS FOR THE BALANCING APPROACH

The assumptions underlying the absolute-priority view and the balancing approach differ on two key points: whether there are duties incumbent on society to promote the general welfare of its members through the conduct of clinical research, and whether there are duties incumbent on individuals to accept minor compromises of their moral interests when necessary for the conduct of important clinical-research activities. The considerations supporting a positive answer to these questions provide grounds for endorsing a balancing approach to the resolution of moral issues in clinical research.

Are there societal duties to support the conduct of clinical research? The argument begins with an assumption shared by defenders of the absolute-priority view and the balancing approach: society has an obligation to establish norms of conduct that prevent persons from causing harm to others. Granting that society has an obligation to control harm-causing practices, the duty to conduct clinical research can be easily established.

The relevance of clinical research to the performance of this societal role focuses on the existence of harmful medical practices. The history of medicine is replete with examples of widely accepted treatments later shown to be injurious, such as high-concentration oxygen therapy for premature infants or gastric freezing for patients with bleeding peptic ulcers. The widespread use of harmful medical practices reflects, in part, extreme difficulties in detecting their inadequacies through uncontrolled observations.[19] When a disease process abates or worsens after medical interventions, it is difficult to determine through uncontrolled observation whether the change has resulted from treatment or from the natural course of the disease. Similarly, the efficaciousness of the treatment cannot be easily separated from the placebo effect of the act of intervention. These problems result in judgments on treatment efficacy and safety that suffer from the fallacy of *post hoc, ergo propter hoc* ("after this, therefore on account of it"). In addition, physicians' bias in favor of a given treatment may result in a pattern of selecting patients for the treatment or in the use of criteria for evaluating results that skew assessment in favor of the preferred treatment. The upshot is that the social control of the use of harmful medical practices requires methods for evaluating therapies that are more dependable than informal observation. These methods are provided by the controlled interventions and observations that characterize clinical trials. Thus, even if we accept only a limited obligation of society to minimize harmful activities, these considerations suggest that society has a duty to sponsor the conduct of clinical research.

Of course, this argument establishes only a limited societal duty to undertake clinical research. This duty pertains to assessing current therapeutic modalities that remain controversial and nonvalidated with regard to their comparative efficacy and safety. It also applies to any forthcoming therapies that achieve widespread acceptance in practice without prior evaluation. However, the argument does not support the existence of a duty to develop innovative treatments for removing or preventing harms to patients that cannot be ameliorated by current therapies. Since much of clinical research is devoted to the assessment of treatment innovations, the argument based on the societal obligation to minimize harmful practices has only limited import.

A further question to be addressed is whether there are societal obligations to remove and prevent harms as well. It is difficult to sustain the claim that society has an obligation to minimize harmful practices but that there are no similar obligations to remove and prevent harms. Not causing harm and removing or preventing harms have precisely the same objective: minimizing the extent of harm that may occur to persons.[20] Moreover, the amount and type of effort required to remove or prevent harms is often no different from that required to control harmful practices. These points are illustrated in the context of clinical research. Protocols that result in new medical treatments and studies designed to evaluate controversial standard therapies are both intended to minimize the extent of harm that might occur to patients. Furthermore, the same process must be undertaken to identify improved treatments or to expose current harmful therapies--formal evaluation of these interventions in well-designed clinical trials. Thus, if society has a role in reducing current harmful practices, then there are strong grounds for asserting that it also has obligations to remove and prevent harms to its members.

An important way in which society can remove or prevent harm to its members involves assuring that they are not deprived, through no fault of their own, of certain basic goods necessary to the pursuit of their life plans. These basic goods include adequate food, clothing, shelter, education, and physical security. Because life-threatening or disabling diseases may also deprive persons of the opportunity to pursue their life plans, safe and effective medical treatment must also be counted as a basic good whose provision by society is required by the obligation to remove or prevent important harms to its members.

Moreover, clinical research has an important role to play in satisfying the latter obligation of society. Adequate medical care serves to remove and prevent the harms caused by seriously disabling and life-threatening diseases. When safe and effective treatment is not available, the societal obligation to remove and prevent harms requires that research be undertaken to develop the generalizable knowledge essential for improving treatment. In this respect, clinical research is similar to projects undertaken to devise procedures or programs to effectively provide other basic goods to persons who are unable to secure these items through their own efforts. This similarity is suggested by the common metaphors that we use in describing societal efforts to improve the availability of basic goods. We engage in "wars" against cancer and other serious illnesses, just as we undertake wars against poverty, illiteracy, and other conditions that deprive persons of the basic goods needed to pursue their life plans.

It might be objected that, if we include effective and safe medical treatment among the basic goods that must be provided to the members of society to remove or prevent important harms, then an unlimited societal duty to continuously expand our store of generalizable medical knowledge is created. Being a limitless undertaking, it would consume all resources available for developing and distributing other basic goods. Providing for other essential needs, however, such as adequate housing and education, also normally creates demands that outstrip available resources. Allocation decisions that limit the portion of total resources distributed to the relief of each type of basic need must be made. In a similar fashion, the portion of total resources devoted to medical research must be balanced against the demands posed by other essential needs. The assertion that there is a societal duty to develop safe and effective treatment for disabling and life-threatening diseases is consistent with, and is not undermined by, the recognition that its fulfillment must be constrained by the need to utilize limited societal resources to provide for other basic needs as well.[21]

Thus, there are strong grounds for claiming that society has obligations to restrict harmful practices, as well as to remove and prevent harms, and that duties to conduct clinical research are generated by these societal functions. This argument does not cover all instances of clinical research. Rather, it establishes a societal duty to conduct clinical research likely to yield generalizable knowledge useful in removing or preventing important harms, such as those caused by seriously disabling or life-threatening conditions. Clinical research not likely to produce such consequences might be desirable but would not be morally obligatory.

The second question requiring our attention is whether there are duties incumbent on individuals to accept minor compromises in the protection of their moral interests when necessary for the conduct of important clinical-research activities. The argument for this claim starts with the widely held view that individuals have limited general obligations of beneficence to remove or prevent important harms to other specific persons when doing so will involve no more than minor costs to their own interests.[22] A stock example is the case of a drowning child who can be easily plucked from the water by a stranger at pool side. Positing this

duty seems reasonable, despite the absence of a special relationship between the parties, because a great harm to a person
possessing intrinsic moral worth can be prevented at little more
than the cost of wet clothes. More generally, "duties of rescue"
provide a social "safety net" to protect the key interests of
individuals when the usual mechanisms implemented by society
(for example, lifeguards at pools) are unavoidably ineffective.

Similarly, when persons organized collectively can remove or
prevent important harms to groups of persons at modest cost to
their own interests, it is reasonable to posit collective duties of
rescue.[23] The logical basis for this extension is the principle
underlying the paradigm cases of duties of rescue. Harms that
deprive persons of important goods needed to pursue their life
plans have sufficient moral significance to justify obligatory
minor compromises in the interests of individuals who are able to
remove or prevent them. It is irrelevant to the application of this
principle whether the needed assistance can be provided by a
single individual or requires groups of persons (such as research
subjects) who are organized collectively. It is similarly irrelevant
whether the assistance is needed by a single individual or by
groups of persons. This principle forms the basis for a large variety
of social programs, involving obligatory sacrifices by individuals
(mainly through taxation), that provide other persons with important goods of which they would otherwise be deprived.

It is reasonable to maintain that collective duties of rescue
apply in the context of clinical research. Deprivation of the basic
good of physical well-being may occur when persons suffer from
diseases or injuries for which safe and effective treatment is
lacking. Clinical research may accomplish the development of
such treatment. Moreover, the design, procedures, or circumstances of these studies may unavoidably require some compromise in the interests of subjects. When these compromises represent only a modest cost to the interests of subjects, the analogy
with duties of rescue suggest that they are morally justified.

The analogy with duties of rescue is often lost because the
rationale for undertaking clinical research is described as "pursuit
of the general welfare." The latter phrase conjures up the image of
a mechanically summed quantity not bestowed on specific individuals. In the context of clinical research, however, pursuit of the
general welfare intimates removing or preventing important

harms that will be visited upon specific, if not now identifiable, persons. The harms to which these individuals may succumb demand moral recognition if we have genuine regard for their intrinsic worth as persons with the capacity to suffer. Thus, respect for their worth as persons requires our collective assistance when it can be rendered at minor cost to our own interests. It follows that there are duties incumbent on individuals to accept minor compromises in the protection of their moral interests as subjects when necessary for the conduct of clinical research that may remove or prevent important harms to others.

One objection to this position is that permitting any compromises to the interests of subjects invites flagrant abuses of their rights and welfare. For example, Robert Veatch asserts that maintaining the absolute priority of respect for personal autonomy serves to "protect ourselves from the dangers of naked utilitarianism."[24] Indeed, it would. His comment suggests a false dichotomy of theoretical and policy alternatives, however: *either* we maintain the absolute priority of respect for personal autonomy *or* we lapse into naked utilitarianism. Between these stark options lies a moral middle ground. We can insist on the priority of full satisfaction of duties to subjects in most circumstances while permitting minor compromises in the protection of subjects' interests when necessary for the conduct of research that may prevent or remove important harms to others. Logically speaking, this latter position is distinguishable from a crass utilitarianism that embraces compromises in protections for the interests of subjects to whatever extent necessary to accomplish clinical-research goals and whenever it is feasible to do so. Factually speaking, adoption of this moral middle ground is not likely to lead to widespread abuses of the rights and welfare of human subjects. Current federal research regulations, now in existence for more than a decade, embody the weighting strategy defended above. There is little evidence that the application of these regulations by IRBs is producing serious violations of the rights and welfare of human subjects that can be characterized as "lapses into naked utilitarianism."

Nevertheless, Veatch is certainly correct that there are moral risks associated with the acceptance of a balancing approach to clinical-research ethics. This weighting strategy requires the exercise of judgment in determining legitimate exceptions to the presumption in favor of full satisfaction of duties to subjects. Key phrases, such as "minor compromises in the requirements of duties to subjects," "prevention or removal of important harms to others," and "necessary for the conduct of research activities," require interpretation. Concern may arise that too much latitude is permitted in determining the extent to which protections for the rights and welfare of subjects may be modified. As Jonsen argues in his essay, however, "The weighing and balancing of principles does not depend on any moral equivalent of the laws of physics. It is done by moral judgment, discretion, prudence or, in Aristotle's idiom, *phronesis.* "[25] A more rigid approach to clinical-research ethics--insisting on the absolute priority of duties to subjects--carries its own risks. It precludes proper recognition of duties of social beneficence requiring us to prevent or remove important harms to others when it can be accomplished at minor costs to our own interests. Thus, the latitude for moral judgment required by the balancing approach is inescapable if, as Jonsen keenly observes, we are to fully acknowledge all dimensions of the moral landscape pertinent to the resolution of moral issues in clinical research.

The foregoing considerations support a balancing approach to the resolution of moral issues that arise in the conduct of clinical research while undermining the plausibility of the absolute-priority view. Moreover, these considerations suggest that something closely akin to the presumptive-weighting strategy is the most defensible species of the balancing approach. In particular, the discussion of duties of rescue suggests that, while pursuit of the general welfare should partly constrain satisfaction of duties to subjects, substantial compromises in subject-related protections should not be tolerated. Compromises in these protections should be permitted only when they are necessary for the conduct of research that may generate knowledge useful in removing or preventing important harms to others. Moreover, these compromises must involve no more than minor infringements on the requirements of duties to subjects. In this manner, the duty of social beneficence to remove and prevent important harms to groups of persons is assigned limited weight in resolving moral issues in clinical research, while correlative compromises in the fulfillment of duties to subjects are narrowly circumscribed.

THE LEGACY OF THE NATIONAL COMMISSION

Critical analyses of the federal research regulations, and the recommendations of the National Commission on which they are based, usually evoke one of two incompatible assessments. On one hand, the suggestion is frequently made today that the recommendations of the National Commission and the subsequent federal regulations are overly protective of the interests of human subjects. According to this view, newer problems encountered in medical research indicate the need to recognize circumstances in which subject-related protections may be modified in order to facilitate the development of generalizable knowledge that is highly important to the welfare of society. For example, Carol Levine has discussed how the duty to secure informed consent poses problems for studies designed to determine HIV seroprevalence in various population groups.[26] If consent were required, unbiased samples (that make it possible to draw defensible statistical inferences regarding population seroprevalence) would be difficult to obtain. Levine argues that there are strong grounds for waiving informed consent requirements for these studies. The reasons cited include the importance of the knowledge to society, the lack of physical risks to subjects because blood drawn for other reasons would be used, and the lack of social risk because identifiers would not be attached to the data collected. I believe that the argument for this conclusion can be sustained using the presumptive-weighting strategy suggested by the federal regulations. Levine's introductory remarks seem to suggest, however, that the philosophical framework of the National Commission's recommendations and the subsequent federal regulations are not sufficiently flexible to embrace her conclusion regarding the seroprevalence studies.

On the other hand, some commentators have maintained that the recommendations of the National Commission and the regulations of the Department of Health and Human Services are not sufficiently protective of the interests of research subjects. According to this view, the recommendations and the federal rules fail in those instances in which any compromises in the fulfillment of duties to subjects are permitted. For example, Diana Baumrind criticizes provisions that allow for the waiver or alteration of consent requirements in research utilizing deception of subjects. She maintains that deceptive practices are wrong "because subjects are deprived of their right of informed consent and are thereby deprived of their right to decide freely and rationally how they wish to invest their time and persons."[27] In her view, baseline rules for protecting the interests of subjects in the exercise of personal autonomy cannot be modified by the potential benefits to society of certain forms of research. However, this assessment does not grapple directly with the critical differences between her framework assumptions and those underlying the federal regulations.

What is common to both types of criticisms is, I think, a failure to recognize that the presuppositions of the National Commission's recommendations and the federal regulations represent a clear departure from previous analyses of moral issues in clinical research. It is assumed that there are duties incumbent on society to conduct clinical research. It is also presupposed that there are duties incumbent on individuals to accept minor compromises of their interests as subjects in order to facilitate the development of generalizable knowledge that removes or prevents important harms to others. More generally, the reports of the National Commission and the federal regulations accept the proposition that there are no moral interests so important that their satisfaction may not be modestly compromised when counterbalanced by tremendous gains along other moral dimensions. These commitments and their supporting arguments undercut the acceptability of an absolute-priority approach to clinical-research ethics. At the same time, they suggest the strong plausibility of a balancing approach like the presumptive-weighting strategy.

An important legacy of the National Commission is this alternative conceptual framework for addressing moral issues in clinical research. A significant current challenge is to apply it systematically to the analysis of moral issues in clinical research, both old and new. It should pay rich dividends in promoting reflective agreement about appropriate norms for the conduct of clinical research.

NOTES

1. See J. Rawls, *A Theory of Justice* (Cambridge: Harvard University Press, 1971), 42-44.

2. See the National Commission for the Protection of Human Subjects of Biomedical and Behavioral Research (hereafter, the National Commission), *The Belmont Report: Ethical Guidelines for the Protection of Human Subjects of Research,* DHEW publication no. (OS) 78-0012 (Washington, D.C.: U.S. Government Printing Office, 1978), Appendix C of this book.

3. P. Ramsey, *The Patient as Person* (New Haven, Conn.: Yale University Press, 1970), 14; P. Ramsey, "The Enforcement of Morals: Nontherapeutic Research on Children," *Hastings Center Report* 6 (August 1976): 21-30.

4. R. McCormick, "Proxy Consent in the Experimental Situation," *Perspectives in Biology and Medicine* 18 (Autumn 1974): 2-20; R. McCormick, "Experimentation in Children: Sharing in Sociality," *Hastings Center Report* 6 (December 1976): 41-46.

5. R. Veatch, "Three Theories of Informed Consent: Philosophical Foundations and Policy Implications," in *The Belmont Report,* Appendix Volume II, by the National Commission for the Protection of Human Subjects, DHEW publication no. (OS) 78-0014 (Washington, D.C.: U.S. Government Printing Office, 1978), 26-1 - 26-66; H.T. Engelhardt, Jr., "Basic Ethical Principles in the Conduct of Biomedical and Behavioral Research," in *The Belmont Report,* Appendix Volume I, by the National Commission for the Protection of Human Subjects, DHEW publication no. (OS) 78-0013 (Washington, D.C.: U.S. Government Printing Office, 1978), 8-1 - 8-45.

6. Of course, the claim that duties to subjects "must always prevail" over pursuit of the general welfare is somewhat ambiguous. It might mean either (1) that these duties should be fully satisfied, or (2) that they should be assigned greater weight than considerations related to the general welfare are. However, the detailed provisions of the *Declaration of Helsinki* support interpretation (1).

References to the *Declaration of Helsinki* are drawn from the 1989 version. For the various renditions of the *Helsinki* doctrine, see G. Annas and M. Grodin, eds., *The Nazi Doctors and the Nuremberg Code* (New York: Oxford University Press, 1991), 331-42. The *Nuremberg Code* is Appendix A of this book; the *Declaration of Helsinki* is Appendix B.

7. Unlike the *Nuremberg Code,* however, the 1975 *Declaration of Helsinki* recognizes the legitimacy of surrogate consent, at least with respect to research involving therapeutic procedures.

8. A modification of this point could be required by paragraph II.5 of the *Declaration of Helsinki,* which indicates that "if the physician considers it essential not to obtain informed consent, the specific reasons for this proposal should be stated in the experimental protocol. . . ." On

its face, this exception is logically inconsistent with paragraph I.9, which requires that "in any research on human beings, each potential subject . . ." must consent to participation. One interpretation of the exception that saves the *Declaration* from inconsistency is that it envisions circumstances in which the well-being of the subject requires the waiving of consent. If this interpretation is correct, then the *Declaration* does not allow pursuit of the general welfare to modify full satisfaction of duties to subjects, but rather permits a paternalistic exception to the informed consent requirement stated in its "Basic Principles."

9. H. Jonas, "Philosophical Reflections on Experimenting with Human Subjects," in *Experimentation with Human Subjects,* ed. P. Freund (New York: George Braziller, 1969), 1-31.

10. For an excellent recent collection of essays on the Nuremberg Doctors' Trial and its implications for the development of research ethics and regulations, see Annas and Grodin, *The Nazi Doctors.*

11. See H. Beecher, "Ethics and Clinical Research," *New England Journal of Medicine* 274 (1966): 1354-60; and M.H. Pappworth, *Human Guinea Pigs* (London: Routledge and Kegan Paul, 1967). On the Jewish Chronic Disease Hospital Study, see J. Katz, *Experimentation with Human Beings* (New York: Russell Sage Foundation, 1972), 9-65. The story of the Tuskegee Syphilis Study is thoroughly dissected in J.H. Jones, *Bad Blood: The Tuskegee Syphilis Experiment,* 2d ed. (New York: Free Press, 1993).

12. For example, see U.S. Public Health Service, "Requirements for Review to Insure the Rights and Welfare of Individuals," revised 1 July 1966, reprinted in H. Beecher, *Research and the Individual* (Boston: Little, Brown, 1970), 293-96.

13. 45 *Code of Federal Regulations* 46, revised as of 8 March 1983.

14. For an earlier analysis of the weighting strategy embedded in the federal regulations, see T.F. Ackerman, "Balancing Moral Principles in Federal Regulations on Human Research," *IRB: A Review of Human Subjects Research* 14 (January-February 1992): 1-6.

15. In the case of persons institutionalized as mentally infirm, the commission suggests that the use of nontherapeutic research procedures involving greater than minimal risk be permitted with subjects unable to consent only if "such risk represents a minor increase over minimal risk" and "the anticipated knowledge (1) is of vital importance for the understanding or amelioration of the type of disorder or condition of the subjects or (2) may reasonably be expected to benefit the subjects in the future." See National Commission, *Report and Recommendations: Research Involving Those Institutionalized as Mentally Infirm,* DHEW

publication no. (OS) 78-0006 (Washington, D.C.: U.S. Government Printing Office, 1978), 16-20.

16. See R. Veatch, *The Patient as Partner: A Theory of Human-Experimentation Ethics* (Bloomington, Ind.: Indiana University Press, 1987), 172-74. See also Veatch's discussion in Chapter 2, pp. 48-51 of this book.

17. F. Roberts, P. Newcomb, and N. Fost, "Perceived Risks of Participation in an Epidemiologic Study," *IRB: A Review of Human Subjects Research* 15 (January-February 1993): 8-10.

18. Indeed, in their survey of subjects subsequent to participation in the epidemiological study, the authors found that 18 percent of the subjects expressed "concern" about the selection methodology and that 8 percent had "reservations" related to the protection of confidentiality. Because there is nothing unusual in the purpose or procedures of this study, these findings suggest that Veatch's third condition for approving such studies--the determination that reasonable persons would not object--could rarely, if ever, be satisfied.

19. H.T. Engelhardt, Jr., "Diagnosing Well and Treating Prudently: Randomized Clinical Trials and the Problem of Knowing Truly," in *The Use of Human Beings in Research*, ed. S. Spicker *et al.* (Dordrecht, The Netherlands: Kluwer Academic, 1988), 123-41.

20. J. Feinberg, *The Moral Limits of the Criminal Law: Harm to Others* (New York: Oxford University Press, 1984), 126-86.

21. See T.F. Ackerman, "Innovative Lifesaving Treatments: Do Children Have a Moral Right to Receive Them?" in *Contemporary Issues in Pediatric Ethics*, ed. M. Burgess and B. Woodrow (Lewiston, N.Y.: Edwin Mellin Press, 1991), 41-56.

22. Feinberg, *Moral Limits*.

23. See R. Goodin, *Protecting the Vulnerable* (Chicago: University of Chicago Press, 1985), 134-44.

24. See Veatch, "From Nuremberg Through the 1990s: The Priority of Autonomy," 57. Veatch does not clarify whether the lapse that his position is designed to avoid constitutes a logical lapse into a moral position conceptually indistinguishable from "naked utilitarianism" or an empirical lapse into widespread abuses of the rights and welfare of subjects that may result from the failure to accept the absolute priority of respect for the personal autonomy of subjects. However, both types of potential lapses are addressed below.

25. A. Jonsen, Chapter 3, pp. 80-81 of this book.

26. C. Levine, "Has AIDS Changed the Ethics of Human Subjects Research?" *Law, Medicine and Health Care* 16 (Winter 1988): 167-73.

27. See D. Baumrind, "The Costs of Deception," *IRB: A Review of Human Subjects Research* 1 (October 1979): 1-4.

5

Changing Views of Justice
after Belmont:
AIDS and the Inclusion of
"Vulnerable" Subjects

Carol Levine

This volume's subtitle reminds us that we stand at the brink of the 21st century. What can we expect? In P.D. James's novel, *The Children of Men*, set in an imagined 21st-century England, the King is under palace arrest, a dictator with the title of Warden rules with a hand-picked Council, and the Archbishop of Canterbury is a woman and a fervent antimonarchist. The Church of England has been superseded by television evangelists, the most popular of whom promises a pleasure-filled afterlife in a kind of eternal holiday on the Costa del Sol.

This state of affairs results from the loss of a future; the last children to be born anywhere in the world--the Omega generation--were born in 1995. Unexplained, universal infertility has created a world without children, and one in which all human life and civilization will eventually disappear. When the protagonist, an Oxford historian, confronts the Warden and the Council about some of the excesses of the regime (such as the mass coerced suicides of the elderly in a ritual called Quietus), one of the Council members defends the need for authoritarian control and says: "Man is diminished if he lives without knowledge of his past; without hope of a future he becomes a beast."[1]

This volume will keep us mindful of the past, in particular of the loss of human life, autonomy, and dignity that is epitomized by the Nazi experiments, but not limited to that horrendous episode. At the same time it will give us directions for a more humane future.

In the late 20th century, historical time has become compressed. The historian in P.D. James's novel specializes in the Victorian era, which lasted through most of the 19th century. *The Belmont Report*, a unifying theme of this volume, has achieved the status of a historical document, already up for reevaluation. Yet it was published in 1978, less than two decades ago.

THE PRINCIPLE OF JUSTICE REVISITED

The Belmont Report represented the culmination of the work of the National Commission for the Protection of Human Subjects of Biomedical and Behavioral Research. In its emphasis on three classic principles of theological and secular ethics--respect for persons, beneficence, and justice--it drew on the centuries-old history of Western thought. In its emphasis on protecting human subjects from harm, coercion, and unconsented experimentation, it reflected the history of the 30 years immediately preceding it.

This emphasis is understandable, given the signal event in the modern history of clinical-research ethics--the cruel and often fatal experiments performed on unconsenting prisoners by Nazi doctors during World War II.[2] American public opinion was shaped by the revelations of unethical experiments such as the Willowbrook hepatitis B studies at an institution for mentally retarded children;[3] the Jewish Chronic Disease Hospital studies, in which live cancer cells were injected into uninformed elderly patients;[4] and, especially, the Tuskegee Syphilis Study of poor black sharecroppers.[5] The single most influential article was written by Henry Knowles Beecher, a respected anesthesiologist, in the *New England Journal of Medicine*. Beecher described a number of studies at major research institutions that placed subjects at risk and failed to obtain informed consent.[6]

Our basic approach to the ethical conduct of research and approval of investigational drugs was born in scandal and reared in protectionism. Perceived as vulnerable, either because of their membership in groups lacking social power or because of personal characteristics suggesting a lack of autonomy, individuals were the primary focus of this concern.

Today the *Belmont* principles are still firmly in place. But there has been a major shift in emphasis and the beginnings of a shift in practice. Investigators, regulators, and institutional review boards (IRBs) are accustomed to examining the risk-benefit ratio (applying the principle of beneficence) and informed consent (applying the principle of respect for persons). But the selection of subjects as a matter of justice has often been considered last and in only one of its aspects--the protection of vulnerable groups from exploitation as subjects. Making justice an equal partner with respect for persons and beneficence does not reduce the likelihood of conflict among the principles or their corollaries; in fact, it adds a layer of complexity.

In *The Belmont Report*, the National Commission stated that justice is relevant to the selection of subjects at two levels--the social and the individual. At the individual level, the National Commission advised that "researchers exhibit fairness: thus, they should not offer potentially beneficial research only to some patients who are in their favor or select only 'undesirable' persons for risky research." At the social level, it said, "distinctions [should] be drawn between classes of subjects that ought, and ought not, to participate in any particular kind of research, based on the ability of members of that class to bear burdens and on the appropriateness of placing further burdens on already burdened persons." Specifically, the National Commission recommended, on the grounds of social justice, that classes of subjects be selected in an order of preference (for example, adults before children), and that some classes of potential subjects (for example, prisoners and the institutionalized mentally infirm) be selected only under certain conditions and perhaps not at all.

AIDS AS A CATALYST

It is ironic that around the same time that *The Belmont Report* was published, the forces of change--in the form of a new disease eventually called AIDS--were already emerging. The first official Centers for Disease Control report from Los Angeles, issued in June 1981, described cases of an unexplained illness in homosexual men who had been treated in the previous 30 months. Although other social, economic, and political forces have contributed to the shift in emphasis in the *Belmont* principles away from protectionism and toward inclusionism, AIDS has been the major catalyst for change.

AIDS took the world by surprise. Disregarding biological and human history, we in the industrialized world had largely come to believe that infectious diseases no longer posed a major threat. Epidemics were, we thought, either relegated to history, curable through one of the miracle drugs of the postwar pharmaceutical armamentarium, or a problem confined to the known diseases of the developing world.

Just as the medical and scientific worlds had to come to terms with the phenomenon of a new and complex retroviral disease, the worlds of law, ethics, and public policy had to grapple with the implications of a communicable disease primarily affecting groups--homosexual men and drug users of both sexes and their children--already stigmatized by mainstream society.

The ethics of research involving human subjects that had developed in the postwar period had focused on individual rights and welfare and on benefits to society through the acquisition of knowledge. It had not been much concerned with threats to public health through communicable diseases, nor with the impotence of medicine to halt or even significantly delay the deaths of large numbers of previously healthy young adults. Some of these young adults and their compatriots refused, in Dylan Thomas's phrase, to "go gently into that good night"; in their "railing against the dying of the light," they accelerated and shaped the deregulation of the drug-approval process that was already underway as a result of pressure from the pharmaceutical industry, legislators, and the public.

The initial demands from people with AIDS and their advocates were based on claims of individual justice and autonomy; that is, sick and dying patients wanted to make their own choices and take their own chances by using unapproved drugs for their lethal condition. The focus was on allowing broader access to ongoing clinical trials by patients who were willing to trade off potentially increased and certainly unknown risk for the possibility, however small, of benefit. Some patients, with the complicity of their physicians, managed to enroll by fudging data or lying outright, a practice well known in cancer trials.[7] Patients who were ineligible for trials because they did not fit the entry criteria or who did not want to be randomized into one of the study groups of a research protocol wanted the option of taking investigational drugs from the trial protocol.

The focus soon broadened, however, to questions of social justice. Groups disproportionately affected by HIV/AIDS--prisoners, drug users, and women (including many members of ethnic minorities)--were excluded from trials, either because of strict protocol entry criteria or because of lack of access to the physicians and healthcare institutions that control research. Interestingly, the initial calls for broadened access often came from those who were included--gay white men--and not just, or possibly not even primarily, from those who were excluded. Many clinicians, desperately seeking therapeutic options, also supported broadened access.

This chapter primarily concerns broadened access. There are, in addition, two other ways in which issues of justice have been reframed since *The Belmont Report*. One trend is an increased emphasis on gaining access to test drugs after a trial is completed but before the drug is approved, and to control the costs of drugs that have been approved, so that they are readily available to the populations that served as the testing ground. The second trend is a demand from the tested populations to have a significant voice in determining not just questions about the design of research but also the fundamental priorities of research. With AIDS, this has taken the form of advocacy for increased research on novel approaches to drug development, trials for drugs to treat opportunistic infections, and a de-emphasis on the profusion of trials involving zidovudine (AZT) and other antiretroviral drugs. Advocates for women's health issues have called for increased research on diseases that affect women throughout the life cycle. If the National Commission for the Protection of Human Subjects of Biomedical and Behavioral Research represented a democratization of the research process by allowing nonscientists--albeit highly experienced professionals in their own right--to enter the inner sanctum, then the past few years can fairly be described as a veritable town meeting.

SELECTING THE LEAST VULNERABLE

Underlying the protectionist view of the selection of subjects is the assumption that research is risky or at least burdensome. If this is true, then subjects should be selected in a way that protects those whose social, demographic, or economic characteristics make them particularly vulnerable to coercion and exploitation.

AIDS has been a catalyst for change, and the absence in recent years of the kind of scandal that came to light with depressing regularity in the 1960s and 1970s removed one barrier to change. The view of research as inherently risky and of research subjects as inherently needing protection has changed in the past several years. The actual physical risk in most research studies appears to be quite low. The President's Commission for the Study of Ethical Problems in Biomedical and Behavioral Research asked three large research institutions to summarize their experience with research-related injuries.[8] Each group found a very low incidence of adverse effects. In one institution, out of more than 8,000 subjects involved in 157 protocols, only three adverse effects were reported, including two headaches after spinal taps. Some of these reassuring results may be due to the vigilance of IRBs and investigators in reducing the likelihood of risk in designing and implementing studies. (There are, nonetheless, sporadic reports of serious injury and death to research subjects.)[9] While risk is an element that subjects always should consider when deciding whether to enter a study, it is now often no longer the paramount issue.

OPENING DOORS AT NIH AND FDA

In arguing for wider inclusion criteria in clinical trials, patient advocates and some clinicians have noted that, in the interest of good medical care, drugs should be tested on the populations that will use them. This belief runs counter to the more traditional research view of subject selection, which focuses on testing drugs in a small, homogeneous population in order to detect differences in efficacy and side effects as rapidly as possible.

The conventional view of appeals for broadened access is that they come from advocacy groups, sometimes noisy and disruptive ones. Yet traditional, even conservative, bodies have stated similar views. For example, the Council on Ethical and Judicial Affairs of the American Medical Association (AMA) declared in its 1991 report, "Gender Disparities in Clinical Decision Making," that "results of medical testing done solely on men should not be generalized to women without evidence that results can be applied safely and effectively to both sexes. Research on health problems that affect both sexes should include male and female subjects."[10]

Advocates' efforts have been given additional weight by the Congressional General Accounting Office (GAO). Examining the inclusion of women in clinical trials, the GAO reviewed the practices of the National Institutes of Health and the Food and Drug Administration.[11] In both instances women were found to be underrepresented. In June 1990, the GAO reported that grant applicants and NIH staff were noncompliant with the agency's stated policy of "encouraging" the inclusion of women as research subjects. Although NIH disagreed with some of the GAO's conclusions, in September 1990 it established the Office of Research on Women's Health "to strengthen and enhance the efforts of the NIH to improve the prevention, diagnosis, and treatment of illness in women and to enhance research related to diseases and conditions that affect women."[12]

In a potentially powerful move, because it brings to bear the power of the federal purse, the *NIH Guide for Grants and Contracts* now *requires* the inclusion of women and minorities. The guide states that grant, cooperative-agreement, and contract applicants:

will be required to include minorities and women in study populations so that research findings can be of benefit to all persons at risk of the disease, disorder or condition under study; special emphasis should be placed on the needs for inclusion of conditions which disproportionately affect them. This policy is intended to apply to males and females of all ages. If women or minorities are excluded or are inadequately represented in clinical research, particularly in proposed population-based studies, a clear compelling rationale for exclusion or inadequate representation should be provided.

Furthermore, any justification for not including women in such studies will be evaluated by the peer-review group assessing the proposal and factored into the final recommendation. No application or proposal for which the justification for exclusion of women is considered inappropriate will be funded unless such a justification is compelling.[13] To date there has been no official accounting of how this policy is working or whether some projects have not been funded because of lack of representativeness.

In Section 492B of the 1993 NIH Revitalization Act, Congress extended this policy by requiring NIH's director to ensure that "each federally funded research project include women and members of minority groups."[14] The NIH director can authorize exceptions. NIH-funded trials must be analyzed to determine whether women or members of minority groups would respond differently to the intervention or agents being studied. Cost is not a permissible consideration in determining whether inclusion is appropriate. Cost may be considered only when the data regarding women or members of minority groups that would be obtained in the project have been or will be obtained through other means that offer comparable quality. This legislative provision does not answer the question of whether transportation, child care, and other types of financial support that will be necessary to enroll women will be considered legitimate trial costs.

An Institute of Medicine study cautions:

neither adherence to quotas in the composition of a study cohort nor the irrational exclusion of a subgroup of people can be supported scientifically. Determining the number of women to be included in a trial should reflect reasonable hypotheses about the relation of treatment efficacy to sex, not global rules about the composition of study cohorts.[15]

The forces of change have not been limited to the NIH. The GAO's review of FDA policies and practices, issued in October 1992, found that although women were represented in every clinical trial of the 53 drugs approved by the FDA in the previous three and one-half years, for more than 60 percent of the drugs the proportion of women in the trial was less than the proportion of women with the corresponding disease. Women were particularly underrepresented in trials of cardiovascular drugs, even though cardiovascular disease is the leading cause of death in women. The report found that the FDA has not "issued specific guidance or criteria for drug manufacturers to use in determining the extent and sufficiency of female representation in Phase 2 and 3 drug trials." The FDA has not defined "representation" nor provided guidance to drug manufacturers for determining when sufficient numbers of women are included in clinical trials to detect gender-related differences in drug response. As a result, pharmaceutic sponsors are uncertain as to what the FDA expects. The focus of challenges to FDA policies has been the agency's 1977 guidelines for the clinical evaluation of drugs. Until the guidelines were revised in mid-1993, women of childbearing age were excluded from large-scale clinical trials until the FDA Animal Reproduction Guidelines were completed, except in cases of life-threatening illness. For Phase 1 studies (to determine pharmacokinetics, the safety of a range of doses, or the mechanism of a drug action) the guidelines stated that "in general, women of childbearing potential should be excluded." For Phase 2 studies (small-scale trials to determine efficacy), women could be included "provided segment II and the female part of segment I of the FDA Animal Reproduction Guidelines have been completed."[16]

Explaining the FDA's decision to revise the guidelines, an FDA working group noted: "In 1993, protecting the fetus from unanticipated exposure to potentially harmful drugs remains critically important, but the ban on women's participation in early clinical trials no longer seems reasonable." The working group cited the scientific benefits of identifying important sex differences in early drug trials, the ethical benefits in terms of enhancing autonomy, and the possibility of reducing the risk of fetal exposure through protocol design (administering a single dose to a woman during or immediately following her menstrual period or after a negative pregnancy-test result). [17]

Even with broadened inclusion criteria, not all patients who want access to promising new agents can be enrolled in clinical trials, either because they fail to meet the inclusion criteria, they live too far away from a research center, or the trials are already closed. Several other mechanisms have been developed, such as the "parallel track," in which qualified patients who cannot enroll in clinical trials may obtain promising drugs through their physicians.[18] Community-based research, especially in cancer and AIDS, has also made clinical trials more accessible to patients. Buyers' clubs make drugs that are on the market in Europe and Asia available to patients, largely without FDA interference.

The main, federally supported, clinical-research effort in AIDS is the NIH-sponsored AIDS Clinical Trials Group (ACTG). Since its inception in 1986, it has generally included fewer people of color and fewer women than the distribution of HIV illness would suggest.[19] As of 22 January 1993, 21,695 people have participated in ACTG trials; 3,645, or 16.9 percent have been African Americans. Yet African Americans account for approximately 29.5 percent of the 249,199 adult or adolescent AIDS cases reported as of 31 December 1992.[20] Hispanic participants are more closely representative: they made up 14.9 percent of the total in ACTG trials and 16.5 percent of all adult and adolescent AIDS cases. These figures, however, represent an increase over minority participation in 1987, which was only 7 percent for African Americans and 11 percent for Hispanics. Women account for 11 percent of AIDS cases and 10.3 percent of ACTG subjects--an increase since 1987, when they made up only 5 percent of trial participants.[21] By comparison, women comprised 7 percent of all reported adult AIDS cases in 1987.[22]

These national figures may be somewhat misleading, since the participation of women and minorities varies considerably at different sites. Some research centers have attracted large numbers of women and minorities while others have low numbers of such subjects. While higher overall participation rates may be sufficient to answer the scientific questions, access for individuals may not have improved.

A newer mechanism offering greater access to clinical trials is the National Institute of Allergy and Infectious Diseases's (NIAID's) Community Programs for Clinical Research on AIDS (CPCRA). Begun in October 1989, the CPCRA involves 17 community-based research programs at about 160 sites in 13 U.S. cities. This program differs from the ACTG by involving primary-care physicians and nurses at community hospitals and health centers, private clinics and practices, and drug-treatment facilities.[23] Because the research setting is more decentralized and primary-care physicians are more involved in setting research priorities, the CPCRA is more likely to recruit minority participants. Of the total enrollment of 6,190 patients (as of 23 January 1993), 57 percent were African American or Hispanic; 19 percent were women, and 38 percent were injection-drug users.[24]

Even in this effort, however, participation by gender and ethnic minority differs considerably by location. Participants in CPCRA trials conducted by the Harlem AIDS Treatment Group in Manhattan are 77.1 percent African American and 41 percent female. In New Jersey, trial participants are quite evenly balanced: 20 percent female, 23.7 pecent Latin/Hispanic, and 44.2 percent African American. The CPCRA trials at the Henry Ford Hospital in Detroit have 39.3 percent African-American subjects but only 9.1 percent women. The Denver CPCRA has a largely white male subject population, with 3.9 percent female subjects. Denver is second (1.4 percent) only to San Francisco (2.4 percent), however, in the percentage of Asian-American participants.[25] Many of these differences can be explained by the local variations in subject populations, but they illustrate that equal access can be quite unequal.

A new NIH program--the NIAID-sponsored Division of AIDS Treatment Research Initiative, or DATRI--provides rapid evaluation of potential new therapeutic agents and regimens. Of its initial 49 subjects, 30.9 percent were people of color.[26]

Other NIH efforts to expand the numbers of minorities and women in its trials include the establishment of ACTG and CPCRA women's health committees to initiate new protocols and improve the recruitment of women. Both ACTG and CPCRA have community advisory boards to increase participation of underrepresented populations and to improve awareness of specific community concerns.

In its 1992 report, *The Challenge of HIV/AIDS in Communities of Color*, the National Commission on AIDS recognized both the underrepresentation of minorities and recent improvements in recruitment and retention. It recommended:

The National Institutes of Health, in conjunction with other appropriate agencies within the Department of Health and Human Services, should intensify efforts to assure access to HIV/AIDS clinical trial information, with regard to trial opportunities, the results of research efforts, and their significance for clinical management. Emphasis should be placed on reaching populations that have had poor or underrepresentative access to clinical trial opportunities. Efforts should include the collection and dissemination of trial-related research and information on new developments in treatment. Dissemination should be carried out in a manner that ensures that information is current, accurate, and comprehensible to target populations and the health professionals who serve them. [27]

This statement is notable for its clear understanding of research as benefit and its advocacy of redressing the imbalance of selection of research subjects.

CHILDREN AS RESEARCH SUBJECTS

Nearly all drugs approved for marketing by the FDA carry a label warning that "this drug is not to be used in children . . ." or "is not recommended for use in infants and young children, since few studies have been carried out in this group. . . ." Pediatricians are forced to extrapolate and estimate dosages for their young patients. As Robert J. Levine has pointed out, "We have a tendency to distribute unsystematically the unknown risks of drugs in children and pregnant women, thus maximizing the frequency of their occurrence and minimizing the probability of their detection."[28]

Protocols involving sick children present particularly difficult choices for investigators, IRBs, primary-care physicians, parents, and foster-care agencies. Investigators typically present information to IRBs to justify the participation of children. Given the ethical imperative to do research, especially on lethal diseases such as HIV/AIDS, an IRB would be hard pressed to justify any delays or significant revisions in a pediatric protocol.

In the past few years, there have been significant advances in pediatric HIV research: notably, studies on AZT, ddI, and ddC. The NIAID now has 15 pediatric AIDS Clinical Treatment Units (ACTUs) within the ACTG. The National Institute of Child Health and Development also has a clinical-trials network, and several other NIH institutes, such as the National Cancer Institute, are also involved in pediatric research. The development of an effective method to prevent maternal-fetal transmission, through the use of anti-retroviral drugs or vaccines, is a high priority nationally and internationally as well.

The public attention on pediatric AIDS has made an impact on pediatric research in other areas. In the fall of 1990, the Pharmaceutical Manufacturers Association published its first survey of drug testing with children. The survey found that 114 pediatric drugs and vaccines were undergoing testing, "although researchers are faced with problems of recruitment, safety and costs for drug testing in children."[29]

The 114 medicines involved 127 research projects, because some of the drugs and vaccines were being tested for more than one use. A quarter of the research projects (32) were for rare diseases; 11 were for genetic disorders, seven each are for HIV/AIDS and growth disorders, and another five were for asthma. Bacterial infections and cancer were the largest categories, with 26 and 24 drugs, respectively. Developing improved DPT vaccines (diphtheria, pertussis, and tetanus) was a high priority. Nine projects dealt with viral infections, including polio, chicken pox, and measles.

Because many of the potential child subjects for HIV/AIDS research are in foster care, their opportunities for participation have been severely limited by the lack of state or agency policies and the reluctance of agency officials to approve the entry of children into trials. A 1990 survey by Judith M. Martin and Henry S. Sacks found that only seven states--Connecticut, Georgia, Illinois, Massachusetts, New Jersey, Texas, and Wyoming--had formal policies. Five states--California, Maryland, New York, North Carolina, and Pennsylvania--had a mechanism making it possible to enroll foster children in trials. In four of these 12 states--Illinois, New York, Pennsylvania, and Wyoming--the biological parent must consent. In 1991, New York City adopted a policy that permits a physician to enroll a child in an approved trial without parental consent if the parent is not available, as long as a "diligent search" has been made to find the parent. Official consent is given by the Commissioner of the Human Resources Administration as the legal custodian of the child.[30]

TOWARD THE 21ST CENTURY

In looking toward the future, we must again be mindful of the past. There still are significant barriers to a full implementation of the principle of justice as exemplified in the selection of research subjects. Two experiences in particular have shaped current attitudes and practices. Two words carry enormous symbolic weight: thalidomide and Tuskegee.

The experience that has most influenced the exclusion of women from research is related to the drug thalidomide: typically it is referred to as the "thalidomide disaster."[31] Thalidomide was synthesized in West Germany in 1954 and approved for marketing in 1958. Its primary use was as a sedative and antidote for nausea in early pregnancy. At least 20 countries approved the over-the-counter sale of thalidomide, including Canada, Great Britain, Australia, and Sweden, but not the United States.

During the same period that thalidomide was being widely distributed, physicians noted an alarming increase in the number of children being born with an unusual and extremely rare set of deformities. The most prominent feature was *phocomelia*, a condition in which the hands are attached to the shoulders and the feet are attached to the hips, superficially resembling the flippers of a seal. By 1962, when sufficient statistical evidence had accumulated to establish thalidomide as the agent causing these deformities, about 8,000 children had been affected. About 35 percent of the women who had received this drug--even a single dose of it-- during early pregnancy bore deformed babies. The harm done to women and their infants by thalidomide was not the result of participation in research; it was the result of inadequate research standards (even by contemporary standards), corporate greed, and physicians' uncritical acceptance of promotional claims. The West German firm that developed thalidomide had had to redefine the nature of "sleep" in standard animal tests to prove that the drug had a hypnotic effect; it ignored early and disquieting reports of side effects--including the very serious neurological complication of peripheral neuritis--and it concealed the number of reported cases of this complication. It used money and influence to counter critical reports with favorable ones. Physicians, too, were at fault in succumbing to aggressive promotional efforts to use a new drug when older, more adequately tested drugs were available.

Animal tests that would have proved that thalidomide was teratogenic were not generally performed at the time. However, those that were available would have clearly established the strong possibility of teratogenicity, and it was well known that drugs could cross the placental barrier and affect the fetus. In fact, a British scientist at the firm that held the distribution license for thalidomide discovered that baby rabbits born to mothers given the drug had the same deformities found in children.

In the United States, a cautious FDA official, Dr. Frances Kelsey--suspecting that thalidomide might cause birth defects--delayed marketing approval, thus lessening the impact on American women. Nevertheless, over 1,200 "investigating" doctors did give their patients the thalidomide made available to them by the drug company that was seeking approval (perhaps in an effort to build physicians' support for the drug). At least 18 thalidomide babies were born in this country as a result, and many more women carrying affected fetuses miscarried.

Dr. Kelsey's caution was well grounded, and the 1962 Kefauver-Harris amendments to the drug-approval laws institutionalized a rigorous preapproval process (Food, Drug, and Cosmetic Act, 1962).[32] Equally important, the powerful emotional impact of the thalidomide experience created an aversion to involving women, especially pregnant women or women of childbearing age, in drug research. Investigators, IRBs, and regulators all approach the inclusion of women of childbearing age in drug trials with considerable caution, if not outright aversion. Only a few IRBs have developed specific policies in favor of inclusion, and these are in community-based HIV/AIDS research settings. For example, in 1989 the Community Research Initiative (CRI, now the Community Research Initiative on AIDS, or CRIA) in New York City developed the policy statement, "Participants of Reproductive Potential." It states:

CRI, in recognition of the continuing exclusion of women from clinical trials, will make every effort not to accept a protocol that treats women and men of reproductive potential differently, unless there is solid scientific basis for that difference. In assessing the legitimacy of exclusion criteria regarding the reproductive potential (including pregnancy), CRI will not necessarily place higher value on the potential risk to offspring than on the potential benefit to the trial participant, as in other situations where the potential benefit to the life and health of the patient is considered to justify some increment of risk to the health of the potential offspring. In making this judgment, the CRI will take into account the availability of alternative therapies for the potential parent which present less risk to potential offspring.

CRI will undertake to ensure that all participants in approved trials will receive adequate information about potential adverse reproductive outcomes.

The IRB of the Whitman-Walker Clinic in Washington, D.C., has also considered the exclusion of women in HIV-drug studies. Its statement declares: "We call on other IRBs to reject participation in any drug trial that excludes women and to join together to demand systematic drug studies of promising drug treatments for pregnant women and women who decline to use birth control methods."[33]

In 1975 Bernard L. Mirkin, Professor of Pediatrics and Pharmacology at the University of Minnesota, posed the options available to society bluntly:

Society may choose to forbid drug evaluation in pregnant women and children. This choice would certainly reduce the risk of damaging individuals through research. However, this would maximize the possibility of random disaster resulting from use of inadequately investigated drugs. In the final analysis it seems safe to predict that more individuals would be damaged; however, the damage would be distributed randomly rather than imposed upon preselected individuals.[34]

The Tuskegee experience presents a barrier of a different sort. This 40-year, Public Health Service sponsored study began in 1932 in rural Macon County, Georgia. Building on both a beneficent motive (using research to replace diminishing funds for syphilis-control programs among poor blacks) and dubious (but then popular) theories about racial differences in disease between blacks and whites, the Tuskegee study enrolled 400 black men with syphilis and 200 members of a control group to study the natural history of the untreated disease. Although the study was originally planned to last only six to nine months, it was extended for 40 years.

The abuses of subjects' rights and welfare during this long period have been well documented: false descriptions of research procedures like spinal taps as treatment; failure to provide currently available therapy and, when it became available, a cure by penicillin; lack of informed consent; the use of burial funds as an inducement to family members to give permission for autopsies.[35] The legacy of Tuskegee is "a trail of distrust and suspicion" that hampers efforts to enroll African Americans in clinical trials as well as to attract them to HIV-prevention and -education programs. Dr. Mark Smith testified to the National Commission on AIDS that the African-American community "is already alienated from the healthcare system and the government and . . . somewhat cynical about the motives of those who arrive in their communities to help them."[36] Stephen Thomas and Sandra Crouse Quinn have asserted in a compelling article that the continuing legacy of Tuskegee "has contributed to Blacks' belief that genocide is possible and that public health authorities cannot be trusted."[37]

Although the details of both the thalidomide and Tuskegee stories may have become distorted in the retelling, they easily fit into powerful beliefs about risks to fetuses, on the one hand, and the existence of officially condoned racism to the point of genocide, on the other.

Moreover, important ethical issues in both instances have not been resolved. There is no resolution of the conflict between American society's failure to provide basic healthcare and HIV/AIDS prevention programs to poor communities of color--a matter of social justice--and the potential coerciveness of using research participation as an entry into the healthcare system. "Why," one African-American woman said to me, "am I in such demand as a research subject when nobody wants me as a patient?"

In redressing the imbalance caused by policies that exclude women without scientific or ethical justification, it is important to remember that women, particularly women who are or may become pregnant, have special moral responsibilities to fetuses that they plan to carry to term, as do investigators and IRB members who develop or approve protocols involving women.

The ethical obligation not to do harm carries particular force when the recipient of the potential harm is an unconsenting fetus, whose future health and welfare may be unalterably affected. Approval by an IRB of a protocol is not an ethically neutral stance: it is an affirmative statement that the choices to be offered to potential subjects, while perhaps difficult to make, are ethically justifiable. Exposing a fetus to serious risk when there are alternative treatments or when the benefits are modest is not, in my view, an ethically justifiable choice.

The potential of harm to a fetus is a morally relevant factor, not least to the mother herself. The vast majority of women see their own primary interests as identical with those of their fetuses. Women do not lightly undertake any medical intervention that will have an adverse outcome on their fetuses; many women in fact may deny themselves optimal medical care in order to avoid risk. Some, however, may exercise their right to choose medical treatments despite known or unknown risks to the fetus.

Some, perhaps most, protocols may not present any known or foreseeable risks to fetuses; for these protocols, there are (as has already been pointed out) no reasons to exclude women, especially those who are not pregnant or do not plan to become pregnant. Some HIV/AIDS protocols may carry the possibility of minimal or even moderate risk to fetuses, but also offer the possibility of great benefit to women. An obvious example would be a life-saving drug or a cure. Another example might be a study involving a drug to treat a debilitating opportunistic infection for which there are no acceptable alternative therapies. In these cases women should not be excluded automatically but should be given the opportunity to make that calculus for themselves, with careful explanation of the risks and benefits.

There remains, however, the small but worrisome category of studies involving drugs that present high risk to fetuses and minimal or even moderate benefit to women. Some would argue that risks to fetuses, as unconsenting participants, must always outweigh considerations of autonomy. Others would argue that there are never any grounds to override a woman's autonomy and to deny her the choice of whether to participate. In this view, valuing a fetus's welfare more highly than a woman's autonomy is objectionable in principle.

Is there a middle ground? Protocols in other diseases may fail to gain approval on grounds of excessive risk to subjects, even when there are potential benefits. Risks to fetuses cannot simply be dismissed as irrelevant, even if one does not grant them rights. But what would constitute serious or excessive risk? Opinions would differ. The administration of zidovudine to pregnant women to see whether it reduces HIV transmission might strike some as posing serious risk to the more than two-thirds of fetuses who would receive a toxic substance *in utero* but be uninfected. Yet such a study has been approved and federally funded. Although the pregnant woman might benefit from receiving the drug, that is not the purpose of the study. In fact, according to the protocol, zidovudine would be discontinued after delivery. Of course the woman might receive it under different auspices.

At the extremes, choices about including pregnant women or women of childbearing age are relatively straightforward. Excluding a woman suffering from a life-threatening condition from access to a potentially life-saving drug on the grounds of harm to an unconceived fetus seems not only unjust but harsh. When the woman is pregnant and her life is in danger, her fetus is equally threatened. At the other extreme, to expose women and their actual or potential fetuses to serious harms when there are alternative therapies or the potential benefits are only trivial honors autonomy at the expense of common sense.

Even if exclusionary barriers related to gender or substance abuse were totally removed, women would still face problems in access to research because of their lack of access to primary healthcare and their special needs for assistance with childcare, transportation, and family responsibilities. Recruitment efforts will have to take into account the multiple roles women play as family caregivers and employees (often in marginal jobs with few opportunities for flexibility). Meeting their own healthcare needs may not be their highest priority; enrolling in research, an alien concept to many, may seem even less important.

The goal is not to convince women to become research subjects, either for their own good or for the good of society, but to make the selection of subjects to undertake the risks and share in the benefits of research more equitable.

Are we headed back to the future? Or can we use the past to create a more just healthcare and research system? As we debate the refining and reinterpretation of the principles of *The Belmont Report*, let us not lose sight of their value as markers of the past and guideposts leading us into the 21st century.

NOTES

1. P.D. James, *The Children of Men* (New York: Alfred A. Knopf, 1992), 98.

2. A.L. Caplan, *When Medicine Went Mad: Bioethics and the Holocaust* (Totawa, N.J.: Humana Press, 1992).

3. D.J. Rothman, "Were Tuskegee and Willowbrook 'Studies in Nature'?" *Hastings Center Report* 12 (April 1982): 5-7.

4. J. Katz, *Experimentation with Human Beings* (New York: Russell Sage Foundation, 1972).

5. J. Jones, *Bad Blood: The Tuskegee Syphilis Experiment*, 2d ed. (New York: Free Press, 1993).

6. H.K. Beecher, "Ethics and Clinical Research," *New England Journal of Medicine* 274 (1966): 1354-60; D.J. Rothman, *Strangers at the Bedside: A History of How Law and Bioethics Transformed Medical Decision Making* (New York: Basic Books, 1991).

7. H.Y. Vanderpool and G.B. Weis, "False Data and Last Hopes: Enrolling Patients in Clinical Trials," *Hastings Center Report* (April 1987): 16-19.

8. The President's Commission for the Study of Ethical Problems in Medicine and Biomedical and Behavioral Research, *Compensating for Research Injuries: The Ethical and Legal Implications of Programs to Redress Injured Subjects* (Washington, D.C.: U.S. Government Printing Office, 1982).

9. See, for example, a report of two deaths in the first days of an NIH trial of a new drug for hepatitis B, and the subsequent cancellation of the study. "Tests of Hepatitis Drug are Stopped as 2 Die," *New York Times*, 9 July 1993, A-10.

10. Council on Ethical and Judicial Affairs, "Gender Disparities in Clinical Decision Making," *Journal of the American Medical Association* 266 (1991): 562.

11. GAO, U.S. Congress, *National Institutes of Health: Problems Implementing Policy on Women in Study Populations*, GAO/T-HRD-90-38, (Washington, D.C.: General Accounting Office, 1990); GAO, U.S. Congress, *Women's Health: FDA Needs to Ensure More Study of Gender Differences in Prescription Drug Testing*, GAO/HRD-93-17, (Washington, D.C.: General Accounting Office, 1992).

12. R.L. Kirschstein, "Research on Women's Health," *American Journal of Public Health* 81 (1991): 291-93.

13. NIH, *NIH Instruction and Information Memorandum OER 90-5 (Inclusion of Minorities and Women in Study Population)*, 12/11/90 (Bethesda, Md.: U.S. Government Printing Office, 1990).

14. U.S. Public Law 103-43, National Institutes of Health Revitalization Amendment, Cong., 1st sess., (10 June 1993).

15. J.C. Bennett, "Inclusion of Women in Clinical Trials--Policies for Population Subgroups," *New England Journal of Medicine* 329 (1993): 288-92.

16. FDA, *General Considerations for the Clinical Evaluation of Drugs* (Washington, D.C.: U.S. Government Printing Office, 1977).

17. R. Merkatz *et al.*, "Women in Clinical Trials of New Drugs: A Change in Food and Drug Administration Policy," *New England Journal of Medicine* 329 (1993): 271-72.

18. "Expanded Availability of Investigational New Drugs through a Parallel Track Mechanism for People with AIDS and Other HIV-related Disease," 57 *Federal Register* 13250-59.

19. The statistics on minority participation are drawn from the National Commission on AIDS, *The Challenge of HIV/AIDS in Communities of Color* (Washington, D.C.: National Commission on AIDS, 1992), 18-22.

20. Data provided by the National Institute on Allergy and Infectious Diseases, *Demographic Summary of ACTG Study Entries from Beginning to 1/22/93*, and *Demographic Summary of CPCRA Participants, 25 January 1993;* cumulative data on the reported number of AIDS cases through 31 December 1992 is from the Centers for Disease Control and Prevention, *HIV/AIDS Surveillance Report* (February 1993).

21. FDA, *General Considerations.*

22. CDC, *HIV/AIDS Surveillance Report* (13 April 1987).

23. FDA, *General Considerations.*

24. Merkatz *et al.*, "Women in Clinical Trials."

25. Community Programs for Clinical Research on AIDS, *Demographic Characteristics of Patients by Unit* (Washington, D.C.: U.S. Government Printing Office, 19 February 1993).

26. FDA, *General Considerations.*

27. National Commission on AIDS, *The Challenge of HIV/AIDS in Communities of Color*, 26.

28. R.J. Levine, *Ethics and Regulation of Clinical Research*, 2nd ed. (Baltimore: Urban & Schwarzenberg, 1986), 240.

29. Pharmaceutical Manufacturers Association, *New Medicines in Development for Children* (Washington, D.C.: Pharmaceutical Manufacturers Association, 1990).

30. J.M. Martin and H.S. Sacks, "Do HIV-infected Children in Foster Care Have Access to Clinical Trials of New Treatments?" *AIDS & Public Policy Journal* 5 (1990): 3-8.

31. The Insight Team of the *Sunday Times* of London, *Suffer the Children: The Study of Thalidomide* (New York: Viking Press, 1979).

32. *Food, Drug, and Cosmetic Act, U.S. Code,* vol. 21, secs. 201-902 (1962, as amended 1980), 321-92.

33. Whitman-Walker Clinic Institutional Review Board, *HIV Drug Studies, Women, and Pregnancy: A Statement from the Whitman-Walker Clinic Institutional Review Board* (Washington, D.C.: Whitman-Walker Clinic IRB, n.d.).

34. B.L. Mirkin, "Drug Therapy and the Developing Human: Who Cares?" *Clinical Research* 23 (1975): 110-11.

35. Jones, *Bad Blood.*

36. National Commission on AIDS, *Hearings on HIV Diseases on African American Communities* (Washington, D.C.: U.S. Government Printing Office, 1990), 19.

37. S.B. Thomas and S. Crouse Quinn, "The Tuskegee Syphilis Study, 1932-1972: Implications for HIV Education and AIDS Risk Education Programs in the Black Community," *American Journal of Public Health* 81 (1991): 1498-1505.

6

Challenges to IRBs in the Coming Decades

Charles R. McCarthy

Public policy requiring institutional review boards (IRBs) to exercise oversight over research involving human subjects is now 31 years old. The process of independent committee review of research involving human subjects in the United States is much older. I have learned, anecdotally, of a precursor IRB at the University of California, Los Angeles as early as 1929. Prior to issuance of the Public Health Service Policy in 1966, at least 16 major research centers had operational committees that reviewed research involving human subjects.

Some of the institutions, including the National Institutes of Health Clinical Center, reviewed only research involving normal, healthy volunteers. Apparently, the reasoning for limiting review was that if physicians believed that research subjects would receive medical benefit from participating in research, their consent could be presumed. Physicians decided whether their patients should or should not participate in clinical studies. Patients trusted their physicians. Few discerned the fact that a physician-researcher has intentions that lie beyond the best interests of the patient.

In a matter of several decades, IRB oversight of research involving human subjects has become a fixture in the research firmament. Our society relies on the IRB to make certain that the rights and the welfare of research subjects, whether they are normal volunteers or patients, are protected in both biomedical and behavioral research.

Although some investigators chafe under the scrutiny of the local IRB, there is little chance of returning to the practices of yesteryear. Oversight by an appropriate and approved IRB, public accountability in research, and recognition of the subject as a full research partner are not only required by law and regulation, but they are values now taken for granted by most of the research community.

Biomedical researchers in this country can be justly proud of the fact that since the Tuskegee study was exposed in 1971,[1] there have been few allegations of abuse of subjects, only a handful of cases where regulatory noncompliance has been documented, and scarcely any documented cases of serious harm inflicted on subjects.

Although the number of research studies involving human beings has steadily increased, (the U.S. Public Health Service--PHS--supports approximately 25,000 projects involving human subjects at any given point in time) the number of cases of noncompliance with regulations has decreased.[2] Consequently, the fraction of research studies in which abuses occur is becoming steadily smaller. All evidence seems to suggest that the system of oversight of the rights and welfare of human subjects, taken as a whole, compares favorably with other regulatory systems in our society. Successful protection has been provided for subjects in a country that continues to be the world's leader in clinical innovation and progress. Although it seems counter-intuitive, historical evidence suggests that sound research design and ethical behavior by researchers go hand in hand.

One might well conclude from the positive record of research involving human subjects that we need to freeze the situation as it is. Critics are few in number and the system is now working better than it ever has. "If the system ain't broke, don't fix it," could be the motto of our time. It might be argued that because the United States has no National Commission, no ethics advisory board, no President's Commission, in fact no standing federal bioethics committee of any kind to guide changes, and because the United States has documented no major human subjects abuses, it needs only to maintain the status quo and all will be well.

A case has been made that our society can utilize committees established by the Institute of Medicine (within the National Academy of Sciences) and state public health boards and commissions to make minor midcourse adjustments in the way that research is conducted. Nothing more is needed.[3]

In my opinion, a *laissez faire* research ethics policy calling for mere maintenance of the present situation would be a serious mistake.

The U.S. Department of Health and Human Services (DHHS) published "Basic DHHS Policy for the Protection of Human Research Subjects," 45 *Code of Federal Regulations* 46, subpart A, the regulations that constituted the basic DHHS policy for the protection of human research subjects, on 26 January 1981.[4] The DHHS also widely publicized and required awardee institutions to utilize the principles set forth in *The Belmont Report* to guide institutional programs for the protection of human subjects and to interpret the new regulations.

When the basic regulations were published, many within the PHS believed that the important task of determining how research involving human subjects ought to be conducted had been completed for all time, and that the regulatory edifice built on the commission's recommendations and guided by *The Belmont* principles would last for generations--perhaps forever.

It is apparent to anyone who looks back on deliberations of the National Commission from the vantage point of 1995, that the work of the commission continues to represent sound ethical thinking relative to biomedical and behavioral research. However, it is equally apparent that much of the work of the commission is time-bound and dated.

Many new biomedical and behavioral research problems have emerged that were not addressed by the commission.[5] The need for identifying additional principles or finding ways to apply established principles to new research problems involving human subjects is becoming more evident each year.

The issues described below constitute my best judgment concerning the nature of new problems that are facing IRBs or that will face them by the time we enter the 21st century.

THE CHALLENGE TO SELF-REGULATION

In the decades of the 1970s and 1980s, a number of DHHS regulatory systems patterned, in whole or in part, after the DHHS regulations for the protection of human subjects were brought into existence. These included the regulation of recombinant DNA activities, the Public Health Service policy on humane care and use of laboratory animals, radiation restrictions, laboratory safety policies, regulation of scientific integrity, and proposed regulations to prevent conflicts of interest.

Although created for different purposes, all of these systems share common elements: (1) they require awardee institutions to regulate themselves; (2) they require awardee institutions to negotiate the details of self-regulation with DHHS by means of a document called an assurance of compliance which, when approved by DHHS, is binding on the institution; (3) they feature a system of shared responsibility that links principal investigators, research institutions, and federal agencies in a common effort; (4) they require awardee institutions to make, or be prepared to make, a public accounting of the results of their efforts at self-regulation; and (5) they rely primarily on mutual trust shared by all the parties to the negotiation of the assurances of compliance. In short, throughout the 1970s and 1980s, the expanding regulatory framework of the DHHS required awardee institutions to establish trust-based, self-regulating, and publicly accountable systems. Generally speaking, this framework has been widely accepted by the public, the Congress, and the biomedical research community. It seems to accommodate well to the culture and independence of academic inquiry.

By the late 1980s and early 1990s, however, ominous questions began to be raised regarding the institutional self-regulating system required by DHHS. First, Mr. Jeremy Rifkin repeatedly charged that DHHS had not established adequate review mechanisms and safeguards to provide appropriate protection for society, the environment, and human subjects against hazards that may be associated with recombinant DNA research. Mr. Rifkin subsequently criticized the ethical aspects of harvesting and using fetal tissue in transplantation research. The Bush administration appointed an *ad hoc* advisory committee to address the question of the use of fetal tissue, then rejected the advice of its own committee and placed a moratorium on the use of fetal tissue in human transplantation research.

Second, radical animal rights groups have resorted to criticism in the media, public demonstrations, destruction of laboratories, harassment of scientists, and lobbying for state and federal laws to prevent or restrict the use of laboratory animals. Many activists find all regulation and use of animals in research to be unacceptable and demand that all such research be terminated.

Recently, animal activists won a major victory in the Washington, D.C. Federal District Court. They persuaded a federal judge to overturn Department of Agriculture Animal Welfare Act Regulations (patterned after the PHS policy on humane care and use of laboratory animals) pertaining to the care of dogs and nonhuman primates. The Animal Legal Defense Fund claimed that the law does not allow institutional review committees and veterinarians to have a role in setting standards for the care of laboratory animals.[6]

Third, a challenge from a different quarter, with potential for uprooting the entire regulatory structure under which biomedical and behavioral research currently functions, has been spearheaded by Democratic Representative John Dingell of Michigan. Mr. Dingell has repeatedly questioned the ability of research institutions to regulate their own research.[7] Most of the cases addressed by the Dingell subcommittee involve accusations of scientific misconduct (such as falsifying, misrepresenting, or stealing data, or engaging in plagiarism).[8] At the heart of the issue Mr. Dingell has raised is the ability of PHS agencies to require awardee institutions to impose sound ethical standards on the biomedical and behavioral research they conduct.

Since all of the regulations identified above are patterned after the DHHS regulations for the protection of human subjects, it follows that if one set of regulations that requires institutions to self-regulate should be discredited, all similar regulations are called into question. *Time* magazine summarized the position taken by Mr. Dingell and others as follows:

The message from Washington is clear: science will receive no more blank checks and will be held increasingly accountable for both its performance and its behavior. . . . Underlying the current furor over funding and fueling Dingell's investigations are the implicit assumptions that science can no longer be fully trusted to manage its affairs and that society should have a larger voice in its workings.[9]

The Dingell criticisms stand in sharp contrast to the history of regulations on research involving human subjects chronicled above. There have been relatively few cases of serious noncompliance with DHHS Regulations for the Protection of Human Subjects over the past decade. The cases that have occurred have been dealt with effectively. The strength of the regulations to deal with noncompliance was manifested in recent findings of non-compliance on the part of the National Institute of Health's (NIH) own scientists, who shipped research materials to foreign collaborators who proceeded to carry out research involving human subjects without required review and approval of a local IRB that mets DHHS standards.[10] In none of these cases was serious physical or psychological harm inflicted on research subjects.

Dingell's challenges contrast with the system of accountability required by the regulations for the protection of human subjects. The Office for Protection from Research Risks (OPRR), which promulgates and implements the regulations on behalf of the Secretary of the DHHS, has been able to uncover noncompliance and to correct it. The OPRR has also played a leading role in promoting the Common Federal Rule for the Protection of Human Subjects. The Common Rule, virtually identical to DHHS regulations, was promulgated by 16 federal departments and agencies in the spring of 1991. The broad acceptance of the system of self-regulation is now a hallmark of the entire U.S. government's approach to the protection of human subjects.[11]

It is possible to predict a protracted and bitter struggle between persons whose views are represented by Mr. Dingell and persons who believe that the system of self-regulation is effective, economical, and well suited to the partnership between the public and the research community. The conflict between those endorsing self-regulation and those who believe that the government should have a system of highly specific rules, enforced by government inspection and backed by severe sanctions, is likely to endure throughout the 1990s.

It also seems reasonable to predict that the Common Federal Rule, administered by the Interagency Human Subjects Coordinating Subcommittee of the Committee on Life Sciences and Health operating under the White House's Federal Coordinating Council for Science Engineering and Technology, will gradually introduce changes into the existing system of institutional self-regulation of protection for human subjects. It is too early to state what the nature of these changes may be, but it is likely that they will include more frequent and more extensive requirements regarding reporting. Surely, opponents of the system will strive to substitute inspection by persons outside of institutions in place of self-regulation. Proponents of the system will introduce greater accountability into the system of self-regulation.

Once again, the burden of proof has shifted to the research community to demonstrate that it can be trusted to manage its own affairs in an ethical, honest, open, and publicly responsible manner. Each generation of biomedical and behavioral scientists will have to prove its credibility in the ever-changing context of new historical development.

IMPLEMENTING THE COMMON FEDERAL RULE FOR THE PROTECTION OF HUMAN SUBJECTS

As noted above, all departments and agencies of the federal government that conduct or support research involving human subjects now function under a common rule. There is no other federal regulation of any kind shared in common by all affected departments and agencies and applicable to all entities that must comply with the regulations. Because the Common Federal Rule was issued in June 1991, it is too early to document the success of this regulatory venture. Questions concerning the equitable implementation of the regulations by all departments and agencies can be legitimately raised now and for many years to come.

The various departments and agencies began this cooperative venture in regulation at many different starting points. The DHHS has 31 years of experience in implementing regulations for the protection of human subjects. The National Science Foundation has been piggybacking on the DHHS regulations for more than 14 years. The Department of Energy has been implementing the regulation as a department policy for about nine years. Some departments, like the Department of Defense, have promulgated regulations that are similar to those of DHHS, but they were not identical. Many departments and agencies are beginning to protect the rights and welfare of human subjects for the first time.

Serious questions remain concerning the ability of all of the departments and agencies to implement the regulations in a consistent manner. This is due to differences in their regulatory experience, their respective functions and missions, their authorizing legislation, and the kinds of research they fund, despite the fact that the regulations must be applied equally to civilian and military subjects and to stable and migrant populations of subjects. Can the Department of Education superimpose the regulations for the protection of human subjects on state-regulated systems of primary and secondary education? Will it be possible for the Agency for International Development to implement the regulations pertaining to research funded by U.S. dollars in foreign sites? Is it really feasible to have to impose standards, common interpretations, and consistent efforts at compliance across the entire federal establishment? If the system needs modification, is it possible to amend the regulations in a timely fashion? Clearances from 16 departments and agencies can take years. How can we make the system current and universal at the same time? These and related questions will be answered in the decade to come.

The ability of the entire executive branch of the federal government to oversee compliance with the Common Federal Rule in a manner that is consistent and equitable, yet flexible and trusting, is an enormous challenge. The challenge can be met only if federal regulators across the spectrum of government and many thousands of awardee institutions, some of them new to the system, understand it and meet it with an equitable and consistent response.

Understanding and motivation are essential characteristics of the system. The challenge of the upcoming decade will be for the government, in conjunction with the research community, to invest in a renewed educational effort to enable the Common Rule to achieve its purposes with minimal disruption of the academic environment.

THE PROBLEM OF DATA AND SAFETY MONITORING IN MULTI-CENTERED TRIALS

When regulations for the protection of human subjects were prepared at various times in the 1970s and early 1980s, the paradigm project for which the regulations were constructed was a trial involving a small cohort of subjects, conducted by a single investigator (or a small team of investigators) at a single institution. The regulations require that a disinterested local committee, an IRB, review and approve ethical aspects of the proposed research project before it can proceed. That approach is now a model for worldwide policies for the protection of the rights and welfare of human subjects.[12]

Although the paradigm case of a small trial conducted by one investigator in one institution under the aegis of one IRB continues to hold for the majority of research projects, it no longer describes many large contemporary research efforts. Typical large clinical trials are characterized by a complex protocol developed by federal scientists working together with colleagues in academia and industry. The protocol is forwarded to multiple research centers for review, approval, implementation, and evaluation. These procedures are conducted simultaneously by many research centers. Each center in turn may forward the protocol to additional research sites (often called satellite institutions) where research involving human subjects is conducted. In such situations, local IRBs no longer have full control over the protocols: (1) because the protocols were not developed by local investigators; (2) because the introduction of significant changes in the research design could cause the sponsor to remove the study from the institution rather than accept modification; and (3) because the IRB that modifies a multi-centered protocol will hear endlessly the argument that the protocol was approved by another institution.

It is customary for an outraged principal investigator to ask, "Why was this protocol good enough for Harvard, or UCLA, or Johns Hopkins, but not good enough for this institution?" IRBs are often unaware that the same arguments are presented to IRBs at the other institutions. A telephone call from one chairperson to another will often confirm that other IRBs can often join forces to require changes in troublesome protocols. The IRB often describes itself as being in a very uncomfortable "take it or leave it" situation with multi-center trials. Since the system was first imposed, IRBs have exercised their authority primarily by asking or requiring investigators to modify protocols. The "take it or leave it" option is inimical to the local autonomy of IRBs. The situation becomes especially difficult if the sponsoring agency or industrial firm is unwilling to compromise with local exigencies. It takes courage for local IRBs to turn down protocols that offer significant revenue and prestige.

Furthermore, since data derived from multi-centered trials are reported to a national data collection center, local IRBs have limited access to the aggregated data and little basis for exercising oversight judgments relative to continuation, discontinuation, or modification of such research projects. This means that the responsibility for protecting human subjects in many cases of multi-centered research projects is shifted to data and safety monitoring committees (DSMCs). Yet data and safety monitoring committees are not currently subject to federal regulations. Responsibility for the rights of subjects continues to be assigned to local IRBs, but exercise of responsibility is often left to DSMCs that do not interact with and are not accountable to IRBs. The membership, functions, procedures, and reporting requirements of such committees are nowhere defined or prescribed. As a result, the protection provided by self-regulation and accountability are often confused and weakened.

Although DSMCs have performed admirably in some instances, they have functioned poorly or not at all in others. For example, DSMCs functioned well when they stopped trial testing for treatment of diabetic retinopathy and research involving administration of AZT for treatment of HIV infection. In both cases the data indicated that it was no longer ethical to deny treatment to subjects in the control arms of studies in which treatment was obviously effective. On the other hand, data and safety monitoring of myocardial infarction studies led to wrangling in committees, replacement of a DSMC chairperson, charges of conflict of interest, and Congressional hearings. The decade of the 1990s will, or at least should, witness greater attention to DSMCs, including clarifications of their responsibilities and relationships to IRBs and a standardization of membership requirements and reporting responsibilities. To avoid overlapping responsibilities and to harmonize the work of such committees with the work of local IRBs is a delicate and daunting problem for funding agencies and the research community in the years just ahead.

This set of problems cries out for leadership by the OPRR and the Interagency Human Subjects Coordinating Committee, as well as cooperation by local IRBs in adapting the system of protection to the reality of multi-centered trials and the need for improved data and safety monitoring.

MOVING BEYOND THE *BELMONT* PRINCIPLES

Although the importance of the principles identified in *The Belmont Report* is seldom seriously challenged (at least in the United States), the adequacy of these principles to deal with all of the ethical questions raised by biomedical and behavioral research remains open to serious question. Although questions concerning these principles are addressed elsewhere in this volume, a few brief remarks are in order here.

The principle of respect for persons places high value on the autonomy of each research subject. However, as it has been understood and applied, it sheds little light on the rights of the family and the community. The principle offers little guidance for those attempting to answer the kinds of questions raised in this volume by Eric Juengst in Chapter 16. How can an IRB ensure respect for all affected by research projects designed to gather information about a family or about a community? Anthropologists and sociologists need to work closely with ethicists to determine how to make the principle applicable to, for example, Native American populations or Mormon or Amish communities. Delicate research into familial tendencies to develop mental illness is not covered by respect for persons as it is currently understood and applied. Furthermore, the principle of respect for persons is difficult to apply in cultures where decisions are made, or are heavily influenced by, heads of families or community leaders. Finally, although the principle calls for special protection for persons whose autonomy is diminished, as presently understood, it rarely provides sufficient guidance concerning situations where substitute consent may be required. These questions are carefully discussed in the new IRB guidebook.[13] They will continue to present both theoretical and practical problems in the years ahead.

As presented in *The Belmont Report,* the principle of respect for persons is to be applied in tension with the principles of beneficence and justice. The Food and Drug Administration (FDA) has, over the past several years, provided for expanded access to investigational drugs that have not yet been approved for marketing.[14] These drugs, available to persons with life-threatening diseases, are eligible for use before all safety data have been evaluated and prior to final establishment of efficacy. Even earlier availability of drugs is provided under the so-called parallel track provisions of the FDA.[15] In the case of AIDS, the application of the principle of beneficence is either diminished or abandoned when new therapeutic agents are made available through expanded access or parallel track mechanisms. In effect, the FDA has said to subjects: "We know you are desperate. We have drugs that might be safe and could be effective for your condition. We have little data to support safety, and virtually none to support efficacy.

You can take the drug at your own risk." Maximizing benefits and minimizing risks plays virtually no role in such a situation.

The wisdom of ignoring or diminishing the role of the principle of beneficence will be a matter of intense debate in the decade ahead. Different views on the importance of beneficence threaten to cleave the unified approach to interpreting the regulations for the protection of human subjects that has characterized the PHS since 1981.

Difficult applications of the principle of justice must also be made in the coming decade. For example, inclusion or exclusion of women of childbearing potential in drug trials is highly controversial at the present time. Some resolution of the question of when and to what extent women of childbearing potential should be included in drug trials seems, at least in part, to be tied to the vexing and divisive debate over the moral status of the human embryo and the human fetus. It can only be hoped that the moral issues associated with abortion will be sufficiently addressed to permit careful application of the principle of justice to the inclusion or exclusion of women of childbearing potential in the testing of drugs.

Just as clarification of the moral status of the fetus could resolve many of the questions related to inclusion or exclusion of women of childbearing potential in drug trials, so too resolution of the moral status of the fetus could clarify present confusion over the nature and extent of permissible research into morning-after drugs, abortifacients, and contraceptives. While it is easy to predict that this debate will continue in the decade ahead, it is not easy to predict what, if any, resolution will come about.

Finding ways to provide minorities with equal access to biomedical research is a problem that is crying out for attention. The present system of recruiting subjects for clinical trials that hold the prospect of benefitting the subjects is often left to referral by the subject's attending physician. However, patients from the lower socio-economic segments of society often lack a relationship with any physician. Who then can refer them to appropriate clinical trials? Statistics bear out the fact that minorities and poor people are underrepresented in research studies today. Clearly, the principle of justice is not being rigorously applied. It takes little clairvoyance to predict that this issue will be a contentious one throughout the next decade. It is hoped that healthcare reform will begin to remedy one of the root causes of underresearching minorities.

Waiving or diminishing the role of the principles of beneficence and justice in life-threatening situations constitutes a situation not foreseen and not addressed by the National Commission for the Protection of Human Subjects or by its successor body, the President's Commission for the Study of Ethical Problems in Medicine and Biomedical and Behavioral Research. Serious attempts to resolve such questions must be made in the decade of the 1990s. The need for a national bioethics deliberative body should be apparent to all who consider these questions.

INTERNATIONAL RESEARCH

The principles identified in *The Belmont Report* are derived, at least in part, from international codes including the *Nuremberg Code* and the *Declaration of Helsinki* (updated several times). Almost universally recognized in the United States, the *Belmont* principles have been slow to win endorsement in foreign countries. Although intended to be universal, their formulation, application, and emphasis on the rights of the individual are distinctly Western, and characteristically American. Science in general, and biomedical and behavioral sciences in particular, recognize no boundaries. Since the American experience includes a rich variety of cultures, it offers evidence that the principles can find universal application.

Can the principles of research ethics find universal acceptance? This question, though not a new one, has special relevance in the decade of the 1990s because of the international dimensions of the AIDS pandemic.

Because of its leadership in biomedical research, the U.S. research community must take the lead in adapting practice to local culture while preserving ethical principles in all parts of the world. This author firmly believes that the principles can be universally, though not necessarily univocally, applied. Adaptation to cultural variants will require ingenuity, patience, and insight on the part of researchers and IRBs, and it will require cooperation from leaders in foreign research sites. Alternative solutions seem to offer only chaos. The local IRB offers the best hope, in my judgment, of finding a reasonable adaptation of the principles to local cultures and subcultures.

TESTING AN AIDS VACCINE

The best hope for a medical solution to AIDS lies in finding one or more effective vaccines that will prevent the spread of this dread disease and in finding immunotherapies that will produce cures or at least prevent death. What, if any, is the role of the IRB in reviewing and approving research conducted partly in a First-World setting and partly in the Third World? The obligation to protect the dignity, the rights, and the welfare of subjects will not be diminished by these challenges, but the present structures for assuring protection of subjects may not be adequate to the task.

Is it possible for the developed nations to identify and test vaccines and therapies on a global scale in an ethical manner? It is currently predicted that test vaccines will render recipients HIV positive, thus offering the possibility that those who test as seropositive because they are infected will be confused with those who test seropositive because they have been vaccinated. What effect will such testing have on our ability to treat AIDS if the vaccines prove to be ineffective or only slightly effective? Will the testing of unproved vaccines be carried out in Third World countries, but the distribution of proved vaccines be limited to developed nations? If not, who will subsidize the enormous cost of immunization in the Third World?

What, if any, is the role of the IRB in reviewing and approving research conducted in Third World settings? What does it mean to refer to an IRB in reference to trials that may be carried out in vast territories by foreign personnel affiliated with no local institution?

Questions that readily arise with respect to AIDS arise in similar, though perhaps less dramatic, fashion with respect to other diseases and conditions. The example of AIDS is chosen as illustrative of the ethical problems that will face a wide spectrum of international biomedical and behavioral research.

COMPENSATION FOR INJURED
RESEARCH SUBJECTS

In 1975, the Department of Health and Human Services impaneled a task force to study its ethical obligations to provide care and compensation for research subjects who are injured as a result of their participation in biomedical or behavioral research.[16] The task force carried out a study that showed that the incidence of serious, long-term injuries to research subjects is very low. Nevertheless, such injuries occur in rare instances. The task force recommended that the department initiate a program for care and compensation of such subjects patterned after the federal workers' compensation system. Action on the recommendations of the task force was considered, but never taken by the department.

In 1981, the President's Commission for the Study of Ethical Problems in Medicine and Biomedical and Behavioral Research recommended that a trial be conducted to determine, among other matters, how much a federal program of compensation would cost the taxpayers of this nation. Upon review of the recommendation of the President's Commission, the department judged that there was no valid and ethical way to conduct a trial of a system of compensation without initiating the very program that was to be tested. Once initiated, it was felt, it could never be terminated and, therefore, it would not be a trial but a full-blown program. No action was taken.

Absence of a federal program for compensation of injured subjects may have a variety of consequences: (1) because injured subjects may be compensated in no other way, the absence of a systematic program of compensation may encourage lawsuits; (2) it may discourage private industry from developing vaccines for fear of litigation and assessment of damages. If a compensation system existed, recipients would be expected to waive their right to sue vaccine manufacturers in return for receiving compensation similar to that provided to injured federal workers. The effect might be the reduction of the likelihood of multi-million dollar judgments against manufacturers of drugs and devices. The demand for compensation for injured research subjects has been raised in each decade since 1960. To date there is no program to compensate injured research subjects. Because the problem is linked to the very nature of research involving risks to the subjects, it is certain to surface again in the decade ahead.

PROFESSIONAL ETHICS

New problems have begun to emerge relative to the professional behavior of research investigators. Some pharmaceutical houses and manufacturers of medical devices have initiated the practice of compensating researchers for testing their products on a *per capita* basis. That is to say, the more subjects that are recruited, the greater will be the pay given to the investigator. This practice, sometimes referred to as bounty hunting, introduces, at the very least, the appearance of conflict of interest on the part of the research investigator.

Another form of bounty hunting occurs when research investigators pay significant sums of money to other health professionals for recruiting subjects for participation in research. This practice suggests that health professionals could have more interest in earning the bounty than in providing the best available care for their patients.

Still another challenge to professional ethics is raised when research investigators establish or invest in industrial firms that will market drugs, biologics, or medical devices undergoing tests conducted by the investigator-investor. Whatever the actual motives of such investigators might be, their potential for making money from the sale of test articles marketed after they have tested them gives the appearance of a conflict of interest.

Sound professional ethics requires researchers to avoid conflicts of interest or even the appearance of conflict of interest. Although sound practices for curbing real or apparent conflicts of interest may emerge, they are not yet well established. In the meantime, it seems reasonable to require all clinical investigators to disclose all matters that could appear to constitute a conflict of interest to the local IRB. The IRB can then decide how much of this information should be disclosed to subjects by way of the informed consent process.

CONCLUSION

All of the issues summarized above should be squarely faced and dealt with by the research community working together with federal agencies, experts in ethics, research institutions, regulators, Congress, and the general public. The integrity of the research enterprise may depend on successful resolution of these and related issues.

NOTES

This chapter is a heavily edited and modified version of an article entitled "Overview: Challenges for the 1990s," in *Emerging Issues in Biomedical Policy: An Annual Review*, vol. 2, ed. R.H. Blank and A.L. Bonnicksen (New York: Columbia University Press, 1993), 156-68.

1. J.H. Jones, *Bad Blood: The Tuskegee Syphilis Experiment* (New York: Free Press, 1981).

2. Information obtained from the Office for Protection from Research Risks, National Institutes of Health, Bethesda, Md.

3. Workshop held by the Congressional Office of Technology Assessment in December 1992.

4. The regulations were identified as "Basic Policy for the Protection of Human Subjects" and published as Title 45 *Code of Federal Regulations* (1981), 8386-91. FDA regulations were published as 46 *Federal Register* (1981): 8958-79. The Common Rule 1991 Version of these regulations appear as Appendix D in this book.

5. J.C. Fletcher and K.J. Ryan, "Federal Regulations for Fetal Research: A Case for Reform," *Law, Medicine and Health Care* 15, no.3 (1987): 126-38.

6. See "Animal Advocates Win Court Ruling," *New York Times*, 26 February 1993, sec. A, 12. *Animal Legal Defense Fund v. the Secretary of Agriculture*. Opinion of Charles R. Richey, U.S. District Judge, Civil Action No. 91-1328 (CRR). Filed 25 February 1993, U.S. District Court, District of Columbia.

7. "Derailing the Due Process," *Washington Post*, 14 August 1991.

8. House Energy and Commerce Subcommittee on Oversight and Investigations.

9. J.M. Nash and D. Thompson, "Crisis in the Labs," *Time*, 26 August 1991, 48-51.

10. See "Findings and Required Actions Regarding Investigation of Noncompliance with HHS Regulations for the Protection of Human Research Subjects Involving the National Institutes of Health Intramural Research Program: Interim Report" (3 July 1991: unpublished report of the OPRR--Office for Protection from Research Risks).

See also the DHHS news release, 19 May 1982, concerning the debarment of Marc J. Straus, M.D. In the debarment proceeding, Dr. Straus acknowledged that false reports were submitted to the Eastern Cooperative Oncology Group; that ineligible patients were used in his studies; that some patients received drug dosages that deviated from the plan of the study; and that some study plans had not been reviewed in compliance with DHHS regulations for the protection of human subjects.

See also the OPRR report (5 February 1985) on the case of Robert P. Gale, who failed to comply with DHHS regulations for the protection of human subjects. See also the unpublished OPRR letter dated 22 November 1989, reprimanding the IRB of Children's Hospital in Boston for a serious error in permitting informed consent to be sought only from one arm of a clinical trial involving the use of extracorporeal membrane oxygenation (ECMO) in neonates in comparison with the standard treatment.

11. See 56 *Federal Register*, (1991): 28003-23 which is reprinted in this book as Appendix D. Using the DHHS regulations as a model, the 16 departments and agencies under the leadership of the DHHS Office for Protection from Research Risks, with approval from the White House Office of Science and Technology Policy and the Office of Management and Budget, simultaneously adopted the DHHS system of awardee self-regulation for the protection of human research subjects involved in research conducted or supported by any of the departments or agencies of the federal establishment.

12. Council for International Organizations of Medical Sciences (hereafter, CIOMS) *Proposed International Guidelines for Biomedical Research Involving Human Subjects* (Geneva: CIOMS/WHO, 1982). The word "proposed" in the title can be misleading. It is intended to convey that the CIOMS and the WHO propose or recommend that this policy be implemented in research projects worldwide. The word "proposed" does not indicate that it is a draft put forward for consideration. CIOMS announced its intention of revamping the guidelines. The first meeting toward this end was held in Geneva in February 1992. See CIOMS Round Table Conference, *Ethics and Research on Human Subjects, International Guidelines: Proceedings of the XXVIth CIOMS Conference, Geneva Switzerland, 5-7 February 1992*, ed. Z. Bankowski and R.J. Levine (Geneva: CIOMS, 1993). The CIOMS Guidelines are reprinted in Appendix F of this book.

13. R.L. Penslar, *Protecting Human Research Subjects: Institutional Review Board Guidebook*, NIH publication no. 93-3470 (Bethesda, Md.: National Institutes of Health Office for Protection from Research Risks, 1993).

14. See 21 *Code of Federal Regulations* 312 (1987), issued by the Food and Drug Administration. 52 *Federal Register* (22 May 1987).

15. See the DHHS Policy entitled "Expanded Availability of Investigational New Drugs through a Parallel Track Mechanism for People with AIDS and HIV-related Disease," 57 *Federal Register* (1992).

16. U.S. Department of Health, Education, and Welfare, *HEW Secretary's Task Force on the Compensation of Injured Research Subjects*, HEW publication no. OS-77-003 (Washington, D.C.: U.S. Government Printing Office, 1977).

PART II

Conflicts of Interest

Introduction to Part II

Harold Y. Vanderpool

Conflict of interest refers to conflicts between basic loyalties that shape human conduct. For professionals, the phrase "conflict of interest" is shorthand for the way various self-interests clash with, and possibly undermine, the professional's prescribed and expected loyalties and roles. In the past, this concept has been frequently used as a way to understand, then control, the often-conflicting personal and institutional loyalties of government officials and lawyers. Government officials are thus required to disclose the sources and extent of their non-government income, and they are often prohibited from receiving outside gifts. Lawyers, too, are required to reveal their personal and financial interests insofar as these might conflict with the interests of their clients.[1] Among other things, worries about how "the commercial spirit has taken such firm hold of the medical research community" have fostered an increasing concern over conflicts of interest in research with human subjects.[2]

Thinking about the ethics of research involving human subjects from the vantage point of conflict of interest generates new insights and perspectives. In particular, conflict of interest fosters critical thinking about how personal and institutional interests clash with, and possibly override or undermine, the ethical principles that are expected of researchers, as discussed and debated in Part I. Obviously, the financial interests and pursuits of individual researchers and institutions can conflict with the principles of protecting research subjects from harm or respecting them as autonomous or self-choosing agents.

Conflict of interest can also be used as a vantage point for undertaking a clear and pointed analysis of the history of human subjects' research. The historical case studies in Chapter 1 illustrate the necessity of prioritizing ethical values and commitments over contending, power-laden values--the aggrandizement of a super race, the enhancement of the capacities of nations to wage war, the advancement of scientific knowledge, the personal fame of innovative researchers, the prestige of universities, and the financial successes of pharmaceutical companies.[3] To translate this perspective into the language of ethical reflection, conflict of interest enables us to identify and morally evaluate the purposes and ends of those who sponsor and conduct research involving human subjects.[4]

The chapters in this Part examine how researchers' possible conflicts of interest include, yet far exceed, commercial issues. The presence and power of multiple, sometimes conflicting interests are ubiquitous to the research enterprise. Researchers' interests include scientific curiosity, altruism, career advancement, fame, travel, honoraria, consultant's fees, and profits from product royalties.[5] Fueling the last four of these rewards are millions of dollars invested by drug companies in sponsored symposia, gifts, honoraria, and paid expenses.[6] Institutional Review Boards' (IRBs) interests include respecting and protecting research subjects, advancing research within their respective institutions, responding to pressures over approving multi-center trials,[7] protecting researchers and their institutions from legal liability, and educating their respective constituencies.

Although considerations regarding "conflict of interest" can sharpen our thinking about the contending and conflicting values in research with human subjects, it can also mislead. It can mislead because the many interests of researchers and institutions may be, in actuality, compatible, rather than conflicting. The various interests at play in clinical research should thus be viewed as *possibly* or *potentially* conflicting.[8] The conflicts in question may be either real or imagined. For example, talented physician-researchers who are well paid to consult with industry can make important, beneficial, and uncompromised contributions toward the development of innovative therapies.[9] Researchers and IRBs alike are challenged to maintain their role-specified ethical priorities on the one hand and to assure the greatest degree of objectivity in research with human subjects on the other. Model policy guidelines for controlling conflict of interest have been developed and endorsed by voluntary groups of researchers, the American Medical Association, and the American Association of Medical Colleges.[10]

Notably, the recently proposed and approved guidelines on controlling conflict of interest by the National Science Foundation and the Public Health Service replace the phrase "conflict of interest" with "objectivity in research."[11] These guidelines deal with the responsibilities of IRBs to control investigator bias due to financial incentives--a task that will increase the workloads of these review boards. Beyond these financially-focused guidelines, other, subtler forms of possible bias are ever present and worthy of attention.[12]

Each chapter in this section breaks new ground and challenges readers to think about how possible conflict of interest impinges on clinical research ethics and oversight. In Chapter 7, John C. Fletcher and Franklin G. Miller deal with the history and ethics of research at its broadest level--the level of a nation's establishing its research agenda and setting forth the parameters of permissible or unpermissible research within that agenda. Deeply concerned about how partisan politics has conflicted and can conflict with scientific freedom and the advancement of critically needed knowledge and therapy, Fletcher and Miller discuss which public institutions ought to be established and how these institutions can keep biomedical research from becoming dominated or co-opted by narrowly focused and conflicting interest groups. In August of 1994, the White House Office of Science and Technology formally proposed that a National Bioethics Advisory Commission should be established. The draft charter for this commission defines its membership and initial priorities, which includes protecting the rights and welfare of research subjects. Fletcher and Miller also set forth a bioethics agenda for the future, an agenda that expands upon the discussion of Charles R. McCarthy in Chapter 6.

In Chapter 8, Stuart E. Lind charts the seven major parties with invested interests in clinical research, and he describes their financial linkages. Lind identifies the many ways that money influences research and becomes a source of ethical concern within IRBs. Throughout, he underlines how most of these issues have never been adequately investigated. Given the many ways and the extent to which researchers and their respective institutions profit in terms of status, influence, and power, why, Lind asks, should monetary matters be singled out as an item of debate with respect to what should be mentioned or not mentioned on consent forms?[13] His concluding discussion on why financial issues have assumed such importance in contemporary clinical research is designed to *decrease* alarm over these recently arising, many-faceted issues.

In Chapter 9, John La Puma addresses new and controversial problems over physicians' conflicts of interest in post-marketing research--research that impacts 75 percent of the revenues of many drug companies, that is being done by large numbers of physicians, that is rarely subject to IRB oversight, and that often is not disclosed to the patient-subjects involved. La Puma describes the conflicts of loyalties inherent to this research (Is it more marketing than research?): conflicts between physicians' maximizing their income, the responsibility of physicians to prescribe the *best* therapy for their patients, clinicians' desires to contribute to scientific knowledge, and the greater costs of newly approved drugs to patients once the research ends.[14] Whether post-marketing research places patient-subjects at risk or not (La Puma argues that it does), ethical questions are raised over how this research is being conducted. La Puma's own survey indicates that, in contrast with a majority of physician-researchers, the majority of patient-subjects want to be informed about such research.[15] La Puma's discussion of alternative ways to address these troubling issues ends with a proposal designed to transform post-marketing research into truly scientific and comprehensive safety trials.

NOTES

1. M.A. Rodwin, "Physicians' Conflicts of Interest," *New England Journal of Medicine* 321 (1989): 1405-7.

2. A.S. Relman, "Economic Incentives in Clinical Investigation," *New England Journal of Medicine* 320 (1989): 933-34, at 934. These

concerns are not registered in *The Belmont Report* and were not extensively recognized even in the mid-1980s. See the brief discussions of R.J. Levine, *The Ethics and Regulation of Clinical Research*, 2nd ed. (Baltimore: Urban and Schwarzenberg, 1986), 151; and A.M. Capron, "Research Ethics and the Law," in *Research Ethics*, ed. K. Berg and K.E. Tranoy (New York: Alan R. Liss, 1983), 21-23.

3. We should be critical of interpreting this history as the story of an ever-greater recognition and appreciation of the weight and worth of ethical principles in the conducting of clinical research. Jay Katz, George J. Annas, and others view the last 20 years of research ethics and regulations as falling short of the ethical principles enshrined in the *Nuremberg Code*. J. Katz, "Human Experimentation and Human Rights," *Saint Louis University Law Journal* 38 (Fall 1993): 20-25; G.J. Annas and M.A. Grodin, "Where Do We Go From Here?" in *The Nazi Doctors and the Nuremberg Code*, ed. Annas and Grodin (New York: Oxford University Press, 1992), 307-14. Others, such as Robert J. Levine in Chapter 10 of this book, view clinical research over the last 30 years as adjusting to ethical principles and pragmatic needs.

4. See the discussion in Chapter 1, pp. 3-6 of this book concerning how ethical analysis includes making discerning judgments about that which is taken to be ultimately good with respect to the purposes and ends of human action.

5. R.J. Porter, "Conflicts of Interest in Research: Personal Gain-- The Seeds of Conflict," in *Biomedical Research: Collaboration and Conflict of Interest*, ed. R.J. Porter and T.E. Malone (Baltimore: Johns Hopkins University Press, 1992), 135-50.

6. Porter includes a chart of over $185 million expended by 17 well-known drug companies on symposia, honoraria, and gifts in 1988. *Ibid.*, 140.

7. B. Freedman, "Multicenter Trials and Subject Eligibility: Should Local IRBs Play a Role?" *IRB: A Review of Human Subjects Research* 16 (January-April 1994):1-6.

8. Porter, "Conflicts of Interest in Research: The Fundamentals," in *Biomedical Research*, 125-126.

9. *Ibid.*, 121-26. Consider also how investigators' interests in career advancement, personal fame, and so on, can (and perhaps inescapably do) serve as motivating factors in researchers' developing innovative therapies for the good of society. The motivating force of fame is boldly expressed in the renowned oath attributed to Hippocrates. This oath ends with the words, "If I fulfil this oath and do not violate it, may it be granted to me to enjoy life and art, being honored with fame among all men for all time to come; if I transgress it and swear falsely, may the

opposite of all this be my lot." L. Edelstein, "The Hippocratic Oath: Text, Translation and Interpretation," *Bulletin of the History of Medicine* suppl. 1 (1943): 3.

10. See B. Healy *et al.*, "Conflict-of-Interest Guidelines for a Multicenter Clinical Trial of Treatment After Coronary-Artery Bypass-Graft Surgery," *New England Journal of Medicine* 320 (1989): 949-50; and American Medical Association Council on Scientific Affairs and Council on Ethical and Judicial Affairs, "Conflicts of Interest in Medical Center/Industry Research Relationships," *Journal of the American Medical Association* 263 (1990): 2790-93. The guidelines of the Association of American Medical Colleges (AAMC) are clear, well-organized, widely used, and readily available in the pamphlet: AAMC, *Guidelines for Dealing with Faculty Conflicts of Commitment and Conflicts of Interest in Research* (Washington, D.C.: Association of American Medical Colleges, 1990). These guidelines were formally adopted in February 1990. As the title indicates, these AAMC guidelines distinguish between conflict of interest and conflict of commitment--the possible conflict between the physician-researcher's academic roles (teaching, research, and/or patient care) and various "outside" activities.

11. "Rules on Conflicts of Interest in Research Mean More Responsibilities for Institutions," *Human Research Report* 9 (September 1994): 1-3. This shift of terminology makes sense with respect to identifying and controlling certain kinds of investigator bias. While "objectivity in research" represents a positive ideal that avoids conveying the impression that the various interests at play are actually in conflict, this phrase fails to capture some of the analytical richness of the phrase "conflict of interest." Conflict of interest (1) does not imply that research has to be objective (arguably, all research is "value infested" and has a subjective component); (2) highlights the notion that many possibly conflicting motives and values can, and at times do, undermine the ethical commitments and the truth-finding purpose of research; and (3) is readily applied to the ways political and social institutions influence, for good or ill, research agendas and how research is conducted.

12. Commenting that the human capacity for self-deceit "is quite extraordinary," Porter discusses several forms of subtler bias. Citing a study that indicates how investigations sponsored by drug companies are much more likely to favor the new drug under development than similar studies by more neutrally situated parties, Porter explores, for example, the impact of researchers' desires to be on a "winning team," their fears of wasting years of effort, etc. Porter, "Conflicts of Interest in Research: The Fundamentals,"131-33. See also Porter's expanded discussion of the many forms of investigator bias in "Conflict of Interest

in Research: Investigator Bias--The Instrument of Conflict," in *Biomedical Research*, 151-62.

13. The U.S. federal guidelines say that informed consent should include "a description of any benefits to the subjects *or to others* which may reasonably be expected from the research." 45 *Code of Federal Regulations* 46.116.a(3) (emphasis by HYV). The significance of this phrase was highlighted by Sanford Chodosh, President of the Board of Directors of Public Responsibility in Medicine & Research (PRIM&R) at the November 1994 PRIM&R Conference in Boston.

14. A strong case can be made for the need for post-marketing research. For example, the FDA has recently changed its rules in the direction of better protection of the confidentiality of those who report adverse effects of recently approved drugs and medical devices. These protections have been made to encourage such reporting. Fears over being drawn into court battles have greatly discouraged such reporting --estimated by one study to represent only 1 percent of "the true number of serious adverse events experienced by patients or subjects each year in the United States." "Federal Agency Will Override State Laws and Rules to Protect Confidentiality Better," *Human Research Report* 9 (March 1994): 1-3. The nature and significance of Phase IV post-marketing research trials is well described in Annex II of the 1993 *CIOMS International Ethical Guidelines for Biomedical Research Involving Human Subjects*, Appendix F of this book.

15. This raises the issues discussed by Robert M. Veatch in Chapter 2, pp. 47-51 of this book.

7

The Promise and Perils of Public Bioethics

John C. Fletcher and Franklin G. Miller

INTRODUCTION

This chapter explores the background of current debate about public bioethics in the United States.[1] Public bioethics is ethical inquiry conducted by a publicly constituted body, which is created and supported by government. Its aim is to identify the major ethical and public policy considerations involved in selected and often controversial issues in the spheres of biomedical research, healthcare, and public health. Its purpose is to examine the history of public bioethics in the United States and to offer recommendations for its future in light of the lessons that can be gleaned from reflecting on this history.

The chapter has four parts. Part one introduces the main themes of the paper: the promise and perils of public bioethics and the role of government in the process. Part two reviews the history of government's role in public bioethics, including the effects of interventions by government in bioethical controversies during a period of neglect of public bioethics. Part three frames the debate about the future of public bioethics and highlights a bioethics agenda now facing the nation. The final part delineates specific recommendations for public bioethics.

THE PROMISE AND PERILS OF PUBLIC BIOETHICS

What is the rationale for public bioethics? A publicly constituted commission of national scope can serve two main purposes.

First, it can offer a forum for developing ethical standards to assure public accountability in biomedical research, healthcare, and public health. In the 1960s and early 1970s, serious abuses of power in publicly funded medical research, described below, indicated to politicians, government officials, religious leaders, and scholars that self-regulation by the medical profession was inadequate to protect the rights and welfare of vulnerable patients and research subjects. A publicly mandated commission with diverse representation was seen as an appropriate vehicle for recommending guidelines for reviewing, monitoring, and conducting research to be incorporated into government regulations.

Second, a national commission devoted to public bioethics can serve the need of government for intelligence and counsel on emerging ethical problems, spawned by advances in scientific knowledge and technology, for the purpose of designing suitable policies. Governments of modern, complex societies act blindly or arbitrarily if they develop policy without being guided by inquiry. The process of policy-relevant inquiry includes fact-finding concerning problems that call for government action and identifying the values at stake in current or prospective policies. The routine modes of government inquiry--hearings, reports in the news media, and public opinion polls--are not adequate to determine the policy implications of complex bioethical problems. Moreover, in a pluralistic society, no religious institutions are positioned to issue authoritative judgments on the ethical dimensions of social problems. Wise policy development with respect to bioethics calls for expert knowledge and analysis to help frame issues relevant to policy and for careful and reflective deliberation to shape recommendations for government action. The process of public bioethics enables government to take advantage of ethical reflection encompassing diverse perspectives and insulated from the pressures of interest-group politics.[2]

The main promise of public bioethics is that it will contribute to the development of sound public policy by timely, well-reasoned analyses of ethical controversies in the spheres of biomedical research, healthcare, and public health. Public bioethics contributes to the formulation of public policies by: (1) clarifying the ethical considerations relevant to an issue of policy, (2) articulating consensus ethical standards for the guidance of policy, and (3) recommending specific safeguards to contain or prevent abuses that have occurred or that could occur when the policy is implemented. A secondary promise of public bioethics is that the ethical analyses and recommendations issued in commission reports will provide valuable guidance to local institutional ethics committees, which focus on protection of human subjects in specific studies, ethical issues in patient care, uses of animals in research, and allegations concerning scientific integrity.[3]

A tertiary promise, harder to discern, is that such commissions provide a new type of public forum within which to negotiate the different interests of medical and scientific professionals and the government, concerning bioethical controversies in the interests of the public. To the extent that the commissions of the 1970s and 1980s succeeded in fulfilling this promise, they forged a new public mechanism for moral discourse and sharing of power among these interests. As the historical review presented below demonstrates, if left unchecked to pursue their agenda, professionals and government officials can dominate and bias policy in the spheres of biomedical research, healthcare, and public health. Public bioethics emerged in the 1970s out of concern about the consequences of unchecked professional power in the conduct of biomedical research. During a subsequent period of eclipse of public bioethics, unilateral government intervention in bioethics controversy created serious problems that might have been prevented or moderated by the presence of a public commission.

Public bioethics is subject to four main perils: political co-optation, bioethics orthodoxy, neglect, and poor performance.[4] This chapter focuses on the first three perils.[5] Forms of political co-optation can range from subtle manipulation to "political capture."[6] Co-optation distorts ethical reflection by imposing partisan political demands or constraints. The peril of bioethics orthodoxy arises to the extent that a narrow ethical perspective controls the inquiry and recommendations of the commission. Neglect of public bioethics occurs when the government sets public policy or intervenes in ethical controversies without being informed by the deliberations of public bioethics commissions. In our view, neither overt political co-optation nor bioethics orthodoxy has characterized the work of an official standing bioethics commission, although the advocacy of particular interest groups are always in evidence.[7] In one instance, however, political controversy over abortion destroyed the capacity of a public bioethics body to function.[8] Examined as a whole, the record of public bioethics has been marked by more promises kept than perils actualized.[9]

Since public bioethics is inquiry done on behalf of government, its promise and perils are inseparable from the pivotal question of the desirable role of government in this domain. We argue in favor of two functions of government in public bioethics, which have been only partially and inconsistently developed in the past. The first function is to be a wise and consistent advocate of public bioethics, in each political season, in the interests of the public. The second function for government is to be a wise user of public bioethics.

THE ROLE OF GOVERNMENT IN PUBLIC BIOETHICS FROM 1966 TO 1993

To understand the past is to gain a standpoint to evaluate the promise and perils of government's future role in public bioethics. The history of public bioethics from 1966 to the present can be divided into three periods. In the first (1966-1973), government played an essentially reactive role by responding to revelations of serious ethical problems in biomedical research. In the second period (1974-1983), government became a proactive advocate of new forms of public bioethics. In the third period (1984-1993), officials within the executive and legislative branches of government neglected public bioethics and intervened unilaterally in bioethics controversies. With no debate in a forum of public bioethics, roadblocks were erected that inhibited what many saw as important progress on problems of human disease, suffering, and behavior. Consequently, these interventions were perceived as unjustified abuses of power and, in some cases, infringements on scientific and academic freedom. Today, officials in the legislative and executive branches are studying proposals to restore one or more public bioethics bodies as well as pondering the proper role of government in public bioethics.

GOVERNMENT AS REACTIVE (1966-1973)

Government became an advocate of public bioethics by slowly and painfully learning that deep reforms were sorely needed to protect human subjects of research. Reports of several scandals and crises in research ethics indicated to key government officials that the discretionary power of investigators to design and conduct clinical research, subject to prevailing norms of professional integrity and informed consent, were not sufficient to protect human subjects.[10] In order to provide a greater assurance of protection, the government in 1966 mandated an impartial process of prior group review of the ethical features of each project designed to involve human subjects. This reform meant that the critical ethical decisions regarding whether research should be undertaken and how it should be conducted were no longer left to the exclusive judgment of investigators. By mandating institutional review boards (IRBs) the government transformed the process of planning and conducting research. Power to make such decisions was shared with others not connected with the research.

Research or reports about specific studies appearing on many lists of scandals are listed in Table 1, beginning with the long-lived Tuskegee Syphilis Study, conducted by the Public Health Service (PHS), and including others.[11]

TABLE 1
Research Ethics Scandals and Reports[12]

Tuskegee (PHS-CDC) Study	1932-1972
Thalidomide and FDA	1962
Jewish Hospital Cancer Study	1963
Baboon-to-Human Heart Transplant	1964
Willowbrook Hepatitis Study	1965
Beecher Article	1966
"Tea Room Trade"	1967
Fetal Research	1973

Even as these scandals unfolded one after another, government still learned slowly and had a large blind spot about the ethics of research in its own institutions.[13] This is most clearly exemplified by the Public Health Service's study of untreated syphilis in Macon County, Alabama, begun in 1932. Initiated and continued without any written protocol, this study was allowed to continue until 1972, well after a period in which the federal government had taken the lead in reforming research ethics. The zeal to reform can be accompanied by blind spots as to the need for reform in one's own institutions.[14]

Awareness grew among some government scientists[15] and members of Congress[16] that ethical problems in research needed more careful attention than could be given in routine peer-review decisions to fund new research. A transition to shared power--between scientists, their interdisciplinary peers, and the public in a practice of prior review--took several years with research scandals exploding along the way. As reflected in Table 1, abuses of power occurred in the hands of investigators who had a monopoly on decisions to initiate and design research. The norms of research could not change until the power to decide about whether and how specific projects should be done was removed from total control of investigators and shared, particularly with IRBs.

GOVERNMENT AS PROACTIVE ADVOCATE OF PUBLIC BIOETHICS (1974-1983)

In 1968, Senator Walter Mondale introduced a resolution to establish a National Commission on Health Science and Society, but the bill failed.[17] In 1972, revelations of the Public Health Service's syphilis study and of research with live fetuses in the context of late abortions increased pressure on Congress to act.[18] Between 1973 and 1978, Congress and the Department of Health, Education and Welfare (HEW) created three public bioethics bodies: the National Commission for the Protection of Human Subjects of Biomedical and Behavioral Research (1974-1978); an Ethics Advisory Board for the Secretary, HEW, (1978-1980); and the President's Commission for the Study of Ethical Problems in Medicine and Biomedical and Behavioral Research (1980-1983).[19]

The reactive period ended with a 1974 public law creating a national commission to examine the ethics of research involving human subjects.[20] It also made the United States the first nation to require that all entities supported by or receiving federal funds submit proposals to conduct research involving human subjects, including the fetus, to prior review by a local IRB with at least one outside member who was not a scientist.

The National Commission's reports and recommendations provided the ethical foundations and rationale for the main approaches taken in research with human subjects in the United States and have had significant influence in other nations. Moreover, the commission's work was largely incorporated, without significant change, into detailed federal regulations to protect human subjects of research.[21] The commission's reports became the basis for public policy on research on fetuses and pregnant women, children, prisoners, and psychosurgery. The scholarly papers and testimony assembled by the commission's staff and contributors were, and still remain, important intellectual documents for scholarship in bioethics.

Members of Congress and leaders in research recognized that there was no clear understanding about the ethical foundations of clinical research. The law mandated the commission to "conduct a comprehensive investigation and study to identify the basic principles which should underlie the conduct of biomedical and behavioral research involving human subjects . . . develop guidelines . . . and make recommendations" especially to protect particularly vulnerable populations of subjects.[22] Pursuant to this mandate, the commission produced *The Belmont Report*, the most thoughtful reflection up to that time on ethical principles that ought to guide research involving human subjects.[23] The conceptual and procedural elements of the commission's work are discussed by Levine[24] and by Jonsen and Toulmin.[25]

The National Commission recommended that it should be succeeded by an Ethics Advisory Board (EAB) to advise the Secretary, HEW, on controversial research proposals and a wide variety of questions in research ethics. The EAB was the first national body to examine *in vitro* fertilization (IVF) research as a treatment for infertility and the possibility of experimentation with an embryo for a non-therapeutic purpose, for example, to study the causes of cancer or infertility. Its report, which favored public funding for IVF research, was never acted upon by a Secretary of the HEW or a Department of Health and Human Services (DHHS) secretary.[26] The EAB did recommend the use of a waiver by the Secretary of the Department to permit research in fetal diagnosis of hemoglobinopathies by fetoscopy, and it debated a scheme for compensating injuries of research subjects.

The President's Commission was established by Congress with a mandate to address broad-based issues in healthcare and research ethics. The mandate was defined so that the commission could initiate studies on its own or by request of the president. Among its 11 reports, the most notable supplied the ethical premises and moral framework to reform the determination of death to include whole brain death,[27] to formulate the evolving consensus on criteria for decisions to forego life-supports (including artificial feeding and hydration) in incapacitated patients,[28] and to lead the way to national policy on recombinant DNA research and the ethical aspects of human gene therapy.[29] The commission's work was widely regarded as timely and valuable on these issues and several others.

Controversy continued among members of Congress in the 1970s as to whether government should fund research in reproductive biology. National debates over abortion fueled this controversy. Other controversial issues emerged about DNA research and the swine flu epidemic. However, during this period, neither Congress nor the executive branch interfered with, intimidated, or threatened the work of the National Commission. Throughout the Nixon, Ford, and Carter administrations, and in the early years of the first Reagan administration, the work of the three commissions was not disrupted or overwhelmed by political concerns. Commission members were able to do their work, and most authorities agree that the quality of their activities was commendable. Despite considerable controversy, government in these years confined itself to the roles of advocate and user of public bioethics.[30]

THE ECLIPSE OF PUBLIC BIOETHICS (1984-1993)

After 1983, when the President's Commission ended, government abandoned the process of public bioethics and the new growth of its twin roles atrophied. Elected and appointed federal officials became major players in bioethics controversies, rather than consistent advocates or users of public bioethics. These officials, moved by fervent, but not critically examined, moral beliefs and political alliances with the pro-life movement, intervened in bioethical controversies without being guided by the process of public bioethics committed to impartial inquiry, informed debate, sharing power, and enlarging foresight.[31] The Reagan and Bush administrations could have continued to advocate public bioethics as a forum for these debates while maintaining a strong moral stance against abortion, embryo research, and on other issues of sexuality. A different strategy prevailed, namely, to discourage or prevent activities under federal control that were not perceived as compatible with the government's moral agenda. Consequently, public bioethics withered in the power struggle about abortion and issues emanating from it.

The Reagan administration failed to recharter an EAB, although requests were made by the NIH director and former DHHS officials.[32] This inaction was contrary to federal regulations requiring that the Secretary of DHHS "shall establish one or more Ethical Advisory Boards."[33] In 1985, passage of the NIH Reauthorization Bill was delayed due to conflict about abortion and fetal research. In this controversy, and lacking an EAB, Congress created a Biomedical Ethics Advisory Committee (BEAC) as part of a set of compromises to pass the bill. Then Democratic Senator Albert Gore, Jr. of Tennessee was a key figure in the negotiations. In the law, Congress banned all investigative fetal research in the context of elective abortion[34] and created a BEAC with a mandate to study the ethics of fetal research and the DHHS Secretary's power to waive the "minimal risk" regulation for such research.[35] The 14-member BEAC was to be an advisory body to a Biomedical Ethics Board (BEB), composed of 12 members of Congress, three each drawn from the minority and majority parties of the Senate and the House. Other mandated topics were human gene therapy and artificial feeding and hydration of dying patients.

After two and one-half years, the BEAC became a reality, but it was unable to function due to internal strife arising from the abortion debate among the Congressional BEB members. Cook-Deegan detailed the 1990 demise of the BEAC.[36] Government's role as advocate of public bioethics in the 1970s had thoroughly atrophied by the end of the 1980s.

In this period, without any prior consultation in a public bioethics forum, government repeatedly intervened in selected bioethical controversies touching mainly on human reproductive issues and sexuality. These interventions occurred in the public sector and in a power vacuum partially created by the neglect of public bioethics. When power is not being shared in the definition, debate, and resolution of specific controversies, government is less constrained to act on its own. Although government was not required by law to consult with any public bioethics body in this period, such direct government intervention in bioethical controversies departed from the practice of prior administrations during the previous decade to employ the process of public bioethics. As a result, government ignored the values associated with the incipient practice of public bioethics. Power used to intervene in bioethical controversies, without being informed by the process of public bioethics, is bound to be perceived by many as abusive. Investigators and clinicians with vested interests in the activities involved will be more willing to accept regulatory limitations if these are the consequence of a process of public deliberation.

Government intervention in this period began with advocacy of proposed "Baby Doe Rules" and the activism of DHHS in that debate.[37] Government also controlled bioethics policy by passive means. Acting not to recharter an EAB meant that no investigative research protocols involving "more than minimal risk" to the fetus and no human IVF research at all could proceed. This brought the NIH's scientific peer review and funding of such activities to a virtual halt.[38] The secondary effects widened to dampen actual and potential research in prenatal diagnosis,[39] the natural history of human genetic disorders and some cancers,[40] fetal therapy,[41] fetal tissue transplant research,[42] and on the drug RU-486 as an abortifacient.[43] These areas of biomedical research touch especially on the lives of women and children.

Government interventions also blocked behavioral studies. Moral opposition, without any public debate, prevented NIH-supported social-psychological studies of adolescents' sexual behavior to understand risk factors for HIV/AIDS.[44] The public health initiative in the AIDS epidemic suffered from government obstruction due to moral opposition to homosexuality and frankness about anal sex and other acts that transmit HIV infection. A respected senior official of the Centers for Disease Control (CDC) charged that the Reagan and Bush administrations' interference in the CDC's response to AIDS caused the agency to commit "public health malpractice."[45] Six years elapsed between the recognition of an AIDS epidemic and Americans' receiving a pamphlet on risk factors from the PHS. The release of the pamphlet required the personal courage of Surgeon-General C. Everett Koop, a bright exception in an otherwise dark period.

A dramatic illustration of unchecked government intervention into research was a moratorium imposed unilaterally on support for fetal tissue transplant research (FTTR) in 1987. As the controversy developed, a degree of moral recklessness can be seen in evasion of a duty to use the legally prescribed public instruments of government to make policy. The premise the Reagan administration adopted for the moratorium was that encouragement of abortion was inseparable from FTTR. An NIH Advisory Panel considered the issues and voted 18 to three, in December 1988, to recommend federal funding of FTTR.[46] The majority argued that FTTR to treat disease was separable from the morality of induced abortion; its premise was that FTTR was a type of cadaveric transplantation.[47] They stressed that society's approval of organ donation after homicide or suicide did not entail moral approval of the cause of death, but a desire to benefit those who would die without transplants. Three panel members dissented due to FTTR's alleged links to elective abortion.

The panel drafted 12 guidelines for federal regulations to guide FTTR and prevent abuses. Dr. Louis B. Sullivan, Secretary, DHHS, rejected the report by letter in November 1989.[48] His action was preceded by no public hearings or prior notices in the *Federal Register*, as required by the Administrative Procedures Act. Extending the moratorium "indefinitely," he based his action on the reason that the administration and Congress opposed any funding of activities by DHHS which "encourage or promote abortion." The moratorium, continued by a possibly illegal action, was lifted by President Clinton on his second day in office.[49]

Other appointed officials also intervened, without consultation with any bioethics body, in bioethical controversy. NIH officials froze funds[50] and later cancelled[51] a NIH-funded conference on behavioral genetics and violence after criticism of the idea of the conference from the Black Congressional Caucus and others who feared undue stigmatization and other consequences.

No public deliberation occurred before this decision, and no justification was given for the appearance of infringement of academic freedom. The NIH's failure to address the question of academic freedom that was inherent in the decision to cancel the conference left an impression of an agency acting with a heavy hand and without foresight as to the consequences. This action was later appealed and the grant restored to the University of Maryland, where authorities felt strongly that their academic freedom had been infringed by these actions.[52] Had the ethical issues embedded in the controversy been debated in a national bioethics forum, it is possible that competing concerns could have been debated, leading to an acceptable compromise.

Worth pondering is whether the heavy handedness involved in some of these interventions, including taking liberties with federal law and infringing academic freedom with no principled arguments, would have been constrained by norms of informed debate, shared decision making, and enlarging foresight that flourished in public bioethics in an earlier period.

In response to government interventions with respect to FTTR and adolescent sexual behavior, Congress created new EABs (not the ones required in federal regulations) in 1993 to prevent the Secretary, DHHS, from making unilateral decisions on moral grounds that block funding for research that has been successfully peer reviewed.[53] This awkward mechanism, which is a product of the controversies of this period, has not been used to date. It did, however, provoke a discussion of the advantages of the *ad hoc* approach to public bioethics.

THE RENEWAL OF PUBLIC BIOETHICS: WHAT IS ITS FUTURE?

THE NATIONAL BIOETHICS AGENDA

The Clinton administration restored freedom to conduct FTTR and studies of RU-486 in the reproductive context. A ban on federal funding of IVF research has ended. The opportunity exists to restore public bioethics in the United States. Meanwhile, a decade's worth of significant bioethical questions need attention. Selection of issues for a national bioethics agenda is an important issue in itself. We propose two criteria to select and

---

TABLE 2
10 Bioethical Issues Facing the Nation

---

1. Issues in Research Ethics
    - Review and evaluate National Commission's legacy on research ethics (no review for 20 years)
    - Research with the cognitively impaired
    - AIDS vaccine trials
    - Testing female contraceptives treated with microbials (vs. STDs/HIV) against condoms
    - Research with human embryos
2. Issues in Healthcare and Public Health
    - Healthcare policy reform
        - Securing access to healthcare
        - Rationing expensive treatments
    - Quality of life and palliative care of the terminally ill
    - Genetic testing and screening (ELSI interface)
    - Issues of personal responsibility for health
    - Organ transplant issues, including availability and xenografts

---

rank issues: need for action in public policy and the prospects for achieving consensus in approaches to the issue.

In Table 2, 10 issues in research, healthcare, and public health are ranked in terms of these criteria. The Office of Technology Assessment's (OTA) list contains 23 issues.[54]

Selected issues in research ethics are noted first. No systematic review of research ethics has been done since the National Commission ended in 1978. Every area of its work and the federal regulations that it inspired need review, such as, policies on IRB review; informed consent; and research with fetuses, pregnant women, children, and prisoners. Another troubling issue is long overdue for national review, namely, the ethics of research with cognitively impaired and/or institutionalized subjects.[55] In terms of issues raised by genetic research, especially in terms of testing families and children, Americans can expect a sea change in their knowledge of health status and the way that medicine is practiced. Preparing for this transformation introduces many issues already under study in the Ethical, Legal, and Social Implications (ELSI) Program of the Human Genome Project. One problem is the lack of an interface between ELSI-supported studies and the public policy process.[56] This opportunity could be provided by a new national commission that could use the knowledge base of the ELSI program.

Among other research issues facing an unprepared nation is early trials of AIDS vaccines with normal volunteers. Another starts with the fact that women around the world are increasingly threatened by AIDS. They need a contraceptive that also provides protection against sexually transmitted diseases, including HIV infection. These microbially treated devices will eventually have to be compared with using condoms, which are known to be effective when used correctly, thus presenting a sharp ethical dilemma. Finally, the United States totally lacks a public policy on embryo and gamete research, even as this work picks up speed and the Human Genome Project marches on. The scope of this task exceeded that of any existing ethics advisory group in the private sector, including the National Advisory Board on Ethics in Reproduction (NABER).[57] For this reason an *ad hoc* NIH Human Embryo Panel was appointed to report to the Secretary, DHHS, and its imminent report will be controversial in permitting human embryo research.[58] It would not be surprising if the task of seeking more consensus in this debate and proposing public policy for federal funding of embryo research were referred to a new commission.

In healthcare ethics, several momentous issues vie for attention. These include access to healthcare (the subject of the last report of the President's Commission) and the ethics of rationing treatments.[59] Is it ethically justified to limit access to expensive treatments due to "personal responsibility," for example, smoking and substance abuse?[60] In the area of death and dying, there is the controversial issue of physician-assisted death.[61] If it is too controversial for the national agenda, the commission could address the ethical issues in palliative care of the dying in America. A final issue is that of the persistent need of sources for organ transplants, including species other than human.

THE CURRENT DEBATE ABOUT PUBLIC BIOETHICS
A debate is now underway in Washington and elsewhere about renewal of public bioethics to address this large national

agenda.[62] There are two options on the table in Washington: to create a new national commission for bioethics, established either by Congress or the president, or to continue the *status quo*, which is to appoint *ad hoc* groups of experts to respond to one issue at a time and then disband. Consensus among key elected and appointed officials exists regarding the need for a body to consider issues in research ethics. There is dispute, however, about what form that process ought to take: for example, a standing national commission or an *ad hoc* approach, that is, a specifically selected group of experts for each task.

Moving to the types of issues that are considered to be broad based, such as some of those listed under healthcare and public health in Table 2, one finds greater controversy in Washington and elsewhere about a national bioethics commission. Some oppose a commission for fear of creating a "bioethics elite" and stress the important work being done by the more than 150 bioethics organizations in the United States.[63] The dominant voice among opponents is fear of the peril of co-optation. In one critic's view, politics inevitably corrupts ethical reflection, and government and institutions always use ethics committees as "cover" for their own self-interests.[64] Another critic is concerned not only about political capture, but also whether a political culture of intense interest groups will itself capsize and sink a standing commission.[65] This concern is also shared by some influential Congressional staffers, who are veterans of the "culture wars" of the 1980s and battles over the free conduct of research. They foresee politicization of a standing body by the abortion issue or its first cousins, fetal and embryo research. A standing commission might be dominated by pro-life or pro-choice forces. Some fear that a standing body might ban valuable research. These views lead them to support the current approach of appointing *ad hoc* expert groups to consider single issues.

AD HOC PANELS OR A STANDING COMMISSION?

Under the *ad hoc* approach, short-lived advisory committees are established for the fact-finding and policy recommendations concerning particular bioethics issues. A public commission addresses a range of issues over an extended period of time. The main argument for the *ad hoc* approach is to prevent politicizing, capture, or stalemating of the process. However, *ad hoc* panels of experts are no less subject to co-optation than standing groups.[66] Co-optation can best be prevented by locating the body in an independent setting and by selecting an experienced chair who is fair, deeply informed about the issues, and willing to resign if necessary to protect the integrity of the process.

More basic questions grow out of the main subject of this chapter. Which form of public bioethics--ad hoc or standing--is better suited to fulfilling the promise and avoiding all of the perils of public bioethics? Which form best serves the proper role of government as consistent advocate and wise user of public bioethics? We contend that one standing and term-limited body could better serve the public and government than several ad hoc groups, especially in view of the large agenda facing the nation. An unreasonable time span would be required to select, staff, and deploy several ad hoc groups. A second and more serious consideration is the learning curve required for the education of members. A crucial quality in public bioethics is appreciation for complex and diverse ethical perspectives required for serious ethical inquiry. Members will learn more and grow faster in their roles by considering several issues rather than only one. The quality and scope of their ethical reasoning is likely to be more inclusive.

A standing body will have more prestige and status in public terms than a series of ad hoc groups. Public participation could be more focused and sustained in a standing group than a number of ad hoc panels. Standing commissions with continuing staff support can provide greater access to the public through more frequent regional hearings than can short-lived ad hoc panels.

OPTIONS FOR A NEW NATIONAL BIOETHICS COMMISSION

At any rate, a period dominated by cautionary appeals for ad hoc panels may be passing, for two reasons. One is the influence of the OTA report, Biomedical Ethics in U.S. Public Policy. Hanna, Cook-Deegan, and Nishimi, who have had extensive experience in public bioethics, had key roles in framing the report. Subsequently, they recommended the appointment of two national bodies, an Ethics Advisory Board (EAB) and a President's Bioethics Commission. They see an EAB serving "at the pleasure" of the

Secretary of the DHHS, to review specific research proposals, and also to serve as a policy forum on substantive issues concerning research with human subjects. Their EAB is a hybrid body combining a function like a national IRB with policy functions like those of a National Commission. These authors also propose a successor to the President's Commission for more broadly based issues in healthcare and health policy.[67] In many ways their proposal fills out the options for Congress in the OTA report.[68]

A second reason for dwindling interest in the *ad hoc* approach is growing uneasiness in Congress and in the executive branch, similar to perceptions in 1973 before appointment of the National Commission. More elected and appointed officials now feel that Congress and the nation are unequipped to deal with the large agenda of issues outlined above and in the OTA report. Two events in 1993 heightened their unease: the embryo cloning report from George Washington University,[69] and the revelation of surreptitious radiation experiments in the 1950s and 1960s.[70] *Ad hoc* panels were created to address these issues, but apprehension remains that the nation's need for public bioethics is too extensive to be optimally met by this approach. In this context, Republican Senator Mark Hatfield of Oregon has introduced a bill to create a National Commission on Biomedical Ethics (NCBE).[71] He is working with Democratic Senator Ted Kennedy and Democratic Representative Edward J. Markey, both of Massachusetts, to review this proposal and move it forward through the legislative process. At the same time, there is a proposal by the Office of Science and Technology Policy (OSTP) of the administration to create a National Bioethics Advisory Commission by executive order. The choices between these two proposals raise the important question of the method of establishing a national bioethics commission.

RECOMMENDATIONS FOR PUBLIC BIOETHICS

In view of current fiscal constraints[72] on federal advisory groups and other considerations, we recommend the establishment by Congress of one national bioethics commission and also the creation of a new, privately supported Institute on Bioethics and Public Policy to aid the new commission's scholarly tasks and to be a clearinghouse for the larger bioethics community and its interests in public policy.

How should a National Bioethics Commission be established? It is clearly more expedient in the short run to act by executive order. After publishing a proposed charter in the *Federal Register* and comment period, the order goes into effect. DHHS could fund the commission by redirecting funds, thus avoiding the Congressional appropriation process. Seeking Congressional approval for the commission's mandate would strengthen it, but it may also slow down the process.

Taking a longer view, a wait may be beneficial in terms of having a commission with greater public stature and perhaps a longer life. In terms of enhanced stature, a Congressional process would provide more systematic review, a greater opportunity for public debate, and broader representative support. A precedent exists in that two notable past commissions were established by Congress. A Congressional process would also be more bipartisan, and if the president appointed the members, both branches of government could be involved.

In terms of longevity, one must reckon with the effect of a presidential election in 1996. In a scenario of a one-term Clinton administration, a commission could be as quickly dismantled by executive action as it was established. Or it could simply not be rechartered by a Republican administration, as was done in the past with the EAB. A commission created by executive order would be chartered for two years beyond initial approval. By contrast, a Congressionally mandated commission would have a longer life, perhaps to the end of the decade. If the commission's term was set by law, a new administration would replace members when their terms expired. This exact situation occurred with the President's Commission after the 1980 election when members with expired terms appointed by President Carter were replaced by members appointed by President Reagan. The commission was able to function well with essentially the same staff and completed its work.

Bioethics was in its infancy in the 1960s and 1970s. Two centers, the Kennedy Institute of Ethics at Georgetown University and the Hastings Center, were the only major resources. The staffs of previous commissions drew heavily on them and the work of selected scholars for papers and testimony to help frame the deliberations of the commissions. Today, there are more than 150 bioethics organizations in the United States, many of them at interdisciplinary centers served by scholars in the nation's universities and academic medical centers.[73] Due to the growth of bioethics as an interdisciplinary field, many more persons and organizations in bioethics can contribute to the significant effort that the nation and the commission need to succeed in the face of a large agenda.

A new commission will also face the fiscal realities of downsizing in government today. It is unlikely to be adequately funded or staffed. For this and other reasons, we believe that the commission's work could be greatly enhanced by the creation of a new, foundation-supported Institute for Bioethics and Public Policy to co-exist alongside the commission for its lifetime. The primary reason for an institute is to provide an organized resource to serve the commission and the public with scholarly ethical analysis and argument concerning issues on the agenda of the commission. In older models of public bioethics, the commissions' staffs selected individual scholars to produce papers and reports for the panel's consideration. Many able and qualified contributors were not selected. This approach may no longer be satisfactory in view of the enormous expansion of professional activity and organizations devoted to bioethics. While respecting the commission's staff's options to select contributors, it could also be an alternative to rely on an institute that aimed to include a broad-based and diverse group of scholars to produce continuing scholarly work in bioethics and public policy.

Another function would be to act as a clearinghouse for bioethics and public policy issues. This would involve the collection and dissemination of documents and information relevant to the commission's tasks and deliberations. Also, the institute's staff could be a resource to interact with the many and diverse bioethics organizations and scholars who will want to make their contributions and positions on the issues available to the commission. These activities could free commission staff from these particular tasks. The more important role, however, would be to assist in the financial support of a broad-based and diverse group of scholars in bioethics to produce the papers and debate in ethics that the commission members will need to consider. An institute could provide a forum for such scholars, as well as support and incentives, to pursue such work.

A third function of an institute would be to participate, from as broad a base as possible, in the process of selection of new issues for the commission's study. Commission staff should undertake this task in an optimal process of consultation. An institute could be one sounding board, among others, in deliberations about the timing and suitability of particular issues. A fourth function is that an institute could study and conduct education about ethical issues with significant public policy implications that are too ill-defined or controversial for the NCBE to put on its own agenda. Two examples are the debates about physician-assisted death, discussed above, and medical futility.[74] Finally, the institute may also serve the development of the profession of bioethics, which today lacks a shared national forum for addressing ethical issues in the public policy arena.

CONCLUSION

This chapter has discussed the rationale for public bioethics in terms of its promotion of accountability and enlarging foresight amidst bioethical controversies. The promise and three of the four special perils of the enterprise were also discussed. The history of public bioethics was traced in three periods from 1966 to the present, as well as the role of government. There are major lessons to be learned from this history. The first is that government, the source of authorization for this process, has twin roles as advocate for and user of public bioethics. Government should pursue these roles consistently to the benefit of the public and medical and scientific groups. Otherwise, the neglect of public bioethics results in a vacuum in which unilateral interventions by government or other interest groups in bioethical controversies are likely to be perceived as abuses of power by the other parties to the process. The locus of authority for public bioethics is the needs and values of modern technological societies for enlarging foresight, sharing power, and accountability in the process of making complex policy decisions in the spheres of biomedical research, healthcare, and public health. The paper also reviewed the current debate about whether public bioethics ought to be pursued in *ad hoc* groups or by a standing commission to be established by Congress or the president. Our argument supports the Congressional approach and also points out the need for a new Institute on Bioethics and Public Policy to serve the commission, the bioethics community, and the public.

ACKNOWLEDGMENT

The authors are grateful to the editor, Harold Y. Vanderpool; to Norman Quist; and to James S. Reitman; for their careful critique and comments on earlier drafts of this paper, which was developed from a talk (by JCF) for a conference sponsored by the University of Texas Medical Branch at Galveston and the Office for Protection from Research Risks, National Institutes of Health, 1 March 1993. Parts of the present paper were given as the 73rd William Beaumont Lecture, sponsored by the Wayne County Medical Society in Detroit, 6 April 1994. JCF is grateful to the society and to Dr. Mark I. Evans for that opportunity.

NOTES

1. Our use of the term "public bioethics" descends from "public ethic" as defined by A.R. Jonsen, "The Totally Implantable Artificial Heart," *Hastings Center Report* 3 (November 1973): 1-4. The most definitive contemporary discussion of this subject is: U.S. Congress, Office of Technology Assessment, *Biomedical Ethics in U.S. Public Policy*, OTA-BP-BBS-105, (Washington, D.C.: U.S. Government Printing Office, 1993).

2. Examples of times when government did not take advantage of this function come readily to mind. In 1972, Congress passed Public Law 92-603 to guarantee end-stage renal disease treatment, irrespective of ability to pay. Moved by emotion and without foresighted debate or advice, Congress thus deprived other candidates for whole organ transplants of life-saving measures. In the same period, no group review preceded initial decisions to screen for carriers of sickle-cell anemia. Screening began in a premature campaign, backed by hastily passed state and local laws, launched without sufficient planning and public education. Confusion can be seen in a medical editorial that referred to screening "22 million Afro-Americans" for a "dread disease." R.M. Nalbaldian, "Mass Screening Programs for Sickle Cell Hemoglobin," *Journal of the American Medical Association* 221 (1972): 500. The rash of lawmaking was reviewed by P. Reilly, *Genetics, Law, and Public Policy*

(Cambridge: Harvard University Press, 1977). A definitive assessment of the moral and social harm done in this period is in National Academy of Sciences, Genetic Screening Programs, *Principles and Research* (Washington, D.C.: National Academy Press, 1975).

Positive examples are a public panel's examination of whether a totally implantable artificial heart ought to be developed. For the panel's report see: U.S. Department of Health, Education, and Welfare, Public Health Service, National Institutes of Health, Artificial Heart Assessment Panel, National Heart and Lung Institute, "The Totally Implantable Artificial Heart: Economic, Ethical, Legal, Medical, Psychiatric, and Social Implications," (Washington, D.C.: U.S. DHEW, PHS, NIH, reprinted 1977. DHEW Publication No. (NIH) 77-191). A good current example is a program (ELSI) of the Human Genome Project to support studies of ethical, legal, and social implications of human genome research. See OTA Report, *Biomedical Ethics*, 8, for a description of the ELSI program and its strengths and weaknesses.

3. J.C. Fletcher, "The Bioethics Movement and Hospital Ethics Committees," *Maryland Law Review* 50 (1991): 859-94.

4. Alan J. Weisbard warned against "bioethics orthodoxy" in public comments during a conference, The Role of Bioethics in Health Care Policy/Broadening the Bioethics Agenda, held in Washington, D.C., 24 May 1994.

5. The task of articulating standards to evaluate the work of public and local bioethics is an important one. One commentator believes that the state of bioethics methodology and evaluation is "completely anarchical." D. Wikler, "Federal Bioethics: Methodology, Expertise, and Evaluation," *Politics and the Life Sciences* 13 (1994): 100-101.

6. The most consistent view expressing the political co-optation theory of public and local bioethics is that of G.J. Annas, *Standard of Care: The Law of American Bioethics* (New York: Oxford University Press, 1993), 1-12.

7. A version of political capture occurred in orders given to the Clinton administration's bioethics task force related to healthcare reform that it could not discuss rationing; see P. Steinfels, "The Clintons Invited 500 Experts to Talk About Health Care. The Task for 30: Think About Ethics," *New York Times*, 2 October 1993; also, see G.J. Annas, "Will the Real Bioethics (Commission) Please Stand Up?" *Hastings Center Report* 24 (January-February 1993): 19-21. This external order to silence a topic should be contrasted with an internal decision by members of the President's Commission not to address selective abortion directly in deliberations and its report on genetic counseling and screening, because of the lack of consensus on the topic. President's

Commission for the Study of Ethical Problems in Medicine and Biomedical and Behavioral Research, *Screening and Counseling for Genetic Conditions* (Washington, D.C.: U.S. Government Printing Office, 1983). It is also an hypothesis that political, rather than ethical considerations, resulted in the NIH Embryo Research Panel having no member opposed in principle to research with human embryos.

8. The Biomedical Ethics Advisory Committee, created by and located in Congress in 1985, is discussed below. Its oversight body, a Biomedical Ethics Board composed of members of Congress, deadlocked along abortion lines over selecting a chairperson, and the enterprise died in 1989, having issued no reports. OTA Report, *Biomedical Ethics*, 12-13.

9. This assessment agrees with the OTA's summation: "Past Federal bioethics efforts have been varied, innovative, and largely successful, but not enduring." *Ibid.*, 38.

10. These two norms--professional integrity and informed consent--are the core of the traditional practices embodied in the *Nuremberg Code*, along with the requirement for previous animal experiments. See P.M. McNeill, *The Ethics and Politics of Human Experimentation* (New York: Cambridge University Press, 1993), 42. *Nuremberg* has no requirement for prior group review. Ironically, the first call for a genuine type of prior group review of research was made by the Berlin Medical Board in 1930, i.e., that there should be "an official regulatory body to which proposals for experiments on man should be submitted." It was not to be implemented due to opposition from leading researchers. N. Howard-Jones, "Human Experimentation in Historical and Ethical Perspective," *Social Science in Medicine* 16 (1982): 1436. This appeal emerged during a bitter debate about the ethics of clinical drug trials in the context of a powerful German pharmaceutical industry. A remarkable set of guidelines on new therapies and human experimentation was released by the German Minister of the Interior on 28 February 1931. These *Richtlinien* (regulations or guidelines) were far more comprehensive and insightful than the *Nuremberg Code*, itself. For example, one guideline stressed that to take advantage of social distress and deprivation was contrary to medical ethics, which is relevant both to the Tuskegee Syphilis Study and to subsequent Nazi experiments. The German physicians at Nuremberg were not judged by the Tribunal against the norms of this document and its legal status in Germany was questioned during the trial. Despite many excellent features, the guidelines made no mention of prior group review, but the idea was clearly alive in Germany in 1930. To date, I have not found evidence of the practice of prior group review before the opening of the Clinical Center at the NIH in 1953, which was still a type of peer review, albeit in a

special group designated for the purpose. Perhaps the oldest source of the norm of peer review for research is in Thomas Percival's code of medical ethics in 1803. He stated that there should not be trials of new treatments without "a previous consultation of the Physicians or Surgeons, according to the nature of the case." For a discussion of Percival's ideas and their relevance to research review, see McNeill, *Ethics and Politics*, 37.

11. This notorious study would be more appropriately named "The Public Health Service Syphilis Study," since the PHS was responsible for it in its entirety, and not the Tuskeegee Institute.

12. On thalidomide see: 89th Cong., 2nd sess. (1966) *Senate Report 1153*, 8-25. On the Jewish Hospital for Chronic Diseases see: E. Langer, "Human Experimentations: New York Affirms Patients' Rights," *Science* 151 (1966): 663-65. On the baboon-to-human heart transplant see: J.D. Hardy, "Heart Transplantation in Man," *Journal of the American Medical Association* 188 (1964): 1132-35. On the Willowbrook Study see: S. Krugman *et al.*, "Infectious Hepatitis Detection of Virus During the Incubation Period and in Clinically Inapparent Infection," *New England Journal of Medicine* 261 (1959): 729-34; S. Goldby, "Experiments at the Willowbrook State School," *Lancet* no. *i* (1971): 749. The Beecher article is: H.K. Beecher, "Ethics and Clinical Research," *New England Journal of Medicine* 74 (1966): 1354-60. On the Tea Room Trade and deceptive social research see: L. Humphreys, *Tea Room Trade: Impersonal Sex in Public Places* (Chicago: Aldine, 1970); D.P. Warwick, "Tearoom Trade: Means and Ends in Social Research," *Hastings Center Report* 1 (1973): 24-38. On fetal research see: "Live Abortus Research Raises Hackles of Some, Hopes of Others," *Medical World News* (5 October 1973): 32-36; V. Cohn, "NIH Vows Not to Fund Fetus Work," *Washington Post*, 13 April 1973.

13. Charles R. McCarthy, former Director of the Office for Protection from Research Risks of the NIH, commented: "It seems to me that . . . for the most part the government was passive, but a few farsighted individuals such as Shannon and Stewart in the Executive Branch, and Ted Kennedy in the Congress, initiated procedures that have matured into a remarkable system. These few individuals were both learners and teachers, but the government as a whole was at best a sleepy, distracted pupil, awakened periodically by a scandal, but otherwise content to 'get by' without having to recite." Personal communication of JCF with CRM, 14 May 1983.

14. The intramural program of the NIH did not have IRBs in the true sense until after the 1974 law, although the Public Health Service required them of others from 1966 on.

15. Two directors of the NIH and two Surgeons-General deserve special mention for raising awareness among their colleagues and in

Congress: James A. Shannon (1955-1968), Robert Q. Marston (1968-1972), Luther L. Terry (1962-1965), and William H. Stewart (1965-1968).

16. Estes Kefauver, Edward Kennedy, Jacob Javits, Abraham Ribicoff, Walter Mondale, and Paul Rogers.

17. U.S. Senate, Committee on Government Operations. National Commission on Health Science and Society, "Hearings before the Subcommittee on Government Research of the Committee on Government Operations," 90th Cong., 2d sess. The commission was to be broadly representative of the disciplines of medicine, physical and social science, law, theology, philosophy, ethics, health administration, and government. In his testimony, Senator Mondale noted that among hundreds of suggestions he received, the areas for study fell into six categories: "transplantation, genetic engineering, behavioral control, human experimentation, public education and professional training, and the interrelationship of basic science, application and diffusion of treatment." (pp. 8-9) The latter issue came to be called "technology transfer."

18. "Live Abortus Research," Medical World News, 5 October 1973, 32-36.

19. Although the Ethics Advisory Board was chartered from 1976-1981, it actually functioned from 1978-1980.

20. National Research Act, U.S. Code, (1974).

21. 45 Code of Federal Regulations 46 (1974).

22. National Research Act.

23. National Commission for the Protection of Human Subjects of Biomedical and Behavioral Research, "The Belmont Report: Ethical Principles and Guidelines for Research Involving Human Subjects," (Washington, D.C.: U.S. Government Printing Office, 1979), included in this book as Appendix C. In our view, any new revision of The Belmont Report needs more careful explication of the ethical significance of the tradition of academic and scientific freedom in the public and private sectors. The original report assumed this tradition without discussing its place in the ethical framework of the document.

24. R.J. Levine, Ethics and Regulation of Clinical Research, 2nd ed. (Baltimore: Urban & Schwarzenberg, 1986).

25. A.R. Jonsen and S. Toulmin, The Abuse of Casuistry (Berkeley, Calif.: University of California Press, 1988), 16-19.

26. U.S. Department of Health, Education, and Welfare, Ethics Advisory Board, Report and Conclusions: Support of Research Involving Human in Vitro Fertilization and Embryo Transfer (Washington, D.C.: U.S. Government Printing Office, 1979).

27. President's Commission for the Study of Ethical Problems in Medicine and Biomedical and Behavioral Research, Defining Death (Washington, D.C.: U.S. Government Printing Office, 1983).

28. President's Commission for the Study of Ethical Problems in Medicine and Biomedical and Behavioral Research, *Decisions to Forego Life-Sustaining Treatments* (Washington, D.C.: U.S. Government Printing Office, 1982).

29. President's Commision for the Study of Ethical Problems in Medicine and Biomedical and Behavioral Research, *Splicing Life* (Washington, D.C.: U.S. Government Printing Office, 1982).

30. Why was this so? K.E. Hanna, R.M. Cook-Deegan, and R.Y. Nishimi distill six elements for any future efforts to restore such forums. They attribute relative success to government and the past bioethics bodies in terms of: (1) the charge to such a body (which will influence its authority or lack thereof); (2) the appointment will influence process; (3) the bureaucratic location; (4) reporting requirements (to whom and how the group reports and in what manner); (5) budget and staffing; and (6) targeted audience(s). In our view, lack of interference and co-optation by government ought to be added to the list. See their article, "Finding a Forum for Bioethics in U.S. Public Policy," *Politics and the Life Sciences* 12 (1993): 205-19.

31. In the controversy on Fetal Tissue Transplantation Research (FTTR), political compromises modified moral beliefs, because newsworthiness was a criterion for how far government intervention would go. The Reagan and Bush administrations did not prevent NIH support of basic research using tissues or cells obtained from fetuses after elective abortion, but it did attack FTTR. Both were possible because of elective abortion. This moral inconsistency was aired by Representative Henry Waxman in House hearings. The Assistant Secretary for Health stated that basic research using fetal tissue was not in danger because it was not likely to be "hyped by the media," which was felt to have an effect on the motivation of women to have abortions. U.S. House Committee on Energy and Commerce. Subcommittee on Health and the Environment, *Fetal Tissue Transplantation Research: Hearing Before the Subcommittee on Health and the Environment of the Committee on Energy and Commerce*, 101 Cong., 2d sess., 2 April 1990, 77-80.

32. Under pressure from Representative Waxman, the Reagan administration published a proposed EAB charter in November 1988. The Bush administration took no action to establish an EAB.

33. 45 *Code of Federal Regulations* 46.204.

34. The Public Health Service Act, as amended by the Health Research Extension Act of 1985, Public Law 99-158, 20 November 1985. This law is reprinted on the inside cover page of the current edition (18 June 1991) of U.S. Department of Health and Human Services, *Protection of Human Subjects*, OPPR Report O-307-551 (Washington, D.C.: U.S. Government Printing Office, 1992) The prominence given to the fetal research guidelines thus dominates the document.

35. 45 *Code of Federal Regulations* 46.211.

36. R. Cook-Deegan, "Abortion Politics Deals Death Blow to Bioethics Body Set Up by Congress," *Kennedy Institute Newsletter* 4 (Fall 1990): 5-7.

37. This period is well reviewed in E.E. Shelp, *Born to Die? Deciding the Fate of Critically Ill Newborns* (New York: Free Press, 1986), 177-201.

38. For a review of NIH's activities in fetal research in this period, see J.C. Fletcher and J.D. Schulman, "Fetal Research: The State of the Question," *Hastings Center Report* 15 (April 1985): 6-12. The OTA reviewed the effect of the "no EAB" intervention on infertility research and found that in this period "investigators indicate that they *do not submit* proposals involving . . . IVF . . . because of widespread awareness of the *de facto* ban on such research." The dimensions of this chilling effect of the moratorium on IVF research are such that NIH estimates that it might receive more than 100 grant applications for human IVF if the Ethics Advisory Board were extant. U.S. Congress, Office of Technology Assessment, *Infertility: Medical and Social Choices*, OTA-BA-358 (Washington, D.C.: U.S. Government Printing Office, 1988).

39. J.C. Fletcher and D.C. Wertz, "Ethics and Prenatal Diagnosis: Problems, Positions, and Proposed Guidelines," in *Genetic Disorders and the Fetus*, 3rd ed., ed. A. Milunsky (Baltimore, Md.: Johns Hopkins University Press, 1992), 823-57.

40. J.C. Fletcher, "Controversies in Research Ethics Affecting the Future of Human Gene Therapy," *Human Gene Therapy* 1 (1990): 307-24.

41. J.C. Fletcher, "Fetal Therapy, Ethics, and Public Policies," *Fetal Diagnosis and Therapy* 7 (1992): 158-68.

42. J.C. Fletcher, "Abortion Politics, Science and Research Ethics: Take Down the Wall of Separation," *Journal of Contemporary Health Law and Policy* 8 (1992): 95-121.

43. C. Anderson and P. Coles, "Drug Debate Expands," *Nature* 348 (1990): 382.

44. "Secretary of Health Ordering a Revision on U.S. Sex Survey," *New York Times*, 8 April 1989; "Sex Survey of Students Angers Conservatives," *New York Times*, 21 July 1991; E. Marshall, "Sullivan Overrules NIH on Sex Survey," *Science* 253 (2 August 1991): 253; J. Palca, "New Watchdogs in Washington," *Hastings Center Report* 23, (March-April 1993): 5.

45. D.P. Francis, "Toward a Comprehensive Prevention Program for the CDC and the Nation," *Journal of the American Medical Association* 268 (1992): 1444-47.

46. National Institutes of Health, Advisory Committee to the Director, *Human Fetal Transplantation Research* (Bethesda, Md.: National Institutes of Health, 1988).

47. J.F. Childress, "Ethics, Public Policy, and Human Fetal Tissue Transplantation," *Kennedy Institute of Ethics Journal* 1 (1991): 93-121.

48. L.B. Sullivan to W.F. Raub, letter, 2 November 1989.

49. The press (P.J. Hilts, "U.S. Aides See Shaky Legal Basis for Ban on Fetal Tissue Research," *New York Times* 30 January 1990, and a letter from Representative Weiss to Dr. Sullivan, 26 January 1990) cited a memorandum from the DHHS General Counsel, saying that the extension of the moratorium was on a "shaky legal base" because it could be a violation of the Administrative Procedures Act that required such decisions to be published in the *Federal Register* and made the subject of rule making. A group of five medical foundations and college associations filed suit on 21 October 1992 in U.S. District Court to overturn the "indefinite moratorium" on FTTR. Their case was based on the unlawfulness of the process by which the moratorium was imposed. M. York, "Fetal Tissue Research Ban Challenged," *Washington Post* 22 October 1992.

50. J. Hogan, "Genes and Crime," *Scientific American* (February 1993): 23-29; L. Duke, "Controversy Flares Over Crime, Heredity," *Washington Post,* 19 August 1993.

51. C. Feldman, "NIH Cancels $78,000 Grant to U-MD Crime Conference," *Washington Post,* 23 April 1993.

52. National Institutes of Health, Grant Appeal: NIH-GA-93-01, 3 September 1993.

53. See OTA, *Biomedical Ethics,* 30. "In the event a Secretary withholds funds, he or she must appoint an ethics board after considering nominations for 30 days; 180 days later, a body must submit a report to the Secretary and Congress. Should the majority of the ethics board recommend that the Secretary not withhold the monies for the research on ethical ground, the research shall be funded unless the Secretary finds that the board's recommendations were 'arbitrary and capricious.' "

54. The OTA report lists 15 issues under biomedical research topics and eight issues in a category described as more "broad-based." *Ibid.,* 29.

55. The National Commission's mandate to develop guidelines in this area was opposed, among others, by the National Institute of Mental Health. Research psychiatrists are generally offended by a premise that mentally ill research subjects are impaired in terms of giving a voluntary informed consent. A moderate alternative is to seek a "durable power of attorney for research decisions" from cognitively impaired subjects, including those who have serious mental illness. The Clinical Center, NIH, pioneered this practice with patients suffering from Alzheimer's disease and other dementias. J.C. Fletcher, F.W. Dommel, and D.D. Cowell, "Consent to Research with Impaired Human Subjects," *IRB: A*

Review of Human Subjects Research 7 (November-December 1985): 1-6. This approach could also be taken in the context of some severe mental illnesses, when at times of more lucidity, patients would be able to execute such directives.

A promising effort to study and innovate in the area of research involving persons with Alzheimer's disease has been funded by the National Institute on Aging (#AG05144), and is headed by Dallas M. High, Ph.D. High describes the scope of this research and its continuity with the earlier Clinical Center policy in "Research with Alzheimer's Disease Subjects: Informed Consent and Proxy Decision Making," *Journal of the American Geriatrics Society* 40 (1992): 950-57.

56. A report of the Committee on Government Operations (H. Rept. 102-478, 102d Cong., 2d sess.) calls for an Advisory Commission on the Ethical, Legal, and Social Implications of the Human Genome Project. There is a real need for policy studies to draw together the implications uncovered by the research funded by the ELSI program.

57. NABER was established in 1990-1991 by joint action of the American Fertility Society and the American College of Obstetrics and Gynecology, because of the vaccum left by the absence of an EAB. Its chairman is Albert R. Jonsen and its executive director is Gladys White, 409 12th St. SW, Washington, D.C. 20024-2188.

58. B. Rensberger, "NIH Panel Looks at Ethics, Standards for Human Embryo Research," *Washington Post,* 7 February 1994.

59. President's Commission for the Study of Ethical Problems in Medicine and Biomedical and Behavioral Research, *Securing Access to Health Care* (Washington, D.C.: U.S. Government Printing Office, 1985).

60. A. Caplan, "Ethics of Casting the First Stone," *Alcoholism* 18 (1994): 220-25.

61. F.G. Miller and J.C. Fletcher, "The Case for Legalized Euthanasia," *Perspectives in Biology and Medicine* 36 (1993): 159-76.

62. See Hanna, Cook-Deegan, and Nishimi, "Finding a Forum." This article was followed in a subsequent issue (vol. 13, 1994) by a "Symposium: Bioethics and Public Policy" with opinions by R.H. Blank, I.H. Carmen, C.B. Cohen, J.C. Fletcher, L. Gilliam (Australia), D. Macer (Japan), D. Mathieu, J. Miller (Canada), E.H. Moskowitz, D. Shairo (Europe), and D. Wikler, followed by a response from the original authors.

63. D. Mathieu, "Another Forum for Bioethics in U.S. Public Policy?" *Politics and the Life Sciences* 13 (1994): 91-92.

64. G.J. Annas, "Will the Real Bioethics (Commission) Please Stand Up?"

65. R.H. Blank, "A National Forum for Bioethics: Attractive but Unworkable or Workable but Unattractive," *Politics and the Life Sciences* 13 (1994): 77-78.

66. For example, conservatives who oppose embryo research in principle will have good reason to object to the report from a NIH Embryo Research Panel without any members who hold this position.

67. Hanna, Cook-Deegan, and Nishimi, "Finding a Forum."

68. OTA, *Biomedical Ethics.*

69. S.K. Miller and G. Vines, "Human Clones Split Fertility Experts," *New Scientist*, (30 October 1993): 7.

70. C.M. Spicer, "Fallout from Government-Sponsored Radiation Research," *Kennedy Institute of Ethics Journal* 4 (1994): 147-54.

71. Senate Report. 1042, described by S. Burd, "Momentum Builds for Federal Panel on Ethical Issues in Science," *Chronicle of Higher Education*, 4 May 1994, A32.

72. Fiscal constraints are extremely important in government today. It is highly dubious if Congress or the administration would permit two bodies, if only for cost-containment reasons. OTA calculated that a standing body to replace the EAB would cost $744,000 annually, or $2,976,000 over a four-year period, and that a term-limited body to replace the President's Commission would cost $1,920,000 per year for four years or $7,680,000. The cost of both groups over four years would be $10,656,000. Also, the Clinton administration has ordered the reduction by one-third of federal advisory bodies.

73. Kennedy Institute of Ethics, *International Directory of Bioethics Organizations* (Washington D.C.: Georgetown University Press, 1994), 20057.

74. Several years of debate about the decision-making process in cases involving medical futility, posed by cases like *Helga Wanglie, Baby L, Baby K*, and other cases involving extensive technology have not led to any consensus about this value-laden topic. See M. Angell, "The Case of Helga Wanglie; A New Kind of 'Right to Die' Case," *New England Journal of Medicine* 325 (1991): 511-12; J.J. Paris *et al.*, "Beyond Autonomy: Physicians' Refusal to Use Life-Prolonging Extracorporeal Membrane Oxygenation," *New England Journal of Medicine* 329 (1993): 354-57; J.J. Paris, R.K. Crone, and F. Reardon, "Physicians' Refusal of Requested Treatment: The Case of Baby L," *New England Journal of Medicine* 329 (1990): 1012-15; G.J. Annas, "Asking the Courts to Set the Standard of Emergency Care: The Case of Baby K," *New England Journal of Medicine* 330 (1994): 1542-45.

8

Financial Issues and Incentives Related to Clinical Research and Innovative Therapies

Stuart E. Lind

INTRODUCTION

Much work in the ethics of human experimentation has focused on issues related to the subjects and the performance of clinical research. Just as there has been a progressive interest in the ethical behavior of public figures, there has been a growing interest in recent years in the behavior of biomedical researchers. Unlike politicians, scientists have not been subject to scrutiny about their private lives as much as they have with regard to actual or alleged misconduct in the performance of their work. As examples of (purported) scientific misconduct have been identified, there has been a tendency for nonscientists to scrutinize more closely the behavior of researchers and to promulgate rules defining scientific misconduct, some of which have not been perceived as reasonable by large numbers of scientists.[1]

There continues to be evolution in thinking and practice concerning the subjects and performance of clinical research, perhaps best exemplified by the essays found in this collection. Over the past decade, however, there has been a new area of concern, investigation, and comment, which has at its center not the subject, nor the investigator-subject dyad, but the investigator him/herself. Those who are interested in this area must grapple with difficult issues not specific to clinical research, but to many human endeavors in which a significant potential conflict of interest exists. It might be thought that biomedical research, growing out of and along with the practice of medicine, would be better equipped to deal with potential conflicts of interest than other fields, since both patients and physicians have long recognized many of the ways in which the physician's interests may conflict with the patient's. Despite a tradition which has been cognizant of such difficulties, biomedical research has not shown itself to be any more advanced in anticipating and handling such conflicts than politics or business.[2]

Thus, a discussion about financial issues and incentives is really a discussion concerning the difficult area of real and perceived conflicts of interest. It would be foolish for me to attempt to answer all the questions related to this topic, so my aim is to use my experiences and insights to catalog areas of potential difficulty for future analyses and discussions. My approach will be to catalog the interactions that may pose problems for those who conduct, oversee, and participate in biomedical research with human subjects and to define areas that are worthy of more attention. Finally, I will consider some reasons why there has been a change in the number and type of financial issues that influence clinical investigation, and I will attempt to place these new concerns within the perspective of changes that have occurred in American society and academic medical centers over the past 15 to 20 years.

Although institutional review boards (IRBs) were founded because of concerns about the basic relationship that characterizes clinical research--that between the investigator and the subject--a variety of other parties now play an important, if sometimes unrecognized role, particularly with regard to financial issues. These include:

1. The Food and Drug Administration (FDA);
2. Third-party payers including private and government insurers;
3. Doctors of patients who might refer the patients to a study;
4. Colleagues of investigators;
5. Supervisors of investigators;
6. Hospitals and their communities of constituents, overseers, competitors; and
7. Manufacturers of drugs and medical devices.

These parties and their interests may interact directly, indirectly, or not at all in any given research study, and the financial considerations that link them may or may not be obvious, although they exist to one degree or another and may be considered by IRBs at various times. This discussion begins by considering the central relationship in clinical research--that between the subject and the investigator (see Figure 1)--and then considers financial questions that arise when other parties are involved.

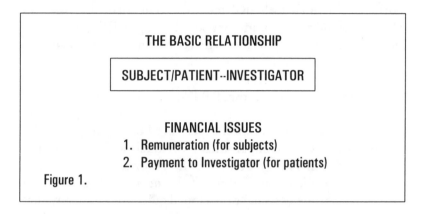

THE BASIC RELATIONSHIP

SUBJECT/PATIENT--INVESTIGATOR

FINANCIAL ISSUES
1. Remuneration (for subjects)
2. Payment to Investigator (for patients)

Figure 1.

FINANCIAL ISSUES RELATED TO THE SUBJECT-INVESTIGATOR RELATIONSHIP

The word "subject" may refer to two different groups of people: those with an illness who might conceivably benefit by participating in a research project (whom I will call patients), and those volunteers (healthy or ill) whose participation in research is used to generate knowledge, without any pretense or hope of benefiting the subject.

ISSUES THAT ARISE WHEN THE SUBJECT IS A VOLUNTEER

There is usually one major financial question that arises when considering the relationship between the healthy volunteer and the investigator: the proper or "appropriate remuneration" for the volunteer's participation in the research project. This may, or should, take into account such factors as the time, effort, risk, and (perceived) unpleasantness of the activities involved. It is always interesting to see the range of individual opinions expressed by IRB members when the question of unpleasantness comes up. It would be interesting to determine what the key factors are in causing an IRB member to say, "*I* certainly wouldn't volunteer for this study!" One's age and financial status are two variables that likely influence a member's reactions.

It is only fair that the question of fair reimbursement be mentioned first, for it has perhaps the longest history in the annals of IRB deliberations.[3] In addition, it provides a window into a central problem that all IRB members live with, the role and influence of individual opinions and values upon IRB operations. This has particular importance when considering financial issues, since each IRB must set its own policies with regard to the various financial issues it considers.

Questions may arise if the IRB feels that the proposed remuneration for the "normal volunteer" is either too large or too small. When the remuneration is perceived to be too great, IRB members often voice concerns that individuals will be coerced to participate.[4] Others may object on the grounds that it is excessively paternalistic for an IRB to determine when remuneration is excessive.[5] Some IRBs have developed guidelines to insure that volunteers receive at least a minimal compensation for their participation, and some have developed lists that describe how much subjects should be compensated for a venous blood drawing, an arterial blood gas drawing, or an EEG examination. As with most of the issues I will discuss, I am unaware of information indicating how widespread or uniform this practice is, nor do we know how IRBs in general cope with the struggle to balance reasonable concern for the rights of research volunteers (including the right to determine what activities they will engage in) with their personal feelings regarding coercion.

ISSUES THAT ARISE WHEN THE SUBJECT IS A PATIENT

When the subject is also a patient, other financial issues may arise. In such circumstances, the investigator may not offer remuneration to the subject, reasoning that the potential for the individual to benefit personally from the study is reason enough for him/her to participate. This is not always the case, however, and individuals with a relatively benign condition (for example, mild to moderate acne) may be compensated for their time in undergoing various tests that the investigator or study sponsor wishes to perform. If the benefit is small, IRB members may feel that additional remuneration is warranted. Some may feel that remuneration should be added to the study because the investigator is otherwise unlikely to recruit enough subjects. Others feel that the benefits are small in comparison with the obligations. This may provoke discussions about the so-called rights of patients to volunteer without adequate compensation and/or the exploitative nature of investigators. Some IRB members believe that inadequate compensation indicates that the investigator is trying to take advantage of subjects who do not realize that they will not sustain any lasting benefit from their participation. As with other discussions of this sort, the lack of data concerning the preferences and values of potential subjects means that IRB members only speak for themselves and not for their constituents or communities.

PAYMENT BY INSURERS FOR RESEARCH CONDUCTED DURING THE DELIVERY OF MEDICAL CARE

In some instances, the patient may pay the investigator for participating in a study conducted during the course of the routine delivery of healthcare. In the most common case, the patient does not pay the investigator directly, but allows the investigator to bill the patient's insurance carrier for medical care, which includes an investigative element. This element may constitute declared research--that which has been submitted to an IRB--or undeclared research, or what I call innovative therapy. Of course, in such circumstances patients do not consider themselves to be paying. In the event that the insurance company recognizes that some element of the patient's care is non-standard, however, patients may find themselves being asked to pay for their participation in a clinical research project. How often this occurs is not known.

IRBs may be told, or may be able to anticipate, that the investigator considers the research plan to be a part of appropriate medical care and plans to submit a bill to the patient's insurance company. Depending upon the makeup of the IRB, arguments may ensue about this proposed course of action. Discussions on such occasions may revolve around the questions of whether practitioners should be encouraged or discouraged to be part-time researchers, or whether the IRB should direct its efforts to saving insurance companies' money for tests and treatments that are not yet standard therapy. At such times some may argue that patients should be fully informed and told of the potential direct costs to them of participating in a study, should their insurance company refuse to cover the costs. If this approach is taken, IRB members may find themselves debating whether dollar estimates should appear on the consent form. In one such discussion I witnessed, where the potential cost to the patient was $25,000 (should the insurance company refuse to pay for any aspect of the hospitalization and treatment), quite a bit of discussion was generated concerning the appropriateness and wisdom of including this worst-case estimate on the consent form. The magnitude of the estimated cost and the difficulty of knowing the likelihood that the patient would have to pay anything finally convinced the IRB to omit such information from the consent form. Because of the potential expense, and the fact that the study involved a new and highly publicized therapy offered in only a few centers nation-wide, the IRB was able to engage the hospital administration in a dialogue that resulted in the latter's agreeing that the hospital would cover the costs should a patient be presented with a bill as a result of the failure of the insurance company to pay. As with most of the financial issues related to clinical research, "hard" information is not available to document how often insurance companies refuse to pay for such treatments, how often patients themselves are asked to pay, and how many institutions foresee such possibilities and guarantee to cover the costs, should third-party coverage not materialize.

Also, as is well known, patients may be excluded from clinical trials of new treatments if their insurance companies require prospective approval of treatment plans and have not classified the treatment as accepted or standard. Finally, it should be noted that the FDA has allowed patients with some kinds of diseases to buy drugs outside of clinical trials prior to the granting of formal marketing approval, although I have no knowledge of this program's successes or problems.

DIRECT PAYMENTS BY PATIENTS

In a small number of instances, the patient may be asked to pay the investigator directly. I have previously reported on a for-profit company that was established to offer novel anti-cancer therapies on a contractual basis to patients who paid the appropriate fees, which ranged from approximately $10,000 to $30,000.[6] While anecdotal reports of private philanthropists who have sponsored research for their own or their relatives' benefit are common, this was the first example of a widely described effort to establish what I have called fee-for-service research. The company's plans and operations were extensively described in a number of national publications and television shows, and its founder stated a number of arguments in favor of such an enterprise.[7] Although the company planned to develop new monoclonal antibody-based therapies with patients' fees, most of its clients came for other treatments, especially after it offered the then-new interleukin-2/LAK cell treatment pioneered by investigators at the National Cancer Institute. Because IL-2/LAK cell therapy was available to only a few patients through National Cancer Institute trials, the company was able to meet patients' demands for access to this treatment and offered this therapy to patients who were not able to enroll on the few clinical studies then in operation. Not only was the company thereby able to sustain itself financially, but its physicians also developed a beneficial modification of IL-2 administration that itself was published in the *New England Journal of Medicine*.[8] Although the company's initial innovative approaches to cancer care have not developed into a proven mode of therapy, IL-2 has been approved by the FDA for limited indications. I was told several years ago that due to disagreements over the direction of the company, the founder left to establish a private research institute, and the company changed its name, although it continued to provide services to cancer patients.

Although the company's approach to patient-funded clinical research engendered significant public discussion, debate about its risks and benefits continues.[9] How many other ventures are proceeding with direct patient payment for research activities is not known. One has led to a number of large-scale clinical trials and considerable scientific controversy. The drug now called tacrine was initially studied in the treatment of Alzheimer's disease by an individual in private practice who reported the apparent benefits of the drug in the *New England Journal of Medicine*.[10] He subsequently wrote about his difficulties in paying for this research, noting that the first 10 patients were treated with funds generated by his private practice. As the number of patients treated with tacrine grew, and grant applications were turned down, additional funding was needed to further the work. The description of the for-profit, patient-funded company devoted to cancer research inspired the investigator to fund his own work in the same way.[11] With a do-it-yourself legal kit, he established a for-profit enterprise, Solo Research, Inc., which used patient fees to carry out the research. Perhaps in response to concerns about the for-profit nature of the company, the investigator reported that he had initiated efforts to establish a non-profit corporation, Solo Non-Profit Research, Ltd., that would allow for ongoing clinical research to be conducted without provoking criticism because of its profit-generating motives.[12]

Although I have written about these issues in a way that might be characterized as finger pointing, I believe that some of the issues raised by the investigators involved in these activities should be considered carefully and with a sympathetic ear. It is not a simple matter for an individual to obtain the funding needed to conduct preliminary studies even if he/she is an established investigator. It is much harder for those who are not well connected with members of the pharmaceutical industry or able to divert funds from other sources. There is also a significant problem when no company is ready and willing to fund the research, despite the experience of the investigators. The inability to obtain funding should not be used as an objective marker of potential benefit or worth of an idea, as evidenced by the fact that the fee-for-service researchers cited above made contributions to their respective medical fields, at least as demonstrated by their ability to generate a peer-reviewed publication.[13]

Although all definitive therapeutic studies seem to be conducted with government or industrial funding that evolves from basic research labs, there will continue to be many advances in medicine made on the basis of observations and ideas of physicians engaged in clinical medicine. Nor should we depend upon drug companies to advance healthcare, since self-interest and internal politics govern their decisions. Asking patients to pay for experimental therapies under defined circumstances, specifically when an estimate of success can be honestly offered that allows the patient the opportunity to make an informed decision, may become an acceptable way to deal with the lack of alternative funding sources.[14]

PROFIT, SCIENCE, AND ETHICAL CONDUCT

While profit may certainly influence how investigators behave vis-à-vis human subjects, profit in clinical research, excluding what some might call trivial, comes in many varieties. It is easy to focus on the monetary profits involved in some types of clinical research.[15] While efforts to minimize the influence of this one type of profit from clinical research are, in my view, appropriate, it should be clearly recognized that there are many other types of incentives, some of which may be more powerful, for individual investigators. Thus, the researcher who is pressured to publish or risk losing a cherished academic position may be more likely to cross the line into unethical behavior than the financially rewarded researcher who knows that everyone is watching, perhaps hoping to see him (and his Mercedes-Benz) run into a (metaphorical) ditch.

It is my view that it is impossible for the IRB to remove either the profit or the profit motive from research, nor should such be attempted. While some might object and believe that research would be better, purer, or more ethical if conducted only by seekers of truth, I feel otherwise. To those who disagree, I recommend a public television show concerning the Tuskegee Syphilis Study, wherein some of the involved investigators continue to expound upon the desirability of clean scientific experiments. A reward-based system coupled to oversight is preferable, in my view, to one concerned mainly with purity of scientific purpose and methods.

PAYING FOR CLINICAL RESEARCH

Payment for clinical research comes from a variety of sources (see Figure 2). Sponsors include:

1. For-profit institutions:
   A. Manufacturers of drugs and medical devices and
   B. For-profit hospitals, treatment centers.

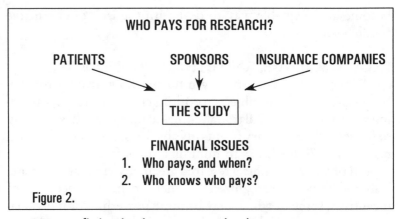

Figure 2.

2. Nonprofit institutions or organizations:
   A. National Institutes of Health; disease-oriented groups such as American Hospital Association, American Cancer Society and
   B. Universities, medical centers, staffs, etc.
3. Insurance companies:
   A. Knowingly or
   B. Unknowingly.
4. Patients.

For-profit institutions commonly pay for clinical research in order to gather data to support an application to the FDA for approval to market a product. The financial issues raised by such sponsorship usually relate to the remuneration offered patients or volunteers and to the monies that are given to investigators who recruit patients for the study.

NOTIFYING THE SUBJECT OF THE STUDY'S SPONSORS

The suggestion that patients should be notified about the sponsor of the research provides an interesting window into the world of IRBs.[16] At face value, arguments in favor of such a policy suggest that such information might influence a person's decision about participating. This information goes beyond the usual factors (such as the procedures, risks, and benefits of participating) used by subjects to make a decision about participation. Unless the proposal is just an attempt to gain control over investigators, some of whom may strike IRB members as personifying the greed and excess said to have gone out of style with the 1980s, then we must consider whether these facts are really relevant for the potential subject, and if so, why?

Although I too oppose greed and excess in investigators, the only reason I can see for adopting such a policy is to discourage the enrollment of patients in a study. Such disclosure would not be likely to push a patient towards enrollment, but could only serve to dissuade him/her from participating by virtue of waving a red flag that warns him or her to be suspicious of the investigator and/or the research. Adoption of such a policy would be likely to make even willing subjects hesitant about participating and suggests that studies put forth by drug companies (or other deep-pocketed sponsors) are somehow different than others, even when the investigator is honest and the study is more than an entry into new markets. Such policies allow investigators with good sponsorships to trade off their sponsorship in a positive way, perhaps to the extent that subjects do not fully analyze the study for themselves, but assume that it must be fine if the government or one branch of the National Institutes of Health has approved it. Manipulating subjects' emotions in order to gain control over investigators seems less honest than simply taxing or seizing research-related income.[17]

WHO SHOULD RECEIVE THE FINANCIAL INCENTIVES OFFERED FOR RECRUITING PATIENTS?

Whether or not one wishes to inform the patient of the study's sponsorship or the incentives available to physicians who recruit them, it is clear that the incentives given to investigators for recruiting may be quite considerable.[18] These funds are often used to pay for a significant number of other projects and/or individuals' salaries. Shimm and Speece have suggested that the availability of such funds, or what we might simply call the profit motive, may pose conflicts of interest for investigators who may be tempted to propose treatments that are either not needed or less beneficial than standard treatments in order to earn the payment.[19] They have proposed that such payments should be directed to a common pool controlled by the medical school dean, which could then be used to fund proposals submitted by all faculty members. Research into the attitudes and practices of IRBs and medical center administrations in this regard would be interesting and helpful to those considering the alternatives.

ANNOUNCED AND SURREPTITIOUS FUNDING OF CLINICAL RESEARCH BY INSURANCE COMPANIES

Recently, insurance company sponsorship of a clinical trial of bone marrow transplantation for women with breast cancer has been instituted. This is noteworthy because insurance companies have heretofore been reluctant to pay for experimental therapy.[20] Although announced third-party coverage of a nonstandard therapy is unusual, insurance company payments have been covering the costs of research projects for many years. This has been mentioned as a concern in the literature, and has been the subject of discussion among IRBs.[21] In a recent article, researchers reported that 23 percent of 196 studies published in 23 journals of internal medicine and neurology during a one-month period in 1991 were unfunded. Of the research examined, 7 percent involved direct clinical costs that were not accounted for by the investigators and which may have been passed on to study participants or third-party payers.[22] It would be interesting to look back in 10 years and determine whether funded or unfunded studies are more likely to lead to lasting benefits or gains.

WHO PROFITS FROM RESEARCH? WHERE DOES THE MONEY GO?

Other parties have financial interests in research with human subjects (see Figure 3). Occasionally, perhaps frequently, investigators find it difficult to recruit patients to their trials. A variety of incentives have been offered to housestaff and other referring physicians to increase such recruitment. This practice of offering finder's fees is a long-standing one that, in the view of some, is benign.[23] Others however, have construed it as immoral and/or a violation of federal law.[24] Such practices are said to be common in clinical practice, although forbidden by professional groups such as the American College of Physicians.[25]

PROFIT IN CLINICAL RESEARCH

Certain high-profile research programs can make a big difference in how a hospital is perceived at the community, state, or

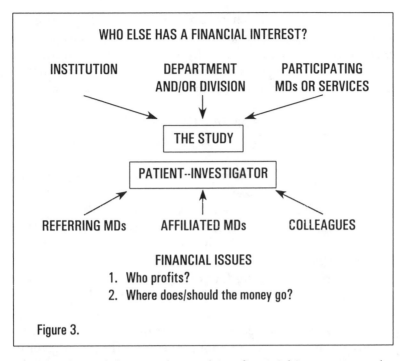

WHO ELSE HAS A FINANCIAL INTEREST?

INSTITUTION   DEPARTMENT   PARTICIPATING
                     AND/OR DIVISION   MDs OR SERVICES

THE STUDY

PATIENT--INVESTIGATOR

REFERRING MDs   AFFILIATED MDs   COLLEAGUES

FINANCIAL ISSUES
1. Who profits?
2. Where does/should the money go?

Figure 3.

local levels, and they can have a large financial impact upon the institution and surrounding community. Clinical research is financially beneficial to institutions because it brings with it overhead charges as well as a certain volume of subjects through hospital facilities. Perhaps the best known example is the transplant program established by Starzl at the University of Pittsburgh, which is said to bring $1 million a day into the city. In addition, it stimulates referrals to the medical center for patients with related disorders. The prestige enjoyed by all associated with a successful research center undoubtedly feeds back to the investigator. Together, all these factors provide incentives for investigators that cannot be monitored or controlled by IRBs.

Thus, investigators profit from their recruitment of patients in several ways. In addition to the money that may be used to pay for dinners, trips, fellows, and research nurses, investigators gain status, influence, promotions, and power as a result of their efforts. Even investigators who do not receive any direct financial rewards or personal recognition in terms of published manuscripts for recruiting patients may be under great pressure to do so because it keeps their institution on the rolls of cooperative clinical trials groups, which in turn keeps superiors in positions of influence and brings dollars into the institution. Given these many incentives, we may ask why we should focus on the cash that flows to investigators, and why we should take pains that its presence be made known to patients in the consent form.

WHY HAVE FINANCIAL ISSUES ASSUMED SUCH IMPORTANCE IN CLINICAL RESEARCH?

A number of factors account for the increased importance of financial matters in the conduct of clinical research over the past two decades. First, there was a growth in the number of people interested in, and capable of, conducting research as a result of the overall growth of medical schools, the size of the classes of students they educate, and the efforts of the NIH to expand research training programs for young physicians, most of whom are not interested in the financially monastic life of the threadbare investigator of old.[26]

Second, it became easier to do research during this period because the measurements no longer required the investigator to spend long hours in the laboratory performing routine tests. The use of machines allowed many measurements of blood and body fluids to be carried out by technicians without oversight of an investigator. Ultrasound, CAT scans, and MRI machines allow for safe and effective examinations of subjects on a repeated basis. In addition to increasing an investigator's productivity, these advances also increased the cost of doing research.

Third, the evolution of molecular biology and biotechnology allowed large quantities of drugs, especially proteins, to be mass produced in a pure form, allowing many more studies to be performed in a short period of time.

Fourth, the explosive growth in techniques of biological research allowed scientists to investigate areas of molecular and cellular biology to a degree never before possible, as exemplified by the Human Genome Project. As a result, it became more difficult for clinical (as opposed to basic laboratory) scientists to gain governmental funding, and clinical research became more dependent upon manufacturers of drugs and medical devices and (surreptitiously) insurance companies.

Fifth, there was a change in the attitudes of many scientists and physicians toward working in industry. Many first-rate people left academia for biotechnology firms, as well as established drug companies. These individuals knew how to motivate academics, many of whom had been placed under increasing demands for clinical service, and were thus particularly interested in obtaining funds by alternative means.

Sixth, clinical research became a means to draw patients to medical centers.

I believe that the efforts of the first and second generations of medical oncologists who tested cancer drugs on their patients as a matter of routine are of particular importance. Because the rise of IRBs mandated an honest approach to patients, the care of cancer patients was moved out of the shadows of surgical wards and into the glare of the consent form. As they fought, with the aid of the news media, to maintain the federal funding that flowed from the 1971 declaration of the war on cancer, the public came to perceive an advantage to participating in clinical research, and the fear of being a human guinea pig began to fade. Because standard anti-cancer therapies were, at best, marginally effective, this subspecialty group of physicians was told that all patients should be entered into clinical trials and that enrollment in a clinical trial provided the patient with the best treatment available.[27] In certain large centers, these physicians recruited a substantial proportion of their patients onto clinical research protocols, thus making research an integral part of their standard medical care. This served to routinize clinical research, not only for their patients, but for students, housestaff, and other physicians, and it created a large incentive for pharmaceutical houses to sponsor clinical trials.

Regardless of whether one believes that the increase in the number of clinical researchers was good or bad, the end result was that clinical research was taken out of the hands of the (relatively) few professional experimenters who dominated clinical research in the 1950s and 1960s and put it into the hands of anyone who could get their protocol approved by an IRB. By allowing many nonprofessional researchers to conduct research while serving as clinicians, these changes moved research into the open so that others, including housestaff and practicing physicians, could witness, judge, and monitor research practices.

We might ask if the conflicts and discussions related to sponsorship, coercion, and the profit motive will be with us forever. Since many of the clashes are related to relative values, and values change over time, it is possible, perhaps likely, that there will be less conflict in future years. Distrust of investigators is implicit in discussions of coercion and the advisability of telling patients who is sponsoring a clinical trial. I would like to think that these attitudes are largely carry-overs from the past. While I certainly recognize that many investigators are interested in minimizing their work or obligations to the IRB, I would like to think that their transgressions are relatively minor, as measured on the large scale provided by the history of clinical research in this country. The questions raised by considering the ways that various financial incentives impact upon the conduct of clinical research are interesting and important and should be the subject of research as well as debate and deliberation.

NOTES

1. M.E. Shapiro and R.P. Charrow, "Scientific Misconduct in Investigational Drug Trials," *New England Journal of Medicine* 312 (1985): 731-36.

2. W. Booth, "Conflict of Interest Eyed at Harvard," *Science* 242 (1988): 1497-98; American Medical Association, Council on Scientific Affairs and Council on Ethical and Judicial Affairs, "Conflicts of Interest in Medical Center Industry Research Relationships," *Journal of the American Medical Association* 263 (1990): 2790-93.

3. M.W. Wartofsky, "On Doing It for Money," in *Research Involving Prisoners: Report and Recommendations,* ed. National Commission for the Protection of Human Subjects of Biomedical and Behavioral Research, DHEW publication no. (OS) 76-132 (Washington D.C.: U.S. Government Printing Office, 1976), 3.1-3.24.

4. R. Macklin, " 'Due' and 'Undue' Inducements: On Paying Money to Research Subjects," *IRB: A Review of Human Subjects Research* 3 (September-October 1981): 1-6.

5. L. Newton, "Inducement, Due and Otherwise," *IRB: A Review of Human Subjects Research* 4 (July-August 1982): 4-6.

6. S.E. Lind, "Fee-for-Service Research," *New England Journal of Medicine* 314 (1986): 312-15.

7. R.K. Oldham, "Patient-Funded Cancer Research," *New England Journal of Medicine* 316 (1987): 46-47.

8. W.H. West *et al.*, "Constant-Infusion Recombinant Interleukin-2 in Adoptive Immunotherapy of Advanced Cancer," *New England Journal of Medicine* 316 (1987): 898-905.

9. J. La Puma, "Researching Non-Profit Research: The Obligations of Hospital Ethicists," *Clinical Research* 37 (1989): 569-73; E.H. Morreim, "Patient-Funded Research: Paying the Piper or Protecting the Patient?" *IRB: A Review of Human Subjects Research* 13 (May-June 1991): 1-6.

10. W.K. Summer *et al.*, "Oral Tetrahydroaminoacridine in Long-Term Treatment of Senile Dementia, Alzheimer Type," *New England Journal of Medicine* 315 (1986): 1241-45.

11. Lind, "Fee-for-Service Research."

12. W.K. Summers, "Fee-for-Service Research on THA: An Explanation" (letter), *New England Journal of Medicine* 316 (1987): 1605-6.

13. West *et al.*, "Constant-Infusion Recombinant Interleukin-2"; Summer *et al.*, "Oral Tetrahydroaminocridine."

14. S.E. Lind, "Can Patients Be Asked to Pay for Experimental Treatment?" *Clinical Research* 32 (1984): 393-98.

15. A.S. Relman, "Dealing with Conflicts of Interest," *New England Journal of Medicine* 310 (1984): 1182-83; A.S. Relman, "Economic Incentives in Clinical Investigation," *New England Journal of Medicine* 320 (1989): 933-34; B. Healy *et al.*, "Conflict-of-Interest Guidelines for a Multicenter Clinical Trial of Treatment After Coronary-Artery Bypass-Graft Surgery," *New England Journal of Medicine* 320 (1989): 949-51; G.D. Lundberg and A. Flanagin, "New Requirement for Authors: Signed Statements of Authorship Responsibility and Financial Disclosure," *Journal of the American Medical Association* 262 (1989): 2003-4.

16. H.M. Spiro, "Mammon and Medicine: The Rewards of Clinical Trials," *Journal of the American Medical Association* 255 (1986): 1174-75.

17. D.S. Shimm and R.G. Speece, Jr. "Industry Reimbursement for Entering Patients into Clinical Trials: Legal and Ethical Issues," *Annals of Internal Medicine* 115 (1991): 148-51.

18. M.J. Finkel, "Should Informed Consent Include Information on How Research Is Funded?" *IRB: A Review of Human Subjects Research* 13 (September-October 1991): 1-3.

19. Shimm and Speece, "Industry Reimbursement."

20. L.N. Newcomer, "Defining Experimental Therapy: A Third Party Payer's Dilemma," *New England Journal of Medicine* 323 (1990): 1702-4.

21. Lind, "Can Patients Be Asked to Pay for Experimental Treatment?"; G.B. Weiss, "Who Pays for Clinical Research?" *Clinical Research*

27 (1979): 297-99; S.E. Lind, "Dilemmas in Paying for Clinical Research: The View from the IRBs," *IRB: A Review of Human Subjects Research* 9 (March/April 1987): 1-5.

22. M.D. Stein, L. Rubenstein, and T.J. Wachtel, "Who Pays for Published Research?" *Journal of the American Medical Association* 269 (1993): 781-82.

23. S.E. Lind, "Finder's Fees for Research Subjects," *New England Journal of Medicine* 323 (1990): 192-95; D.J. Higby, "Finder's Fees for Research Subjects" (letter), *New England Journal of Medicine* 323 (1990): 1716.

24. D. Hsia, "Finder's Fees for Research Subjects" (letter), *New England Journal of Medicine* 323 (1990): 1710-11.

25. *American College of Physicians Ethics Manual*, 3rd ed., cited in *Annals of Internal Medicine* 117 (1992): 947-60.

26. R.G. Petersdorf, "Academic Medicine: No Longer Threadbare or Genteel," *New England Journal of Medicine* 304 (1981): 841-43.

27. R.D. Gelber and A. Goldhirsch, "Can a Clinical Trial Be the Treatment of Choice for Patients with Cancer?" *Journal of the National Cancer Institute* 80 (1988): 886-87.

9

Physicians' Conflicts of Interest in Post-Marketing Research: What the Public Should Know, and Why Industry Should Tell Them

John La Puma

INTRODUCTION

The goals and methods of post-marketing research are unknown to many scholars, patients, and sometimes even to the physicians who voluntarily participate. Yet, post-marketing research represents an enormous and expensive effort by the pharmaceutical industry to market and study medications and procedures approved by the U.S. Food and Drug Administration (FDA) for clinical use.[1]

Most post-marketing research is conducted by practicing physicians on "me-too," or duplicative drugs. Sales of duplicative drugs--patented, nearly identical medications manufactured by competing companies--now comprise up to 75 percent of the revenues of large drug companies.[2] One five-year Phase IV study on gemfibrozil and high density lipoprotein (HDL) cholesterol is reported to have cost $137 million.[3]

Here, I will describe post-marketing research in its usual form and tell why it has remained a hidden financial conflict of interest for medical practitioners. I will then chart the key ethical issues that such research presents for physicians who are invited by industry to be investigators. I will suggest several ways in which the identified issues might be resolved, both at the micro level of doctor and patient, and the macro level of industry, medicine, and government.[4]

I will conclude by suggesting that industry take the lead in informing patients of the goals and objectives of most post-marketing trials. Industry, medicine, and government may together wish to restructure the aim and focus of post-marketing research in the United States, as prescribing decisions shift from individual physicians to managed-care formulary groups.

WHAT IS POST-MARKETING RESEARCH?

The FDA divides research into four phases: clinical pharmacology (I), clinical investigation (II), clinical trials (III), and post-marketing clinical trials (IV).[5] Phase IV research at its best is "the systematic detection and evaluation of adverse events under customary conditions in ordinary medical practice."[6]

There are two types of post-marketing research. The first type is "commitments"--that is, research that comprises an ongoing commitment to the FDA from the manufacturer. Commitments are usually requested by the FDA, and their timely completion may be a required condition of continued, or even accelerated, approval.

Phase IV research is only sometimes required. For example, when a drug is approved under FDA's accelerated approval regulations, a Phase IV study may be required if there are unanswered clinical questions which the FDA considers important, for example, concomitant use with other medications, or an incomplete safety profile.[7]

Such commitments and required reviews often seek to understand essential, missing scientific data describing a new drug's actions and rare adverse effects. Physician participation in such Phase IV research is not analyzed here.

Analyzed here is the other type of post-marketing research--"seeding" studies. By far the most prevalent type of post-marketing research, seeding studies are usually company-sponsored, observational cohort studies without a control group, conducted in the outpatient setting.[8] Their primary purpose is familiarization of physicians and patients with new drugs that are being marketed. Like other forms of promotion, post-marketing research influences physicians' drug choices and formulary recommendations.[9]

Most post-marketing investigators are physicians practicing in private offices or other outpatient settings. These physicians are investigators in the broad sense in that they add to data collection, rather than in the more technical sense of closely and systematically examining and inquiring. Physicians are invited by pharmaceutical company sponsors to complete an information sheet for each patient enrolled. The sheet varies in length and detail from one trial to the next. Some investigators enroll their own patients, and others rely on other physicians to refer subjects. Investigators record the pertinent data, mail it to the sponsor or to a sales representative, and collect what is often a per capita fee for patient enrollment.

In turn, the pharmaceutical sponsor will pay for the patient's initial supply of medication, laboratory examinations, and office visit, and will pay the physician for his or her time and effort. Institutional review boards (IRBs) seldom review the research protocol, even when it is sent to the investigator. Informed consent may or may not be obtained from the patient. Many post-marketing physician-investigators may not consider postmarketing trials to be truly research, as the medications prescribed are approved for the very purpose they are dispensed.

It is uncertain whether the data collected in post-marketing trials is usually published in the peer-reviewed medical literature, but if it is, it does not appear regularly in widely circulated mainstream medical journals. One review of 31 British post-marketing studies performed under voluntary guidelines found that more than one-third had been abandoned before completion.[10] The review also found only one important new safety hazard in all 31 studies.

The real value of post-marketing research, then, does not appear to reside in the prestige of publication. Instead, the value of the research to its sponsor involves the process of distributing the drug, in word-of-mouth benefits about the drug among physicians, and in sales representatives' easier access to physicians.[11]

PREVALENCE

How prevalent is such research, and how often do practicing physicians perform it? To answer these questions, we recently reported a preliminary analysis in abstract form and presented the data in two scientific meetings. We pretested and then distributed parallel questionnaires to 269 consecutive general internal medicine outpatients and to all 733 members of the active medical staff of a suburban community teaching hospital.[12]

Of 733 eligible medical staff, 394 (54 percent) responded; 144 of the physicians responding (36 percent) had been asked by a drug company to enroll patients in a post-marketing clinical trial of an FDA-approved new drug; 106 (27 percent) had done so.

In at least one suburban middle-class community, then, more than a third of the responding physicians had been invited, and more than three-fourths of those invited had accepted industry's invitation to participate in post-marketing clinical trials.

CHARTING OF ETHICAL ISSUES

What ethical issues does post-marketing research present for physicians who are compensated by industry to enroll patients and gather data? The central issues are dual loyalty, whether post-marketing trials count as research, accountability, truth telling, informed consent, and patient advocacy. Several of these issues have been previously discussed, but they are analyzed here in relation to the underlying issue of physicians' conflict of interest.[13]

The chief problem for post-marketing researchers centers on their own recognition of their financial conflict of interest.[14] Professional organizations have identified physicians' inability to recognize, or once recognized, to neutralize their own financial conflicts of interest in research.

Some professional organizations have attempted to keep their members accountable by asking them to tell others about their financial sponsorship. This idea of accountability is an appeal to conscience: if one's colleagues know about it, or if the investigator must commit it to paper, then its plainness on the page may give the investigator sufficient moral pause.

The American Federation for Clinical Research suggests that its members inform colleagues about a project's funding source when results are presented or published as research.[15] Harvard University now requires its faculty investigators to disclose their funding sources to the dean. Several researchers[16] and two American Medical Association (AMA) councils[17] have created industry consultancy and stock ownership guidelines for physicians to reduce even the appearance of conflict of interest in research.

Yet these sets of guidelines, and others--AMA guidelines to informed consent to medical research,[18] recent FDA criteria for investigators,[19] and even the detailed and stringent four-part British regulations[20]--do not tell investigators whether to inform the patient about their own financial ties.

The problem is simply this: A physician who is paid twice for a patient visit--by the patient's insurer and by industry, who is given free samples and reimbursed for laboratory examinations, all to prescribe a new approved drug, will be tempted to use the post-marketed drug in place of alternative medications. A physician who is paid once for a patient visit--by the patient's insurer--for prescribing an existing approved drug has no such temptation.

In fact, the new drug may not be the best, safest, or most effective for the patient. But in providing the drug, the physician behaves as if he or she is contributing to the greater good (via research), is adequately treating the patient's condition, and is maximizing his own income. Post-marketing research suggests that physicians can achieve all of these results with a single prescription, yet any one may conflict with the others.

Note that there are no extra direct costs to the patient for the doctor's choice, and indeed, the patient receives several free items for which he or she would otherwise pay, were he or she not enrolled--all to the good. Once the patient runs out of samples, however, the physician writes a prescription for the same drug, and the drug company now has a paying customer. So, the financial conflict of interest is not limited to the physician and patient, but extends to all other patients who will use the new drug. They must bear the new drug's price, already likely to be higher than that of standard therapy and now boosted by the cost of post-marketing research.

Note also the ways in which this conflict of interest gives rise to moral issues relating to informed consent. The patient is often unaware that there is a financial conflict of interest; that he or she is in a research trial; that he or she is taking a drug for which there is necessarily an incomplete safety profile; that the physician is paid twice for seeing the patient; or that the drug company's purpose in providing samples is to market the drug through the physician, and to familiarize both the physician and patient with the drug. Patients may also be unaware that other, less expensive alternative medications may exist that are equally, if not more, safe and effective than a full prescription of the drug undergoing post-marketing research.

Financial conflict of interest in post-marketing research, at least as it is presently conducted and understood, thus raises issues of fairness for physicians. For physician-investigators, moral responsibility should be thought of both as an obligation to patients as a population, as well as to an individual patient-subject. Acting with others in mind is consistent with changes in modern medical ethics toward considerations of justice.[21] Yet such changes highlight conflicting loyalties and dilemmas of informed consent to research risk.

CONFLICTING LOYALTIES

The fundamental conflict for the participating physician is that when serving the patient, the physician is also serving three other masters. They include two payers (the patient's insurer and the research's sponsor) and a patient population–the group which, in theory, will benefit from the results of post-marketing research.

The dilemmas involved in balancing one's moral obligations to a payer and to a particular patient have been well discussed elsewhere.[22] These tensions will likely worsen with the market-place changes created with the debate on health reform, especially as the doctor-patient relationship becomes more political.[23]

Yet the dilemmas of fairness to others encountered by the physician-investigator engaged in post-marketing research appear as complex, if not more so, as dilemmas of proportionality experienced by physicians, faced with balancing out and rationing medical services.[24] Owing a simultaneous duty to both the research sponsor and an unseen, future population of patients is one ball in the air too many for most physician-investigators. Charged with loyalty to one patient at a time in the office and to the needs of his or her other patients yet to come, physicians quadruple their loyalties.

INFORMED CONSENT FOR RESEARCH RISKS

Aside from the financial conflicts of interest faced by investigators, does post-marketing research pose health risks to patients that are significant enough to require the patient's informed consent?

Although controversy continues over the necessity of informed consent for low-risk and even no-risk research, federal guidelines allow informed consent to be waived when certain groups of research subjects face "minimal" risks, that is, risks no greater than those encountered in daily life.[25]

The risks post-marketing research pose are, of course, those known about the administered drug itself, and those that approved standard therapy might entail. Because the drug's safety profile is not yet complete, patients risk the unknown side effects of a medication that is ostensibly under research. Yet its physical risks to the patient are, relatively speaking, likely to be minimal, and patients are readily persuaded to participate in these research trials.[26]

There is another risk, however, which informed consent might be required to alleviate, the risk incurred from the physician's conflicting loyalties.[27] Because the patient does not know that his or her physician works not only for him or her and for his or her payer, but also for an unseen industry employer, the patient needs to be able to weigh the possibility that the physician is prescribing medication for reasons other than its medical indication.

Such risks have been identified in recent indictments of a pharmaceutical company, its distributor, and a pediatric endocrinologist who prescribed the company's synthetic growth hormone, allegedly accepting over $1.1 million in research kickbacks.[28] In addition, the U.S. Inspector General has recently issued a fraud alert, threatening criminal prosecution and warning industry and physicians to be wary of research kickbacks, misleading protocols, and bogus post-marketing arrangements.[29]

As dramatic as these allegations have become in the press, the largest risk patients face in post-marketing research is the potential loss of trust in their physicians.[30] On the one hand, participation in post-marketing research tests the practitioner's loyalty, responsibility, and integrity. On the other hand, patients can and do suffer emotional and psychological harm when they feel betrayed, and those harms may well result in behavioral change, that is, voting with their feet.

Practitioner integrity was regarded as the foundational concept of research ethics by Henry K. Beecher, who, among others, believed that integrity served as a means of self-policing the profession, as well as a way to eliminate abuses until then unrecognized.[31] Practitioners' integrity has proved insufficient, however, to resolve the problems posed by physician self-referral, necessitating federal regulations and guidelines and the policing of ownership of laboratories and investments. Whether such extrinsic regulation will prove necessary to regulate post-marketing research remains to be seen.

ASSESSING THE NEED FOR INFORMED CONSENT

Informed consent for post-marketing research could include providing information about investigators' compensation and financial ties. Such disclosure could counteract the physician's natural tendency to steer eligible patients toward a medication that also rewards the physician, other things being equal. Disclosure might also foster a more trusting physician-patient relationship. Furthermore, if disclosure meets an objective test criterion for informed consent--whereby information given represents what reasonable patients would consider important--it could establish a uniform level of information given to all patients.

As indicated above, consent to research is not an ethical absolute. It can be, and is, omitted in certain contexts, for example, if the research poses minimal harm, or if the research is performed with members of a population (such as children) who cannot give consent themselves but must rely on the surrogate consent of others.

Since post-marketing research embraces these examples, why not omit informed consent altogether? After all, informed consent seems to work best for those of us who are fortunate enough to be schooled in ways to ask questions well, confident enough to ask them when we want to know more, and well-heeled enough to employ a lawyer to ask them if the well-heeled do not like the answers they hear. For many, perhaps most research subjects, informed consent is not likely to safeguard their interests.

Further, informed consent for post-marketing research would presumably focus on informing patients of investigators' financial ties. Although including financial information in dialogues about informed consent with research subjects has been considered, no nationally recognized precedent exists.[32] Such information has not been included in the policies and guidelines of professional associations or government agencies, or even in ethical codes or mandates. It is unknown whether information about physician-investigator remuneration would influence patients to enroll or decline enrollment in research. Empiric analyses of this question eluded a computer-based review of the medical ethics literature.[33]

To describe patients' and physicians' attitudes about informed consent and physician-investigator financial ties to a research sponsor, we performed the survey described previously. A majority of physician-respondents (64 percent) found it acceptable to be paid a fee by the drug company for each patient enrolled. A majority of patient-respondents (57 percent) did not find it acceptable, a statistically significant difference. Fewer physicians (75 percent) than patients (86 percent) believed a physician should inform a patient if the physician is paid for enrolling the patient. This difference between physicians and patients was also significant. Most physicians (67 percent) and patients (69 percent) thought physicians might enroll patients just to pocket the fee.[34]

These data indicate that patients want information about and have concerns about the remuneration of physicians when they consider taking part in a research study of a new drug.[35] Physicians and patients in our survey appeared to agree that financial ties to the research sponsor should be part of patients' informed consent to the research.

PHYSICIAN FEES FOR POST-MARKETING RESEARCH

How much compensation is too much? The AMA's Council on Ethical and Judicial Affairs decided that a $100 gift to physicians from industry was maximal--an arbitrary determination.[36] The Health Care Financing Administration recently proposed rules to curb physician managed care bonuses that create "substantial financial risk," limiting the amount of income at risk to 30 percent or less.[37] Many patients already believe that physicians as a group are overpaid, and that any more than nominal amounts is inappropriate.

Physicians and patients in our survey appeared to disagree over whether physician remuneration is acceptable in post-marketing research. It is little wonder that physicians want to be paid for their efforts. They perform a marketing service for the pharmaceutical company, which has made its way into the intimacy of the medical office, right next to the doctor's tongue blade and work station. The patient surely knows that the samples of new medication he or she will take home are just a spinoff of the physician's bargain. But why has the physician bargained with the company? To provide indigent patients with those samples? To see patients he or she might otherwise be unable to afford to see? Or to enhance the stock and consultancy positions he or she may hold with the pharmaceutical sponsor?

These are provocative questions of motive and intent, yet they beg the underlying question: Is any compensation appropriate for post-marketing research? The defensibility of compensation can, for example, be derived from lost opportunity: while physicians are completing forms and finding samples, they are not generating other revenue, and such research involves direct and indirect costs. Provided that the study is scientifically valid, remuneration for paperwork completed, time spent, and complexity of patient data gathered seems reasonable. Yet to reward work that does not meet scientific research standards--presently the easy majority of post-marketing research--is to endorse the moral position that marketing and promotion are responsibilities as professional as those of taking care of patients' medical needs.

All in all, physicians may find informing patients of their conflicts of interest both difficult and inadequate. Even if physicians disclose their conflicts of interest to patients, their conflicting loyalties will not be erased.[38]

FIVE IDEAS FOR RESOLVING
CONFLICTS OF INTEREST

Several ideas are suggested here to keep physicians from having personal financial interests in research that create conflicts of interest with patient care.

One idea calls for the creation of an intradepartmental or intra-institutional mechanism to collect pharmaceutical dollars awarded for research. The money would pay for the physician's and the institution's direct costs associated with the study, and the remainder would become part of a department-wide or institution-wide pool. Faculty from the department or institution could submit research proposals to be peer reviewed, and the fund could pay for the most meritorious proposals.[39]

A second idea would permit post-marketing research to continue in its second form, but would regulate the development of drugs. For each duplicative drug, a nonduplicative drug that meets an important clinical need is researched, developed, and marketed. This would require much greater oversight of the pharmaceutical industry than currently exists.

A third idea suggests examining the models of healthcare systems in other countries in which post-marketing surveillance systems are well developed. There is an international need to assess post-marketing research rigorously and systematically.[40] In Britain, for example, Phase IV trials are managed centrally by a research foundation funded by pharmaceutical sponsors. The data are public knowledge and open to public scrutiny, irrespective of the results and sponsorship.

A fourth idea proposes that industry itself forego physician rewards for post-marketing research. Industry may have incentives to do this, since it can then appeal more directly to consumers without paying doctors to be middlemen. As industry strives to align itself with healthcare reform, it can be clear, honest, and straightforward with its customers by telling them what they are paying for and why.

Finally, managed care may change the face of post-marketing research, as it has other parts of medicine. Industry might attempt to specialize, with some companies producing only, for example, oncologic and gastrointestinal drugs, and others concentrating on vascular and cardiac medications. Managed-care formulary groups will try not to stock duplicative drugs. Industry itself may shake out duplicative medications, and this will create the opportunity for pursuing the scientifically legitimate goals of post-marketing research.

OTHER ALTERNATIVES

Other possibilities exist, and while logical, may be less effective than those above. They include the following.

First, enforce IRB review. Although Phase IV research is research on approved drugs, FDA regulations require IRB reviews of all research.[41] Yet, most pre-marketing research is done in the outpatient setting, and few outpatient clinics, accountable health plans, or even multi-site, managed-care organizations have IRBs. Many physicians do not belong to an organization with an IRB. Although one IRB has reported requiring investigators to tell prospective subjects how much investigators are paid per patient, this policy is uncommon.[42] Post-marketing protocols are seldom submitted to IRBs, and IRBs are unlikely to see them in the future.

Second, create a supervisory intermediary body. Most scholars will argue that the last thing science needs is another intermediate body. Yet, the supervision of clinical research may be beneficial both scientifically, to regulate and improve the quality of the data produced from post-marketing research, and morally, to return the public trust.[43] Such an intermediary might be similar to the institutionally centered foundation alluded to earlier, created with pooled industry dollars.[44] The intermediary would be supported by both pharmaceutical sponsors and the interested federal agencies.

Third, abandon post-marketing research altogether. Much good has arisen from Phase IV research, yet it has grown out of control and become primarily a marketing venue and a series of safety trials rarely, if at all. Still, post-marketing research could be reengineered to capture the work that patients and industry need.

TOWARD SCIENTIFIC POST-MARKETING RESEARCH

What could transform post-marketing research into the comprehensive safety trials it might be--so that legitimate, scientifically rigorous efforts to detect and then clarify unsuspected beneficial effects and adverse reactions might be undertaken? Two modern forces could do this: healthcare reform with its emphasis on controlling costs, and managed care with its emphasis on efficiency.

The medical profession and industry would have a small window of opportunity at the very beginning of major healthcare reform. Already, financial incentives have emerged to change post-marketing research. These incentives are not related to physicians' remuneration for research, but to the rise of managed-care formulary groups. Changes in post-marketing research designed to improve its scientific defensibility and clinical utility may occur if the present goals, methods, and results of post-marketing research become public knowledge.

Making the transition to scientifically oriented post-marketing research may not be as hard as it might seem, since rigorous scientific criteria for post-marketing research, with their precedent in pre-marketing research, have already been proposed. Stephens suggests seven characteristics for scientifically sound post-marketing studies:

1. Retrospective collection of data and use of large databases;
2. A control group at least half as large as the study drug group;
3. A specific aim to the study with details regarding its statistical power;
4. Independent oversight by a clinician/epidemiologist, a pharmacologist, and a statistician;
5. At least one-year follow up for drugs of long-term usage;
6. Signed informed consent for all prospective studies; and
7. Rigorous protocol-drive follow up of dropouts and deaths.[45]

Adherence to these criteria would transform post-marketing research from promotional studies to promising scientific ones of real value to industry, patients, and physicians. If the quality and content of post-marketing research improved, it might attract academically trained investigators who are able to differentiate between marketing protocols and medical research protocols. Improved quality might also promote the study of nonduplicative drugs and encourage physicians to recognize and avoid self-interest in prescription and referral practices.[46]

CONCLUSION

In its 1994 Policy Summary Update, the Canadian Medical Association wrote, "A pre-requisite for physician participation in industry-sponsored research activities is evidence that these activities are ethically defensible, socially responsible, and scientifically valid."[47] At present, these burdens are not met by the vast majority of post-marketing research studies.

Ethically, dilemmas of informed consent and questions of conflicting loyalty confuse physicians. Socially, industry-sponsored post-marketing research unnecessarily increases the cost of all pharmaceuticals to patients, often promoting drugs that resemble other drugs, which are already available. Scientifically, post-marketing research protocols usually are designed not to test a null hypothesis. They usually lack control groups, do not undergo IRB review, and are designed to change physicians' prescribing habits--not with peer-reviewed scientific data, but with covert compensation.

Industry's moral duty is to make available a safe, effective product at a reasonable price for most patients. This duty is called into question by the very existence of current post-marketing research. Physicians should help industry make available post-marketing research methods and results to an enquiring public, eager to reduce its healthcare costs without rationing services. Industry and physicians together should work to detect even rare adverse drug reactions, to minimize financial conflicts of interest, and to maximize patient information about both. Post-marketing research represents an opportunity for industry to create a new moral space within its corporate culture and to resolve conflicts of interest for participating physicians.

NOTES

1. W.A. Ray, M.R. Griffin, and J. Avorn, "Evaluating Drugs after Their Approval for Clinical Use," *New England Journal of Medicine* 329 (1993): 2029-32.

2. G. Kolata, "Pharmacists Paid to Suggest Drugs: Some Doctors Dislike a Link with the Manufacturers," *New York Times,* 29 July 1994.

3. B.W. Richard, A. Melville, and L. Lasagna, "Postapproval Research as a Condition of Approval: An Update, 1985-1986," *Journal of Clinical Research and Drug Development* 3 (1989): 247-57.

4. J. La Puma and J. Kraut, "How Much Do You Get Paid if I Volunteer? Suggested Institutional Policy on Reward, Consent, and Research," *Hospital and Health Services Administration* 39 (1994): 193-203.

5. R.J. Levine, *Ethics and the Regulation of Clinical Research,* 2d ed. (Baltimore-Munich: Urban & Schwarzenberg, 1986).

6. G.A. Faich, H.A. Guess, and H.M. Kuritsky as reported in M.D.B. Stephens, "Marketing Aspects of Company-sponsored Postmarketing Surveillance Studies," *Drug Safety* 8 (1993): 1-8.

7. S. Nightingale, conversation with author, 4 January 1994. The FDA's regulations are given in 21 *CFR* 314.5000 and following.

8. Stephens, "Marketing Aspects."

9. M.M. Chren and C.S. Landefeld, "Physicians' Behavior and Their Interactions with Drug Companies: A Controlled Study of Physicians Who Requested Additions to a Hospital Drug Formulary," *Journal of the American Medical Association* 271 (1994): 684-89.

10. P.C. Waller *et al.,* "Review of Company Postmarketing Surveillance Studies," *British Medical Journal* 304 (1992): 1470-72.

11. R.C. Noble, "Physicians and the Pharmaceutical Industry: An Alliance with Unhealthy Aspects," *Perspectives in Biology and Medicine* 36 (1993): 376-94.

12. W.J. Rhoades *et al.,* "Should Disclosure of M.D. Renumeration Be Part of Informed Consent to Research on New Drugs?" (paper presented by Rhoades at the 16th Annual Meeting of the Society for General Internal Medicine, Washington, D.C., 29 April 1993).

13. J. La Puma, "Patient Enrollment in Seeding Studies: Questions of Ethics for Practicing Physicians," *American Journal of Public Health,* (in press).

14. M.M. Chren, "Independent Investigators and For-Profit Companies: Guidelines for Biomedical Scientists Considering Funding by Industry," *Archives of Dermatology* 130 (1994): 432-37.

15. Federation for Clinical Research, "Guidelines for Avoiding Conflict of Interest in Research," *Clinical Research* 38 (1990): 239.

16. R.J. Levine, "New International Ethical Guidelines for Research Involving Human Subjects," *Annals of Internal Medicine* 119 (1993): 340-41.

17. American Medical Association, Council on Scientific Affairs and Council on Ethical and Judicial Affairs, "Conflicts of Interest in Medical Center/Industry Research Relationships," *Journal of the American Medical Association* 263 (1990): 2790-93.

18. American Medical Association, Council on Ethical and Judicial Affairs, "Conflicts of Interest: Biomedical Research," in *1992 Code of Medical Ethics--Current Opinions* (Chicago: American Medical Association, 1992).

19. D.A. Kessler, "Drug Promotion and Scientific Exchange: The Role of the Clinical Investigator," *New England Journal of Medicine* 325 (1993): 201-3.

20. Joint Committee of the ABPI, BMA, CSM, RCGP, "Guidelines on Postmarketing Surveillance," *British Medical Journal* 296 (1988): 399-400.

21. S.M. Wolf, "Health Care Reform and the Future of Physician Ethics," *Hastings Center Report* 24 (March-April 1994): 28-41.

22. D.P. Sulmasy, "Physicians, Cost Control and Ethics," *Annals of Internal Medicine* 116 (1992): 920-26; M. Angell, "The Doctor as Double Agent," *Kennedy Institute of Ethics Journal* 3 (1993): 279-86.

23. J. La Puma, "Anticipated Changes in the Doctor-Patient Relationship in the Managed Care and Managed Competition of the Health Security Act of 1993," *Archives of Family Medicine* 3 (1994): 665-71.

24. P.T. Menzel, "Some Ethical Costs of Rationing," *Law, Medicine & Health Care* 20 (1992): 57-66.

25. 45 *Code of Federal Regulations (CFR)* 46 is in this book's Appendix D.

26. H.M. Spiro, "Mammon and Medicine: The Rewards of Clinical Trials," *Journal of the American Medical Association* 255 (1986): 1174-75.

27. G.J. Agich, "Human Experimentation and Clinical Consent," in *Medical Ethics*, ed. J.F. Monagle and D.C. Thomasma (Rockville, Md.: Aspen, 1988), 127-39.

28. M. Freuedenheim, "Caremark Is Indicted in Kickbacks--Genentech Executive Also Charged in Sales," *New York Times* 5 August 1994.

29. D.M. Gianelli, "Drug Makers Warned: Some Promotions Are Kickbacks," *American Medical News* 5 September 1994, 10-11.

30. D.S. Shimm and R.G. Spece, "Industry Reimbursement for Entering Patients into Clinical Trials: Legal and Ethical Issues," *Annals of Internal Medicine* 115 (1991): 148-51.

31. H.K. Beecher, "Ethics and Clinical Research," *New England Journal of Medicine* 274 (1966): 1354-60.

32. M.S. Jellinek, "IRBs and Pharmaceutical Company Funding of Research," *IRB: A Review of Human Subjects Research* 4 (October 1982): 9; S. Lind, "Finders' Fees for Research Subjects," *New England Journal of Medicine* 323 (1990): 192-95; M. Rodwin, "Physicians' Conflicts of Interest: The Limitations of Disclosure," *New England Journal of Medicine* 321 (1989): 1405-9.

33. P.A. Singer, S. Miles, and M. Siegler, "Computer Searches of the Medical Ethics Literature," *The Journal of Clinical Ethics* 1 (Spring 1990): 195-98.

34. J. La Puma and W.J. Rhoades, "Should Physician Remuneration Be Part of Informed Consent to Postmarketing Clinical Trials?" (paper presented by Rhoades in abstract form at the Sixth Annual National Meeting of the Society for Medical Decision Making, Triangle Park, N.C.: October 1993).

35. J. La Puma *et al.*, "Should Disclosure of Physician Remuneration Be Part of Informed Consent to Research?" *Clinical Research* 41 (1993): 578A.

36. K.B. Johnson and D. Orentlicher, "Guidelines on Gifts to Physicians from Industry: An Update," *Food and Drug Law Journal* 47 (1992): 445-58.

37. *Federal Register*, 14 December 1992.

38. M.A. Rodwin, *Medicine, Money and Morals* (New York: Oxford University Press, 1993).

39. La Puma and Kraut, "How Much Do I Get Paid if I Volunteer?"

40. A.J. Gordon and R.J. Petrick, "Worldwide Regulations for Manufacturers on Clinical Safety Surveillance of Drugs," *Drug Information Journal* 26 (1992): 1-15.

41. FDA Rules and Regulations, *Federal Register* 46, 27 January 1981; *CFR* 56: 101-5.

42. R. Roizen, "Why I Oppose Drug Company Payment of Physician/Investigators on a Per Patient/Subject Basis," *IRB: A Review of Human Subjects Research* 10 (January/February 1988): 9-10.

43. Chren, "Independent Investigators and For-Profit Companies."

44. J.P. Kassirer and M. Angell, "The Journal's Policy on Cost-Effectiveness Research," *New England Journal of Medicine* 331 (1994): 669-70.

45. Stephens, "Marketing Aspects."

46. L.S. Milner, "Ethical Considerations in Clinical Cancer Research: The Need for Disclosure of Financial Compensation," *Journal of Oncology Management* 2 (1993): 36-41.

47. Canadian Medical Association Policy Summary, "Physicians and the Pharmaceutical Industry (Update 1994)," *Canadian Medical Association Journal* 150 (1994): 256a-256c.

PART III

Controversy Over
Cross-Cultural Research

Introduction to Part III

Harold Y. Vanderpool

The chapters in this section debate a highly controversial issue: whether the basic ethical principles of research articulated in the West ought to be required of clinical research jointly conducted by developed and developing nations. After the sides of this debate are described, its implications will be identified and related to current trends and future directions.

Does requiring non-Western nations to abide by, for example, *The Belmont Report's* accent on autonomy constitute "medical ethics imperialism," whereby a Western and possibly disruptive ethical standard is forced upon certain cultures? This view is maintained by Robert J. Levine in this section's Chapter 10 and Nicholas A. Christakis in Chapter 11, both of whom oppose requiring all research subjects in non-Western cultures to be treated as autonomous individuals.

Or does the requirement of individual or first-person informed consent display justifiable esteem for persons in all cultures and preserve a core of human rights that should be honored universally?[1] This perspective is maintained by Carel B. IJsselmuiden and Ruth R. Faden in Chapter 12.

The implications of this debate are far-reaching. It challenges us to reexamine the philosophical underpinnings and ethical principles of contemporary Western research ethics and to grapple with the following concerns: How should the ethics of international biomedical research--in particular, jointly conducted research between Western sponsors and non-Western host nations--be formulated?[2] How should clinical research be conducted with subcultural enclaves within nations with diverse cultural traditions?[3] To what extent should existing U.S. federal regulations--as overseen, for example, by the National Institutes of Health's (NIH's) Office for Protection from Research Risks (OPRR)--be revised and/or further spelled out?

CURRENT U.S. REGULATIONS AND POLICIES

To begin with the last of these questions, the U.S. federal regulations of 1991 specify that its policies are required for "research conducted, supported, or otherwise subject to regulation by the Federal Government outside the United States."[4] The OPRR's latest (1993) guidebook defines the purview of this requirement as follows: "The Regulations for the protection of human participants in research apply to all research involving human participants that is conducted or supported, in whole or in part, by DHHS [the U.S. Department of Health and Human Services] in foreign or domestic settings. Note that *any* support provided by DHHS . . . may trigger applicability of the regulations."[5]

This guidebook further specifies that it is unacceptable for foreign sites to regulate their research solely according to the principles within the *Declaration of Helsinki* or some other international code. Instead, all sites must rely on "protections that are at least equivalent to those afforded by DHHS regulations" in 45 *Code of Federal Regulations (CFR)* 46.[6] The guidebook adds that, "international guidelines, such as the Declarations of Helsinki . . . are a good place to start, but do not describe the specific procedures through which those principles are to be realized."[7] The "specific procedures" in question involve, for example, incorporating the several elements of informed consent both on consent forms and in the procedures used to secure the consent of human subjects.

These points indicate that the OPRR has been requiring virtually "chapter and verse" compliance with the U.S. federal regulations before it approves partially or fully funded DHHS research abroad.[8] For about two years, however, the OPRR has begun to negotiate somewhat more flexible assurance of compliance agreements with certain foreign and domestic (such as American Indian) sites. This includes the OPRR's now allowing research-conducting institutions to use "the Belmont Report, the Declarations of Helsinki, or another appropriate code . . . or statement of principles" as its basic ethical guideline, and, for example, allowing institutions to paraphrase federal consent requirements in ways that closely approximate those that are specified in 45 *CFR* 46.116.[9]

Although OPRR's recent flexibility and openness do not require foreign sites to fulfill the letter of U.S. federal law, this flexibility is exercised as if the principles of Western research ethics are universally valid and required of DHHS-sponsored cross-cultural research. OPRR's requirement of "protections that are *at least equivalent* to those afforded by DHHS regulations" is apparently narrowly construed as virtually synonymous with existing U.S. research ethics and regulations.[10] In comparison, the authors in this section are debating a far more revisionist agenda--the use of guidelines and ethical principles that are *morally* equivalent, but at points *fundamentally different* from those presently operative in the West.

INTERNATIONAL CODES AND GUIDELINES

International codes and guidelines for the ethics of research with human subjects include the *Nuremberg Code,* the *Declaration of Helsinki,* and the Council for International Organizations of Medical Sciences (CIOMS)/World Health Organization's (WHO) *International Ethical Guidelines for Biomedical Research Involving Human Subjects.*[11] The 1993 *CIOMS/WHO Guidelines* were "designed to be of use, particularly to developing countries, in defining national policies on the ethics of biomedical research, applying ethical standards in local circumstances, and establishing or redefining adequate mechanisms for ethical review of research involving human subjects."[12]

Notably, CIOMS's commentary on the general ethical principles underlying its guidelines lists and summarizes the same principles contained in *The Belmont Report*: respect for persons (including respect for autonomy), beneficence, and justice.[13] The *CIOMS/WHO Guidelines* 1 through 3 also stipulate elements of informed consent that closely parallel the basic elements of informed consent in the U.S. federal regulations.[14]

Even in guideline 8, which deals with research involving subjects in underdeveloped communities, the *CIOMS/WHO Guidelines* hold that "every effort will be made to secure *the ethical imperative* that the consent of individual subjects be informed" (emphasis added). *CIOMS's* commentary on this guideline holds that, "All reasonable efforts should be made to obtain the informed consent of each prospective subject . . . to ensure that the rights of prospective subjects are respected." This includes clearly telling each subject "everything that would be conveyed if the study were to be conducted in a developed community." The service of "a reliable intermediary such as a trusted community leader" is mentioned as a useful means to ensure that prospective subjects have been adequately informed and have given their consent, not as a substitute or proxy for such consent.[15]

These points show that *CIOMS/WHO Guidelines* rest upon and appeal to the ethical principles that are outlined in *The Belmont Report* and that underlie the U.S. federal guidelines. These guidelines and principles are to be respected and upheld along with respect for each "community's customs and traditions"[16] and along with the review and approval of the research in question by "a national or local ethical review committee or its equivalent" in the host nation.[17]

Enter the debates in this section. IJsselmuiden and Faden argue that the just-sketched principles and guidelines on informed consent ought to be universally honored.[18] In contrast, Levine views the accent on informed consent in these guidelines as "excessively influenced by the legacy of *Nuremberg*."[19] Similar to Levine, Christakis doubts that individual informed consent is an ethical or cultural universal. And he argues that if cross-cultural or multinational negotiations of ethical differences can arrive at a consensus, deviations for international standards (presumably those also set forth by *CIOMS/WHO*) can be set aside.[20]

RESEARCH ETHICS: PLURAL, RELATIVE, OR UNIVERSAL PRINCIPLES?

The differing positions of the authors in this section are predicated upon divergent views of ethics and ethical reasoning. Levine holds to a modified version of casuistry, in that he accents flexible and practical moral reasoning within particular situations, yet believes that universal or transcending moral rules are discoverable.[21] Critiquing the *Nuremberg Code* and the *Declaration of Helsinki*, as time-limited and ethically flawed, Levine reproves *Nuremberg* and *Helsinki* fundamentalists, who appeal to these texts as if they are infallible scripture. He favors the CIOMS/ WHO guidelines over the *Nuremberg Code* and the *Declaration of Helsinki*, in part because the *CIOMS/WHO Guidelines* rest upon "transcending moral rules" that can be shorn of Western bias.[22] Levine explains why he credits the *Nuremberg, Helsinki,* and *CIOMS/WHO* documents with an ascending order of validity and why even the *CIOMS/WHO Guidelines* need to be further clarified and changed.

Skeptical that universal or transcending ethical principles exist, Christakis advocates ethical pluralism, which he views as steering between "the autocracy of universalism and the anarchy of relativism."[23] Christakis argues that the ethical universalism that underlies international codes and guidelines of research ethics is problematic for several reasons: it conflates technological superiority with moral superiority, displays disrespect for understandings of personhood in most regions of the world, and so on. Ethical relativism is equally problematic, but for different reasons, including its inability to censure reprehensible practices or to provide guidance when ethical conflicts occur. Christakis indicates how his notion of ethical pluralism both respects the varying ethical norms of respective cultures and fosters negotiated compromises over moral differences. He believes that these compromises can be reached via the types of *procedural* guidelines he charts--in contrast to the compromise-negating, *content-based* ethical standards of present international codes.

IJsselmuiden and Faden believe that certain ethical principles, obligations, and commitments should be regarded as absolute or universal. And they argue, in particular, that first-person informed consent should be adhered to in cross-cultural research. Parallel to the wording of and commentary on the *CIOMS/WHO Guidelines*, they propose that Western elements of informed consent can and should be sensitively translated into the language, symbolism, and mores of non-Western cultures.[24] They oppose ethical pluralism's position that cultures should be regarded as morally different, but equal. This, they argue, can foster sexual abuse, exploitation by Western researchers, and "a system of ethical apartheid."[25] In contrast to Christakis, they view first-person informed consent as supportive of the worth and value of persons and as symbiotic with "a total strategy for human development" that includes the life-enhancing goals of medicine.

ETHICAL PERSPECTIVES

Like other areas within medical ethics, the topics and approaches in this section bristle with theoretical and practical ethical issues, only a few of which will be identified here for purposes of clarification and challenge. These issues can engage moral philosophers as well as medical ethicists, clinical researchers, and IRB members.

For the sake of clarity and understanding, what is the meaning of ethical relativism or ethical pluralism? All, or at least nearly all, ethicists agree that moral decisions are relative to their historic, social, and cultural circumstances, and that it is not possible to uphold moral rules or principles (such as not lying or not harming) without exception.[26] Consider, for example, how informed consent was regarded in the United States[27] and is still regarded in certain Western settings[28] as either rightfully overruled or highly delimited in clinical research when consent required/requires the revealing of a dire, psychologically harmful diagnosis of cancer. In such cases, ethical principles that are considered universally valid are counterbalanced with other, equally weighty *prima facie* principles.[29] Historical and contextual relativism in this sense should not be regarded as a form of *ethical* relativism. Definitions of ethical relativism include these two viewpoints: First, that *the basic moral principles* of individuals and cultures are different and conflicting; and, second, that no rationally convincing *methods* are discoverable that can show why one cluster of moral principles is preferable to another.[30] Christakis's ethical pluralist position rests on the first of these perspectives, denies that it leads to skepticism about ethics, and holds that it is amenable to negotiated solutions over ethical differences and conflicts. Christakis's commitment to negotiated solutions represents a partial rejection of the second, just-listed definition of relativism, in that he believes that rational methods can give rise to ethically agreeable outcomes.

Christakis's ethical pluralism bears similarities with the ethical relativism advanced by David Wong, who regards some of the moral duties of respective cultures as fundamentally different from others. Wong nevertheless affirms that "the argument from diversity" (the existence of deep and wide disagreements between the moral beliefs and behaviors of cultures) "does not support relativism in any simple or direct way."[31] Wong then summarizes how his form of ethical relativism can both censure some moralities (for example, those of fascist societies) and recognize the validity of only "adequate moralities" that "must promote the production of persons capable of considering the interests of others."[32]

Those who favor some version of ethical universalism or absolutism--that universally valid and applicable ethical principles are discoverable--may well ask whether Christakis's and Wong's positions logically rest on certain universally shared moral norms.[33] Christakis's ethical pluralism opposes moral abuses--including the abuse of minors and minorities; requires norms of equality in moral negotiations and the conduct of research; and forbids exploitative research that offers no benefit to host cultures. Wong's ethical relativism opposes moralities that aggravate interpersonal conflict, and he approves of only those moralities that promote the nurturing and care of persons capable of considering the needs of others.[34] In spite of the controversy, these positions appear to point toward underlying agreements between the authors in this section: that universal or transcending moral principles should serve as moral prerequisites for conducting cross-cultural biomedical research involving human subjects.

NOTES

1. M. Angell, "Ethical Imperialism? Ethics in International Collaborative Clinical Research," *New England Journal of Medicine* 319 (1988): 1081-83.

2. The most notable international initiative in this regard is that of the CIOMS in collaboration with the WHO. The final text (defined as

its preamble and 15 guidelines) of the CIOMS/WHO principles is included as Appendix F in this book. Text and commentary are available in the booklet, CIOMS, *International Ethical Guidelines for Biomedical Research Involving Human Subjects* (Geneva: CIOMS, 1993).

3. Consider, for example, the way the "three ethical principles" of *The Belmont Report* (this book's Appendix C) are being adjusted by the U.S. Indian Health Service for research with American Indian, Alaskan Native, and Canadian First Nations communities. A working group at the November 1994 Public Responsibility in Medicine and Research meetings in Boston was presented with documents containing these adjustments by William L. Freeman, Director of Research Programs in the Indian Health Service, Albuquerque, N.M.

4. 45 *Code of Federal Regulations (CFR)* 46.101.b. These regulations are given in full in Appendix D.

5. OPRR, *Protecting Human Research Subjects: Institutional Review Board Guidebook* (Washington, D.C.: U.S. Government Printing Office, 1993), 2-6.

6. 45 *CFR* 46.101.b.

7. OPRR, *Protecting Human Research Subjects*, 2-8.

8. These approvals are predicated upon the OPRR's making an Assurance of Compliance agreement with each foreign site--usually a "single-project" assurance agreement. These assurances are discussed in Chapter 1, note 48.

9. These points and quotations are taken from OPRR's "International Human Subjects Assurance" forms and directions. I thank Dr. Melody H. Lin, Director, Division of Human Subject Protections, OPRR, for her comments and assistance on interpreting these documents and describing OPRR's recent approaches.

10. This is normal and expected for the OPRR, the mandate of which is to see that existing federal guidelines are followed. Nevertheless, the meaning and practical import of the OPRR's "at least equivalent" rule of thumb deserve critical scrutiny. If a foreign site's elements of informed consent must be *at least equivalent* to those outlined in 45 *CFR* 46.116, can any one of these outlined elements be omitted without adding one or more equally "weighty" elements that are not listed? But, if the term "equivalent" is interpreted as "more or less equal," what elements can be disregarded? Perhaps more importantly, does an ethical equivalence standard permit a "greater honoring" of one ethical principle (e.g., a higher benefit-harm probability or an unusual degree of justice) to replace or largely discount another (e.g., consent)?

11. These codes and guidelines are provided in this book's Appendices A, B, and F. Although these three sets of codes and guidelines are

the most notable and influential international codifications, others have been developed and utilized. A brief discussion of other international formulations is found in CIOMS, *International Ethical Guidelines for Biomedical Research Involving Human Subjects*, 5-7. See also the Bibliography on International Research Ethics and Guidelines compiled by the OPRR, *Protecting Human Research Subjects*, 6-71 through 6-74.

12. CIOMS, *International Ethical Guidelines*, 7.

13. *Ibid.*, 10-11.

14. The *CIOMS/WHO Guidelines* explicitly require the "elements" of consent found in 45 *CFR* 46.116.(a).(1) through (6) and (8), and even more explicitly outline aspects of communication and understanding that need to be fulfilled. These guidelines further add the requirement "that therapy will be provided free of charge for specified types of research-related injury." Although the *CIOMS/WHO Guidelines* do address the "additional elements of informed consent" in *CFR* 46.116.(b), they do not mention that consent can be altered or waived under the circumstances specified in *CFR* 46.116.(d).

15. CIOMS, *International Ethical Guidelines*, 27. Note that Robert J. Levine interprets *CIOMS/WHO's Guidelines* 8 and 15 more broadly, that is, as allowing for "certain behaviors that are ethically acceptable in one cultural context," but which "may be unacceptable in another." For Levine, this includes the possibility of not uniformly requiring informed individual or proxy consent in some cultural contexts. See Levine, Chapter 10, pp. 239, 243 of this book. Levine nevertheless recognizes that, as stated, the *CIOMS/WHO Guidelines* on informed consent closely conform to Western standards, and that, as such, they need to be revised.

16. CIOMS, *International Ethical Guidelines*, 27.

17. Guideline 15 of the *CIOMS/WHO International Ethical Guidelines*.

18. In a previous publication, IJsselmuiden and Faden criticized the proposed *CIOMS/WHO Guidelines* as "not helpful," because they are "sufficiently vague to allow for virtually any method of obtaining consent." They have not specified how the *CIOMS/WHO Guidelines* should be altered. C.B. IJsselmuiden and R. Faden, "Research and Informed Consent in Africa--Another Look," *New England Journal of Medicine* 326 (1992): 830-34, especially 830.

19. Robert J. Levine, Chapter 10, p. 255 of this book.

20. Christakis, in Chapter 11 of this book. See also N.A. Christakis and R.J. Levine, "Multinational Research" *The Encyclopedia of Bioethics*, revised ed. (New York: Simon & Schuster Macmillan, 1995), 1780-87.

21. Casuistry is discussed in Chapter 1, note 16 of this book, and is explicated by Jonsen in Chapter 3 of this book.

22. The quote is from CIOMS, *International Ethical Guidelines,* p. 26. Robert J. Levine discusses why these transcending rules need to be further explored and explicated.

23. Christakis, Chapter 11, p. 276 of this book.

24. See guideline 15 and the CIOMS commentary in *International Ethical Guidelines,* 27.

25. IJsselmuiden and Faden, Chapter 12, pp. 289, 291 of this book.

26. See the discussion of Arthur J. Dyck, *On Human Care* (Nashville: Abingdon, 1977), 116-19.

27. In keeping with the broadly shared belief and practice that cancer patients should be benevolently shielded from knowing their diagnosis (because of fears over the severe reactions that patients or patient-subjects would undergo), the American Medical Association's 1966 "Ethical Guidelines for Clinical Investigation" held that "In exceptional circumstances and to the extent that disclosure of information concerning the nature of the drug or experimental procedure or risks would be expected to materially affect the health of the patient and would be detrimental to his best interest, such information [respecting voluntary consent] may be withheld from the patient. In such circumstances such information shall be disclosed to a responsible relative or friend of the patient where possible." American Medical Association, "Ethical Guidelines for Clinical Investigation" (1966), reprinted in the *Encyclopedia of Bioethics,* ed. W.T. Reich (New York: Free Press, 1978), 1773-74, quotation from 1774. The beliefs and practices of the time were surveyed and analyzed by D. Oken, "What to Tell Cancer Patients," *Journal of the American Medical Association* 175 (1961), 1120-28.

28. See, for example, M. Baum *et al.,* "Ethics of Clinical Research: Lessons for the Future," *British Medical Journal* 299 (1989): 251-53. This article concludes that review committees can decide when "the principle of non-maleficence should override that of autonomy" in particular clinical trials and that "all patients should retain the option to abrogate their responsibility and right to autonomy," 253.

29. See the discussions in Chapter 1, note 15, and by Veatch, Chapter 2, pp. 51-54 of this book.

30. Dyck, *On Human Care,* 121-34.

31. D. Wong, "Relativism," in *A Companion to Ethics,* ed. Peter Singer (Oxford: Basil Blackwell, 1991), 442-49, quotation at 444. Wong asserts that to substantiate ethical relativism, the argument from diversity predicated on anthropological studies would also have to prove that "objectively correct or incorrect [moral] judgments" do not underlie this diversity. He thus comments that, "Moral relativists must chart some other more complicated path from the existence of diversity to the

conclusion that there is no single true or more justified morality" (445). In their analysis of ethics and cultural diversity, some contemporary non-relativists distinguish between customary morality (the local customs and attitudes identified by cultural anthropologists), common morality (ordinarily shared moral principles that transcend customary morality, but are not yet related to rational theories), and coherent models or theories of moral justification. See, e.g., T.L. Beauchamp and J.F. Childress, *Principles of Biomedical Ethics*, 4th ed. (New York: Oxford University, 1994), 5-6, 44-7, 100-11; and Dale Jamieson, "Method and Moral Theory," in *A Companion to Ethics*, 476-87.

32. Wong, "Relativism," 446-47.

33. Although the terms universalism and absolutism are often used interchangeably, the term universalism is preferable in that it does not connote that some moral principles or duties must be absolutely observed without exception. See note 29 above and the discussion to which it refers, and the discussion of Beauchamp and Childress, *Principles of Biomedical Ethics*, 32-37.

34. Wong, "Relativism," 446.

10

International Codes and Guidelines for Research Ethics: A Critical Appraisal

Robert J. Levine

This chapter is concerned with international codes and guidelines that offer guidance for the ethical conduct of research involving human subjects.[1] The major documents to be considered are the *Nuremberg Code*, the World Medical Association's (WMA) *Declaration of Helsinki*, 1964 and 1975, and *The International Ethical Guidelines for Biomedical Research Involving Human Subjects* developed by the Council for International Organizations of Medical Sciences (CIOMS) in collaboration with the World Health Organization (WHO); these will be referred to respectively as *Nuremberg*, *Helsinki*, and *CIOMS Guidelines*.

There is a continuing controversy as to which, if any, of these three documents should be considered most authoritative in cases of inconsistencies. This paper will not refer further to this controversy. At this point I shall simply state my perspective on this issue; evidence to support this perspective will be presented subsequently. I believe these international documents should be considered a progression with each succeeding document superseding its precursors. Those who wrote *Helsinki* and *CIOMS Guidelines* were aware of the work of their predecessors. To a considerable extent they found their predecessors' work very useful and drew heavily on their accomplishments. But also, they each found the work of their predecessors imperfect or incomplete and were motivated to a large extent to correct the imperfections or supply the deficiencies they detected.

The authors of *Helsinki* were concerned with the fact that *Nuremberg* did not provide adequate guidance for most of the research activities carried out by medical doctors using humans as research subjects. Thus, they found it necessary to add provisions for authorization by proxy consent of the use of children and others lacking the capacity to consent for themselves. It was also necessary to provide guidance for the conduct of research in which risk could be justified by expected therapeutic benefit to the individual subject and not solely "by the humanitarian importance of the problem to be solved by the experiment" (*Nuremberg*, principle 6 in this book's Appendix A).

The *CIOMS Guidelines* explicitly acknowledge the influence of *Nuremberg* and *Helsinki*. Indeed, *CIOMS* quite modestly states that its guidelines are designed to provide guidance for the correct application of the principles of *Helsinki*, particularly when research is initiated by researchers and sponsors in technologically developed countries and carried out in developing countries. However, as we shall see, the *CIOMS Guidelines* clearly depart from *Helsinki's* requirements in several substantial respects. Justification of these departures are offered at several points. For example, "the Declaration [of Helsinki] does not provide for controlled clinical trials. Rather, it assures the freedom of the physician 'to use a new diagnostic or therapeutic measure, if in his or her judgment it offers hope of saving life, reestablishing health or alleviating suffering.' "[2]

In this chapter, I shall examine the continuing controversy between adherents to the position of ethical universalism and those committed to the position of cultural pluralism. As we shall see, the authors of *Nuremberg* and *Helsinki* each believed that their documents were universally applicable. Each asserted principles that they intended and earnestly believed to be universal. I shall present evidence to refute these claims of universal validity. I shall argue that the *CIOMS Guidelines* are more successful than their predecessors in reaching global applicability.[3] Their success may be attributed to two of their accomplishments: First, unlike *Nuremberg* and *Helsinki*, they recognize the legitimacy of a limited degree of cultural pluralism. Second, the *CIOMS Guidelines* avoid *Nuremberg's* errors of omission and *Helsinki's* logical imperfections. The chapter concludes with recommendations for future efforts to improve international guidelines for the ethical conduct of research involving human subjects.

ETHICAL UNIVERSALISM OR PLURALISM?

In the course of the recent international dialogue on healthcare, ethics, and human rights it has become increasingly clear that some participants in the dialogue are firmly committed to ethical universalism and some others to ethical pluralism.[4] Ethical universalists believe there is a universal set of ethical principles that are applicable to all human beings regardless of their situations in particular cultures. The task of the moral philosopher, then, is to discover those universal principles that apply in all times and in all places. Ethical pluralists, by contrast, recognize that all ethical principles are developed in the course of discussions held within particular cultures and that these discussions necessarily reflect the unique histories and other circumstances of particular cultures. On this view, ethical principles are invented rather than discovered. Pluralists further acknowledge the inevitability and recognize the legitimacy of variation across cultures of ethical norms and principles. In recent years, participants in the debate have engaged in name-calling with pluralists labeling universalists "ethical imperialists," and universalists branding pluralists "cultural relativists."

CLAIMS OF UNIVERSALITY IN THE INTERNATIONAL DOCUMENTS

Michael Grodin concludes his important article on the historical origins of *Nuremberg* by calling it "an attempt to provide a natural law based on a universal set of ethical principles."[5] That this vision was shared by *Nuremberg's* authors is indicated by the judges' statement in its preface: "*All* agree, however, that certain basic principles must be observed in order to satisfy moral, ethical and legal concepts" (emphasis added). Immediately following this sentence are the 10 principles of the code. Another statement by the judges, which follows the principles, further reflects their belief in the universality of the principles:

Obviously all of these experiments ... were performed in complete disregard of international conventions, the laws and customs of war, the general principles of criminal law as derived from the criminal laws of all civilized nations. . . . Manifestly, human experiments under such conditions are contrary to 'the principles of the law of nations as they result from the usages established among civilized peoples, from the laws of humanity, and from the dictates of public conscience.'[6]

This statement grounds the argument advanced by some commentators that the authors of *Nuremberg* considered it a natural law document.[7]

Helsinki asserts its claim to universality in its introduction by reference to two other documents: "The Declaration of Geneva of the World Medical Association *binds the physician* with the words, 'The health of my patient will be my first consideration,' and the International Code of Medical Ethics declares that, 'A physician shall act only in the patient's interest when providing medical care which might have the effect of weakening the physical and mental condition of the patient' " (emphasis added; see Appendix B of this book for the *Helsinki Code*). Later in the introduction, *Helsinki* refers to its "recommendations as a guide to *every physician* in biomedical research involving human subjects" (emphasis added).

In the *CIOMS Guidelines*, immediately preceding the preamble, there is a passage entitled "General Ethical Principles." These are the familiar "basic ethical principles" first introduced into a public policy context in the United States in 1978 by the National Commission for the Protection of Human Subjects of Biomedical and Behavioral Research: respect for persons, beneficence, and justice. At no point in the guidelines is there any further reference to these principles.

Because *CIOMS Guidelines* are particularly concerned with research carried out by investigators from developed countries involving as subjects residents of developing communities, its authors were obliged to come to terms with cross-cultural variations in ethics. Like *Nuremberg* and *Helsinki*, the *CIOMS Guidelines* also aspire to worldwide applicability. However, unlike *Nuremberg* and *Helsinki*, they do not assert the universal validity of a set of rules that either prescribe or proscribe specific behaviors. Rather, they recognize the legitimacy of a limited amount of ethical pluralism. According to the commentary under guideline 8: "Investigators must respect the ethical standards of their own countries and the cultural expectations of the societies in which the research is undertaken, *unless this implies a violation of a transcending moral rule*" (emphasis added).

The *CIOMS Guidelines*, unlike *Nuremberg* and *Helsinki*, recognize that certain behaviors that are ethically acceptable in one cultural context may be unacceptable in another. They recommend procedures that may be followed to reach agreements about what types of behavior would be considered ethically acceptable in cases in which the norms of the investigators' culture differ from those of the host country. In the commentary on guideline 15, CIOMS states that: "[E]thical review in the external sponsoring country may be limited to ensuring compliance *with broadly stated ethical standards,* on the understanding that ethical committees in the host country will have greater competence in reviewing the detailed plans for compliance in view of their better understanding of the cultural and moral values of the population in which the research is proposed to be conducted" (emphasis added).

Reasons for this recommendation are elaborated further in the commentary under guideline 8:

> The *ability to judge* the ethical acceptability of various aspects of a research proposal requires a *thorough understanding of a community's customs and traditions.* The ethical review committee must have as either members or consultants persons with such understanding, so that the committee may evaluate proposed means of obtaining informed consent and otherwise respecting the rights of prospective subjects. Such persons should be able, for example, to identify appropriate members of the community to serve as intermediaries between investigators and subjects, to decide whether material benefits or inducements may be regarded as appropriate in the light of a community's gift-exchange traditions, and to provide safeguards for data and personal information that subjects consider to be private or sensitive (emphasis added).

ARE THE INTERNATIONAL DOCUMENTS GLOBALLY OR UNIVERSALLY APPLICABLE?

Nuremberg is clearly an American creation. As stated by Telford Taylor in the opening statement of the prosecution on 9 December 1946: "The charges against these defendants are brought in the name of the United States of America. They are being tried by a court of American judges."[8] In drafting the *Nuremberg Code,* the judges relied heavily on the testimony and advice of two American physicians who were also experienced researchers, Andrew Ivy and Leo Alexander. Indeed, major portions of the final document were drafted by these two consultants.[9]

In passing, it is worth noticing that in the United States, in recent years, any policy-making body comprised exclusively of white, upper middle-class men would be regarded as highly suspect, even if its mandate were limited to determining real estate zoning rules. In the late 1940s, by contrast, such homogeneously male and white groups commonly issued pronouncements on what could be considered proper behavior for all "civilized people." This is not to say that *Nuremberg* is necessarily incorrect in any respect merely because only white American men participated in its conception. One wonders, however, just whom might they have considered "uncivilized."

Doctors Ivy and Alexander relied on resources that they believed elaborated universally applicable ethical principles. These included the Oath of Hippocrates, which they quoted incorrectly in at least two respects: First, they said it was the source of the dictum commonly regarded as the first principle of medical ethics, *primum non nocere* (first, or above all, do no harm). The closest approximation of such a statement in the Hippocratic writings is found in *Epidemics*: "As to diseases, make a habit of two things--to help, or at least to do no harm."[10] Second, they strongly implied that the oath of Hippocrates covered the ethics of research involving human subjects, although research is not mentioned either in the oath or anywhere else in the Hippocratic corpus. Other authorities on whom they relied either implicitly or explicitly were all writers situated in the tradition of Western civilization including Thomas Percival (British), William Beaumont (American), Claude Bernard (French), and several pre-World War II German writers.[11] Alexander also cited several American reviews and court decisions as important grounds for his ethical perspectives.[12]

An even more serious problem was that the consultants, particularly Ivy, attempted to convince the judges that the principles they were recommending--and that became the *Nuremberg Code*--were already employed to guide the conduct of research involving human subjects in the United States and elsewhere in the "civilized world." This is clearly an error. With the possible exception of Andrew Ivy himself, I am aware of no investigator (myself included) who was actively involved in research involving human subjects in the years before 1964 who recalls any attempts to secure voluntary or informed consent according to *Nuremberg's* standards.[13] Normal volunteers were usually advised that they were being asked to participate in research, and there was usually a presentation of the major risks and in some cases, particularly for the more intelligent or curious, the intended benefits. Patients, however, were rarely advised if and when some additional procedures that were not clinically indicated were performed to serve the goals of research, even when these presented non-trivial risks.

According to Grodin, Ivy attempted to mislead the tribunal by giving false testimony about the ethical standards that were in place in the United States at the time the Nazi experiments were performed:

> It appears that Dr. Ivy studied the tribunal prosecution's pretrial records and exhibits and then reported his views on the ethics of human experimentation to the American Medical Association's trustees, who *subsequently* incorporated his guidelines into the *Journal of the American Medical Association*. . . . In cross examination, the defense readily discovered the lack of . . . published substantive standards on human experimentation in the United States . . . prior to 1946. [emphasis added][14]

This point notwithstanding, the standards to which Ivy referred were, with some alterations, incorporated into the *Nuremberg Code*.

At this point it should be clear that *Nuremberg* is not an accurate account of standards that can be accepted as universal regardless of the intentions of its authors. Let us now consider *Helsinki*. Sharon Perley and her colleagues have published a comprehensive overview of the influence of the *Nuremberg Code* on subsequent development of international and national guidelines for the conduct of research involving human subjects.[15] They provide convincing evidence that *Nuremberg*, though nowhere mentioned in the *Declaration of Helsinki* or any of its early drafts, "greatly influenced" the development of the declaration. "Although nowhere documented, this . . . conclusion has been

reached by almost all commentators [on] medical research ethics."[16]

In 1953, the World Medical Association's Committee on
Medical Ethics began its discussion of the problems presented by
medical research. At that time, it recognized

a need for *professional* guidelines designed *by physicians for physicians* (as
opposed to the *Nuremberg Code*, which was formed by jurists for use in
a legal trial). Moreover, it was recognized that experiments must be
classified into two groups: "experiments in new diagnostic and therapeutic methods" and *"experiments undertaken to serve other purposes than
simply to cure an individual."*[emphasis added][17]

As will become clear shortly, it is the second of these two
recognitions that led to the development of a major flaw in
Helsinki, an error in logic that undermines its validity in any time
or place. Therefore, there is little need to examine in detail its
claim to universality. It is, however, worth considering briefly
some similarities and differences between *Nuremberg* and *Helsinki*.

Perhaps because the writing of *Helsinki* was "greatly influenced" by *Nuremberg*, it continues to require consent for the
authorization of research involving each and every individual
subject; in this way it continues the American perspective.[18]
While *Nuremberg* referred to "voluntary consent," with "informed" being one of its elements, *Helsinki* calls it "informed
consent." Unlike *Nuremberg*, *Helsinki* recognizes the validity of
proxy consent in situations in which the subject lacks the capacity
or legal competence to consent. Alexander had proposed to the
judges at Nuremberg that they include provisions for consent by
the next of kin for "mentally sick patients"; they declined "probably because they did not apply to the specific cases under trial."[19]

As mentioned earlier, *Nuremberg* seemed to have little or no
influence on the actual conduct of research even in the United
States, the nation that instigated its promulgation. By contrast,
publication of *Helsinki* in 1964 effected change almost immediately. Shortly thereafter, investigators found that, on the occasion
of submitting abstracts of their work for consideration for presentation at conventions such as those of the American Federation
for Clinical Research, they were obliged to sign statements that
their work had been conducted in accord with the *Declaration of*

Helsinki. Similar statements were required of authors when they submitted reports of their work for publication in medical or scientific journals.

In the United States, the first federal policy statement on the protection of human subjects was issued by the Surgeon General of the United States Public Health Service on 8 February 1966, less than two years after promulgation of *Helsinki.*[20] In the same year, Henry Beecher's classical exposé, "Ethics and Clinical Research," was published in the *New England Journal of Medicine.*[21] I believe that the availability of a document that set forth specific criteria for ethical justification of research involving human subjects enabled Beecher and others who published exposés in the late 1960s and early 1970s to do so. For the first time, there was an official document created by physicians and endorsed by many medical organizations to use as a measuring stick. Now one could state, "This is a violation of article I.5 of *Helsinki,*" rather than, "I think this is wrong because it allows the interests of science and society to prevail over those of the subjects."[22]

As noticed earlier, *Nuremberg* may reflect an excessively American bias owing to the composition of the group that wrote it. *Helsinki* was drafted by a committee of physicians who recognized a need for professional guidelines designed by physicians for physicians. This may account for its focus on assuring that physicians have the freedom to use new therapeutic and diagnostic modalities if, in their judgment, they offer important advantages over standard therapeutic and diagnostic measures. It may also account for the fact that, even in its most recent revision in 1989, *Helsinki* does not require approval by a research ethics committee.[23]

The group that developed the *CIOMS Guidelines* was distinctly heterogeneous with regard to gender, race, nationality (both developed and developing countries) and profession ("representatives of ministries of health and medical and other health-related disciplines, health policy makers, ethicists, philosophers and lawyers").[24]

The *CIOMS Guidelines* come closer to global validity than did its predecessors. There is, for example, a distinct departure from the uniform requirement for informed individual or proxy consent based on recognition that in some cultures individual informed consent cannot be accomplished. There is, moreover, a systematic repudiation of the illogical constructs that undermine the validity of *Helsinki*. And yet, as I shall discuss shortly, more work needs to be done to make this document even more widely applicable.

THE PROBLEM OF EXPLOITATION

Universalists argue that there must be universal standards to prevent exploitation of residents of technologically developing countries. Universalists correctly point out that most therapeutic innovations are developed in industrialized nations. Investigators from these countries may go to technologically developing countries to test their innovations for various reasons. Some of these reasons are good (for example, some of the diseases for which they wish to develop therapies exist only or primarily in developing countries), and some of them are not (for example, to take advantage of the less complex and sophisticated regulatory systems typical of developing countries). Moreover, universalists observe that once the innovations have been proven safe and effective, economic factors almost always limit their availability to citizens of the country in which they were tested. Requiring investigators to conform to the ethical standards of their own country--or to those embodied in the *Declaration of Helsinki*--when conducting research abroad is one way to restrain exploitation of this type. Universalists also point to *Helsinki* as a widely accepted universal standard for biomedical research that has been endorsed by most countries, including those labeled technologically developing. This gives weight to their claim that research must be conducted according to universal principles. Furthermore, the complex regulations characteristic of technologically developed countries are, in general, patterned after *Helsinki*.

Marcia Angell, in a particularly incisive exposition of the universalists' position, suggests this analogy:

Does apartheid offend universal standards of justice, or does it instead simply represent the South African custom that should be seen as morally neutral? If the latter view is accepted, then ethical principles are not much more than a description of the mores of a society. I believe they must have more meaning than that. There must be a core of human rights that we would wish to see honored universally, despite local variations in their superficial aspects. . . . The force of local custom or law cannot justify abuses of certain fundamental rights, and the right of self-determination, on which the doctrine of informed consent is based, is one of them.[25]

Pluralists join with universalists in condemning economic exploitation of technologically developing countries and their citizens.[26] Unlike the universalists, however, they see the imposition of ethical standards for the conduct of research by a powerful country on a developing country as another form of exploitation. In their view, it is tantamount to saying: No, you may not participate in this development of technology, no matter how much you desire it, unless you permit us to replace your ethical standards with our own. Pluralists call attention to the fact that *Helsinki*, although widely endorsed by the nations of the world, reflects a uniquely Western view of the nature of the person. As such, it does not adequately guide investigators in ways to show respect for all persons in the world.[27]

Pluralists argue that it is unnecessary to assert the universal validity of specific substantive standards. The issue of how to treat persons with respect, for example, is not resolved by insisting on universal requirements for informed consent. It is better to address this issue as has been done in the *CIOMS Guidelines* through the promulgation of "broadly stated [international] ethical standards" with the expectation that the details of compliance with these broadly stated standards will be worked out on a case-by-case basis by ethical committees in the host country that have a high degree of understanding of what it means to treat a person with respect in the community in which the research is to be conducted.

The problem of exploitation of developing countries may also be dealt with satisfactorily, as has been done in *CIOMS Guidelines*. In guideline 8, for example, there is a prohibition against undertaking research involving subjects in underdeveloped communities unless, (1) it could not be carried out reasonably well in developed communities and, (2) the research is responsive to the health needs and priorities of the community in which it is to be carried out. There are several additional requirements specified to minimize the likelihood of exploitation of developing communities and their individual members. In particular, the

CIOMS Guidelines require review *and approval* of all proposed research by ethical review committees in both the initiating and the host countries, while *Helsinki*, article I.2, requires only "consideration, comment and guidance" by an independent committee "in the country in which the research experiment is performed." *Nuremberg* is silent on the matter of ethical review, placing all responsibility for upholding ethical standards on the investigator.

Moreover, *CIOMS Guidelines* include detailed accounts of the responsibilities of research sponsors including pharmaceutical companies and other institutions to assure, for example, "that any product developed through . . . research will be made reasonably available to the inhabitants of the host community or country at the completion of successful testing. Exceptions to this general requirement should be justified and agreed to by all concerned parties before the research begins" (commentary under guideline 15).

THE RELEVANCE OF EMPIRICAL DATA

Although the tension between universalism and pluralism is not likely to be resolved soon, there is one point on which adherents to each of these positions can and do agree. Any attempt to develop guidelines for ethical conduct must be grounded in a thorough and accurate understanding of the culture or cultures in which the guidelines are to be applied; otherwise, the guidelines will not accomplish their objectives. In an article in which they question the validity of the first set of international guidelines promulgated by CIOMS in collaboration with WHO, *Proposed International Guidelines for Biomedical Research Involving Human Subjects*,[28] IJsselmuiden and Faden recognize the importance of a thorough understanding of the cultures that will be affected by guidelines.[29] However, they claim that virtually all recent commentary on research ethics in developing countries, particularly those in Africa, relies on anthropological data that are out of date. For this reason they challenge the reliability of many recommendations offered by recent commentators--especially those who endorse informed consent policies and practices in developing countries that differ from those prevailing in developed countries as do the *CIOMS Guidelines*.

The anthropological studies IJsselmuiden and Faden characterize as "outdated" were published as recently as the 1980s. IJsselmuiden and Faden claim that such studies become obsolete so rapidly largely owing to the extensive recent "urbanization, education and industrialization" of the African population. Their claim is at odds with one conclusion reached by the symbolic anthropologist, Emiko Ohnuki-Tierney, based upon her field studies in modern urban Japan. Ohnuki-Tierney's data afford a convincing refutation of the assumption that modernization or urbanization undermines the symbolic realm of the people, the structure of their meaning and thought.[30]

THEORETICAL CONSIDERATIONS
Ruth Macklin argues:

Something is amiss if ethical theory allows only ... two alternatives: an ethical relativism that reduces to radical subjectivism, an 'anything goes' morality; or an ethical absolutism that posits the existence of moral commands obligatory for everyone, but neither universally acknowledged nor clearly articulated. I think there is an alternative to these two unacceptable philosophical positions. One way of spelling out that alternative lies in an analysis of the concept of moral progress.[31]

Macklin argues that unless we have some "basic normative principles," we can make no judgments as to whether our society advanced or regressed when we, for example, abolished slavery or accorded to women the right to vote. Moreover, we have no basis for saying whether a society that tolerates apartheid or torture of prisoners is more or less "advanced" in a moral sense than one that does not. Agreement on such basic normative principles "does not require a prior acceptance of some particular absolutist ethical theory . . . to make cross-cultural or transhistorical judgments about comparative degrees of moral progress.[32]

Macklin proposes two basic normative principles, *humaneness* and *humanity*:

Humaneness: One culture, society, or historical era exhibits a higher degree of moral progress than another if the first shows more sensitivity to (less tolerance of) the pain and suffering of human beings than does the second, as expressed in the laws, customs, institutions, and practices of the respective societies or eras.

Humanity: The more advanced society would show "more recognition of the inherent dignity, the basic autonomy, or the intrinsic worth of persons."[33]

Macklin makes it clear that these basic normative principles, indeed even "ultimate moral principles," can be compatible with very different normative standards in different societies. In fact, interpretation of the same basic principle can give rise to rules calling for opposite behaviors in two societies that differ in relevant respects. For example, consider a principle of utility that requires a maximization of people's happiness and minimization of unhappiness. In a society with very limited resources, considerations of utility could give rise to a rule requiring that elderly people be allowed to "die when they can no longer contribute to economic production. . . . In a society of abundance, however, old people can easily be supported when they are no longer productive."[34] In such a society it would tend to maximize happiness if all people could be assured of support in their declining years.

While I agree with Macklin's conceptual approach, I must express reservations about her principle of humanity, particularly with her identification of "recognition of . . . the basic autonomy" of human beings as a criterion for the evaluation of a society's moral progress. Macklin and I agree that one leading candidate for what she calls "an ultimate moral principle" is the Kantian categorical imperative (also known as the principle of respect for persons): "So act as to treat humanity, whether in thine own person or in that of any other, in every case as an end withal, never as a means only." The key concept is that persons are never to be treated only or merely as means to another's ends. When one goes beyond this level of formality or abstraction, the principle begins to lose its universality. When this principle is elaborated to require, for example, that all persons are to be treated as self-determining, it loses its relevance to some cultures in which individual self-determination is less highly valued than it is in the United States.[35]

American universalists would argue that persons in such cultures must be educated; they must be taught to value self-determination as much as we do. Some might add that they must learn to value and protect the right to be self-determining or else they will remain vulnerable to exploitation by those who have decision-making authority. Pluralists counter this argument by pointing out that the society seems functional as it is. If we impose on it our ethical standards, it may have a destructive effect on the culture. Furthermore, we should show respect for a society by allowing it to be self-determining.

In the specific context of research involving human subjects, there are some research and development activities that must be carried out in order to be responsive to the urgent health needs of persons who live in societies in which self-determination is not merely not highly valued: it is considered anti-social. There are, for example, certain tropical diseases that exist only or primarily in such societies. It seems inappropriate to say to persons in such societies that we will conduct research addressed to your health problems but only if you allow us to replace your ethical standards with our own. In my view, the conduct of such research in such populations with appropriate committee review, but with consent procedures that may fall short of the requirements of Western civilization, is responsive to the universally applicable requirement to refrain from using persons merely as means to the ends of others.

The *CIOMS Guidelines* reflect what I consider a satisfactory compromise position holding that some ethical standards are universal while recognizing the legitimacy of some degree of ethical pluralism. As noticed earlier, *CIOMS Guidelines* refer to universal principles as "transcending moral rules" without explicating what these rules are.

The recognition in *CIOMS Guidelines* that some moral principles are universal and that various cultures may develop very different rules to uphold the universal principles is implicit in their suggestion, referred to earlier, that the responsibility of ethical review committees in the external sponsoring country, " . . . may be limited to ensuring compliance with *broadly stated principles*, on the understanding that ethical committees in the host country *will have greater competence in reviewing the detailed plans for compliance in* view of their better understanding of the cultural and moral values." (emphasis added)

An inevitable feature of any document that aspires to global validity is that the fundamental principles must be stated at such a level of abstraction that they do not seem to prescribe or proscribe very many behaviors. Further, such documents must necessarily have mostly procedural norms (which prescribe procedures for determining what actions are considered ethically acceptable in specific contexts) and relatively few substantive norms (which prescribe actions that must be performed in contexts that are defined, if at all, only in general terms).

ERRORS IN THE INTERNATIONAL DOCUMENTS

Nuremberg and *Helsinki* each contain statements that do not accurately reflect contemporary understandings of research ethics. In this section, examples of these errors and their unfortunate consequences are presented to those who have an interest in sponsoring, conducting, or reviewing research involving human subjects.

SITUATION IN TIME, PLACE, AND CONTEXT

A statement made by Fletcher and Schulman in their critique of U.S. federal policy is germane to our topic: " . . . if Federal policies on research with human subjects are understood as a moral code, it is necessary to keep their provisions under critical evaluation. Moral codes that cannot be tested and examined in the light of actual choices usually wither and die, because they lose relevance to ever new scientific questions."[36]

One important problem with the international documents is that they reflect the concerns and perspectives of the time in which they were written and of the individuals by whom they were written. I shall focus on *Nuremberg* to illustrate the nature of this problem.

Nuremberg was not addressed to the entire field of research involving human subjects as that field is currently understood. This document was written in response to the atrocities performed by Nazi physician-researchers during the Second World War. Its first principle--"The voluntary consent of the human subject is absolutely essential"--was and is clearly relevant for experiments of the sort that were assessed by the Nuremberg Tribunal. This principle is undoubtedly appropriate for research activities in which risk of physical or psychological injury is

presented to healthy, competent adults by procedures or interventions that do not hold out the prospect of direct benefit to the
individual subjects. It is not appropriate, however, for randomized clinical trials of new, or old drugs involving children, for
example. Moreover, it is not appropriate for research in the field
of epidemiology involving no contact with individual humans
apart from examining their medical records or computerized
databases. Further, it is inappropriate for most research activities
designed to evaluate innovations in programs or policies.[37]

In 1966, the United Nations General Assembly adopted the
International Covenant on Civil and Political Rights of which
article 7 states: "No one shall be subjected to torture or to cruel,
inhuman or degrading treatment or punishment. In particular, no
one shall be subjected without his free consent to medical or
scientific experimentation." In context, it is clear that biomedical
research was perceived in the 1960s as a type of torture or cruel,
inhuman, or degrading treatment.[38] This is the same perspective
that informed the drafting of *Nuremberg*. But this is not the way
most thinking people envision biomedical research today.[39]

Most people who sponsor, conduct, or regulate research
understand the historical origins and intentions of such statements in *Helsinki, Nuremberg,* and the International Covenant on
Civil and Political Rights. As they perform in their professional
roles, they apply such requirements only where such application
is appropriate. However, serious problems are often created when
naive persons get involved in the process. Among the adverse
consequences of their involvement are occasional requirements
by research ethics committees of extremely burdensome and
unwarranted consent procedures for research involving record
review or program evaluation. In some cases such naivete has
resulted in unduly restrictive state or national regulation.[40]

Other types of problems may be caused by commentators
who are not naive. I am referring to the *Nuremberg* fundamentalists, most of whom are academics who have credentials that
appear to establish their credibility as experts in bioethics, who
criticize ethically sound research programs or policies as being in
violation of the *Nuremberg Code* or the International Covenant
on Civil and Political Rights. Often such critiques compare the
program or policy with the activities of Nazis because it is, after

all, the *Nuremberg Code* that is being violated.[41] Such criticisms are most typically found in newspapers and on television and occasionally in academic journals.[42] Such comments often cause a great deal of consternation on the part of lay readers and their representatives in legislative bodies.

CONCEPTUAL ERRORS

Problems are also created by conceptual errors in some of the international documents. One such error can be exemplified by placing one article of *Helsinki* developed for clinical research (II.6) in immediate proximity to one developed for nonclinical research (III.2).

II.6. The physician can combine medical research with professional care, the objective being the acquisition of new medical knowledge, only to the extent that medical research is justified by its potential diagnostic or therapeutic value for the patient.

III.2. The subjects should be volunteers--either healthy persons or patients for whom the experimental design is not related to the patient's illness.

These statements have several unfortunate and unintended consequences. First, many types of research cannot be defined as either clinical or nonclinical. Consider, for example, a placebo-controlled, clinical trial of a new drug. Certainly, the administration of a placebo for research purposes is not "justified by its potential diagnostic or therapeutic value for the patient." Therefore, according to *Helsinki*, this is nonclinical, and those who receive the placebo must be "either healthy persons or patients for whom the experimental design is not related to the patient's illness." This, of course, is unreasonable. Another unfortunate consequence is that a strict interpretation of *Helsinki* would lead us to the conclusion that all rational research designed to explore the pathogenesis or epidemiology of disease is to be forbidden. Because it cannot be justified as prescribed in article II.6, it must be considered nonclinical and therefore can be done only on healthy persons or patients not having the disease one wishes to investigate. This cannot be what those who drafted *Helsinki* intended.[43]

How could those who drafted *Helsinki* have made such errors? The most plausible explanation I can think of is that, as noticed earlier, the WMA, in creating the category they call clinical research, was concerned primarily with assuring the freedom of the physician "to use a new diagnostic or therapeutic measure, if in his or her judgment it offers hope of saving life, reestablishing health or alleviating suffering" (*Helsinki*, article II.2). The class of activities contemplated under the rubric of clinical research in *Helsinki* is what has come to be called in the United States by such names as "compassionate use," "treatment use," "expanded access," and others. This class does not include controlled clinical trials.

Such errors as I have identified in *Helsinki* must be corrected. If we knowingly violate some of its standards routinely as, for example, when we design or conduct a placebo-controlled clinical trial, how can we insist that researchers comply with those of its other articles that are reasonable? The authority of the entire document is undermined if its errors are not corrected.

Helsinki, like *Nuremberg*, is also often cited inappropriately by commentators who may or may not be naive.[44] One recent example is the publication of a paper by Rothman and Michel which brands all or most placebo-controlled clinical trials unethical because they are in violation of *Helsinki*.[45]

Those who inappropriately appeal directly to *Nuremberg* or *Helsinki* as the ultimate source of ethical guidance have done a lot of damage by causing unnecessary confusion and consternation. Such damage could be limited if they appealed instead to the *CIOMS Guidelines* acknowledging the fact that the narrow focus of *Nuremberg* and the conceptual errors of *Helsinki* have been largely rectified by the *CIOMS Guidelines*.

RECOMMENDATIONS FOR FUTURE DEVELOPMENTS

I hope that I have presented sufficient evidence to persuade the reader that the *CIOMS Guidelines* represent a substantial improvement over their predecessors, *Nuremberg*, *Helsinki* and CIOMS's own *Proposed International Guidelines*. I am concerned that at this point it might seem to the reader that I believe that all the problems associated with the development of international ethical guidelines for the conduct of biomedical research involving human subjects were identified and resolved by those who drafted the *CIOMS Guidelines*. I do not intend to leave the reader with this impression. More work remains to be done.

Like all ethical codes, the *CIOMS Guidelines* must be the object of constant critical evaluation. They must be revised from time to time in the light of actual experience and in response to problems that arise as they are applied to specific cases. If this is not done, then we may expect them to become outdated and irrelevant.

Some issues that must be considered and dealt with in future revisions of *CIOMS Guidelines* are anticipated in their background note: "Certain areas of research do not receive special mention in these guidelines: they include human genetic research, embryo and fetal research, and fetal tissue research. These ... areas [are] in rapid evolution and in various respects controversial. . . . [Hence] it would be premature to try to cover them in the present guidelines."[46]

And, of course, there will be additional issues that we are now incapable of anticipating, just as in 1964 the authors of *Helsinki* could not anticipate the current dominance of the randomized clinical trial as the preeminent research strategy for validation of new therapeutic modalities, much less the intractable disputes that would subsequently be incited with the introduction of therapeutic fetal tissue transplantation.

I believe that there are some concepts in the *CIOMS Guidelines* that now, less than two years after their publication, should be reconsidered. For example, guideline 8 on research involving subjects in underdeveloped communities requires that "every effort will be made to secure the ethical imperative that the consent of individual subjects be informed." The only example provided in the commentary of a permissible exception to this rule is "when because of communication difficulties investigators cannot make prospective subjects sufficiently aware of the implications of participation to give adequately informed consent." Even in such cases the "investigator is required to ensure that each prospective subject is clearly told everything that would be conveyed if the study were to be conducted in a developed community."

In other words, it is necessary to thoroughly inform subjects even if there is nothing in their experience that could prepare them to grasp the meaning of, for example, Western concepts of disease causation. Subjects must invariably be informed "that they are free to refuse to participate . . . without loss of any entitlement." This rule is to be applied even in cultures in which departure from the course of action decided upon by the community is almost literally unthinkable. Such provisions in the *CIOMS Guidelines* suggest that this document continues to be excessively influenced by the legacy of *Nuremberg*.

The *CIOMS Guidelines* should also be revised to explicate the "transcending moral rules" to which they refer. The "general ethical principles" referred to in this document are not entirely satisfactory. For example, the version of the principle of respect for persons set forth in the *CIOMS Guidelines* is limited in its applicability by its focus on "respect for autonomy," a priority of Western civilization. As noticed earlier, respect for persons is a more universally valid principle when stated in terms of a prohibition of using human beings only or merely as means to another's ends.

Finally, for reasons I have argued elsewhere, I believe it would be very helpful to include cross-cultural anthropologists in the continuing process of evaluating, criticizing, and revising international ethical guidelines.[47] Other participants in the process of developing international guidelines, in their attempts at conducting dialogues across cultural boundaries, often inadvertently and unknowingly create confusion by relying on literal translations without awareness of the underlying symbolic and idiomatic meanings. This is why I believe we need the expert assistance of anthropologists in making our attempts at cross-cultural communication go beyond mere literal translation to the level of shared meanings.

NOTES

1. Parts of this paper are adapted or excerpted from the following three previous publications of the author: R.J. Levine, *Ethics and Regulation of Clinical Research*, 2nd ed. (Baltimore, Md.: Urban & Schwarzenberg, 1986); R.J. Levine, "Informed Consent: Some Challenges to the Universal Validity of the Western Model," *Law, Medicine & Health*

Care (1991): 207-213; R.J. Levine, "The International Dialogue on Health Policy, Ethics and Human Values: Recommendations for the Next Decade," *Poverty, Vulnerability, and the Value of Human Life: A Global Agenda for Bioethics. Proceedings of the 28th CIOMS Conference* (Geneva: CIOMS, 1994), 234-42.

The author was co-chair of the steering committee of the group that developed the CIOMS/WHO *International Ethical Guidelines for Biomedical Research Involving Human Subjects.*

2. CIOMS/WHO, *International Ethical Guidelines for Biomedical Research Involving Human Subjects.* (Geneva: CIOMS, 1993) The preface and guidelines of this booklet are printed in this book's Appendix F.

3. In this article the term "universal" refers to principles and guidelines that are thought to apply in all human societies and in all historical periods. Other terms such as "global" or "world-wide" refer to principles and guidelines that are thought to apply to all human societies but not in all historical periods. The authors of global guidelines expect them to require periodical revision.

4. N.A. Christakis and R.J. Levine, "Multinational Research," *Encyclopedia of Bioethics,* revised ed., (New York: Simon & Schuster Macmillan, 1995), 1780-87.

5. M. Grodin, "Historical Origins of the Nuremberg Code," in *The Nazi Doctors and the Nuremberg Code: Human Rights in Human Experimentation,* ed. G.J. Annas and M.A. Grodin (New York: Oxford University, 1992): 121-144, at 137.

6. As quoted in G.J. Annas and M.A. Grodin, eds., *The Nazi Doctors and the Nuremberg Code,* 104.

7. S. Perley *et al.,* "The Nuremberg Code: An International Overview," in *The Nazi Doctors and the Nuremberg Code,* 149-173, at 152.

8. T. Taylor, "Opening Statement of the Prosecution, December 9, 1946," in *The Nazi Doctors and the Nuremberg Code,* 67-93, at 67.

9. Grodin, "Historical Origins of the Nuremberg Code," 134-147.

10. A.R. Jonsen, "Do No Harm," *Annals of Internal Medicine* 88 (1978): 827-32.

11. Grodin, "Historical Origins of the Nuremberg Code," 124-32.

12. *Ibid.,* 126.

13. H. Wigodsky and S.K. Hoppe, "Humans as Research Subjects," in *Birth to Death: Biology, Science and Bioethics,* ed. D.C. Thomasma and T. Kushner (Cambridge: Cambridge University, 1995), in press.

14. Grodin, "Historical Origins of the Nuremberg Code," 134.

15. Perley *et al.,* "The Nuremberg Code: An International Overview."

16. *Ibid.,* 158.

17. *Ibid.*, 157.

18. I do not mean to imply that a requirement for informed consent is uniquely American. The philosophical basis of informed consent is more properly characterized as a product of Western civilization. Even American writers typically refer to Europeans as the source of the philosophical grounding for the informed consent requirement. However, the uniform requirement for informed consent to research and to medical practice developed earlier in the United States than in other nations. This, I believe, reflects the great emphasis placed on individualism and self-determination in the American social definition of the "person." See Levine, "Informed Consent: Some Challenges to the Universal Validity of the Western Model."

There is further cause for concern about imposing an American perspective on the development of international guidelines. As anthropologist Willy De Craemer has observed, in his summary statement on the American perspective:

> Taken as a whole, our [American] conception of personhood has at least one major paradoxical attribute. Although it places a high positive value on a universalistic definition of the worth, dignity, and equality of every individual person, it tends to be culturally particularistic, and inadvertently ethnocentric. To a significant degree, it rests on the implicit assumption that ideas about personhood are common to many, if not most, other societies and cultures. Beyond that, it assumes that the American way of thinking about the person represents the way men and women of all societies and cultures should and do think about personhood when they are being supremely rational and moral.

W. De Craemer, "A Cross-Cultural Perspective on Personhood," *Milbank Memorial Fund Quarterly-Health and Society* 61 (Winter 1983): 19-34.

19. Grodin, "Historical Origins of the Nuremberg Code, 136.

20. Levine, *Ethics and Regulation of Clinical Research*, 323.

21. H.K. Beecher, "Ethics and Clinical Research," *New England Journal of Medicine* 274 (1966): 1354-60.

22. It is overly simplistic to think that the publication of a single document had a direct cause and effect relationship on the work of Beecher and the USPHS Surgeon General. It is clear that Beecher was aware of the activities of the World Medical Association and was in communication with WMA before publication of *Helsinki* (Perley *et al.*, "The Nuremberg Code: An International Overview," 155). Also, those who were preparing the Surgeon General's memorandum were aware of

Beecher's activities. And yet I believe that awareness of the WMA project, which began in 1953, and anticipation of its effect had direct influences on both Beecher and the USPHS Surgeon General.

23. Physicians are accustomed to professional autonomy and to professional self-regulation. See R.C. Fox, *The Sociology of Medicine: A Participant Observer's View* (Englewood Cliffs, N.J.: Prentice Hall, 1989). The privilege of and responsibility for self-regulation were accorded to the medical profession by various national and state governments, because it was recognized that the profession had a monopoly on a large body of esoteric knowledge. Since persons outside the profession could not master this large body of knowledge, governments had no real alternative to allowing medical professionals to be self-regulating. In exchange for this authority, the medical profession was expected to use its esoteric knowledge exclusively for the benefit of society and its individual members.

In the 20th century, there has been an increasing recognition that not all of the physician's professional activities are grounded exclusively, or even primarily, in esoteric knowledge. In the context of research involving human subjects, this recognition has given rise to the participation of persons other than physicians in creating rules such as those requiring informed consent and equitable selection of subjects.

For the same reason, persons who are not physicians have been appointed to membership on research ethics committees to ensure that research is planned and conducted in compliance with the rules.

24. CIOMS/WHO, *International Ethical Guidelines for Biomedical Research Involving Human Subjects*, 6.

25. M. Angell, "Ethical Imperialism? Ethics in International Collaborative Clinical Research," *New England Journal of Medicine* 319 (1988): 1081-83.

26. N.A. Christakis, "Ethical Design of an AIDS Vaccine Trial in Africa," *Hastings Center Report* 18 (June/July, 1988): 31-37; N.A. Christakis, "Responding to a Pandemic: International Interests in AIDS Control," *Daedalus* 118 (1989): 113-14.

27. Levine, "Informed Consent: Some Challenges to the Universal Validity of the Western Model."

28. CIOMS/WHO, *Proposed International Guidelines for Biomedical Research Involving Human Subjects* (Geneva: CIOMS, 1982).

29. C.B. IJsselmuiden and R.R. Faden, "Research and Informed Consent in Africa--Another Look," *New England Journal of Medicine* 326 (1992): 830-34.

30. E. Ohnuki-Tierney, *"Illness and Culture in Contemporary Japan: An Anthropological View"* (Cambridge: Cambridge University Press, 1984).

31. R. Macklin, "Universality of the Nuremberg Code," in *The Nazi Doctors and the Nuremberg Code*, 240-76, at 242.

32. *Ibid.*, 242.

33. *Ibid.*

34. *Ibid.*, 244.

35. Levine, "Informed Consent: Some Challenges to the Universal Validity of the Western Model."

36. J.C. Fletcher and J.D. Schulman, "Fetal Research: The State of the Question," *Hastings Center Report* 15 (April 1985): 6-12.

37. J. Lynn, J. Johnson, and R.J. Levine, "The Ethical Conduct of Health Services Research: A Case Study of 55 Institutions," *Clinical Research* 42 (1994): 3-10.

38. The concept reflected in article 7 of the International Covenant on Civil and Political Rights was actually drafted at about the same time as *Nuremberg* as the Universal Declaration of Human Rights, which was adopted by the United Nations General Assembly in 1948.

39. R.J. Levine, "The Impact of HIV Infection on Society's Perception of Clinical Trials," *Kennedy Institute of Ethics Journal* 4 (1994): 93-98.

40. P. Riis, "The Danish Brain Collection and its Important Potentials for Future Research," *IRB: A Review of Human Subjects Research* 15 (November-December 1993): 5-6; C.G. Westrin, "Ethical, Legal and Political Problems Affecting Epidemiology in European Countries," *IRB: A Review of Human Subjects Research* 15 (May-June 1993): 6-8.

41. A.L. Caplan, "The Doctors' Trial and Analogies to the Holocaust in Contemporary Bioethical Debates," in *The Nazi Doctors and the Nuremberg Code*, 258-75.

42. R.J. Levine, "Commentary on E. Howe's and E. Martin's 'Treating the Troops,' " *Hastings Center Report* 21 (March-April 1991): 27-29.

43. Levine, *Ethics and Regulation of Clinical Research*.

44. There are *Helsinki* fundamentalists as well as *Nuremberg* fundamentalists.

45. K.J. Rothman and K.B. Michels, "The Continuing Unethical Use of Placebo Controls," *New England Journal of Medicine* 331 (1994): 394-98.

46. CIOMS/WHO, 1994: *International Ethical Guidelines for Biomedical Research Involving Human Subjects*, 7.

47. Levine, "The International Dialogue on the Health Policy, Ethics and Human Values."

11

The Distinction Between Ethical Pluralism and Ethical Relativism: Implications for the Conduct of Transcultural Clinical Research

Nicolas A. Christakis

INTRODUCTION

Transcultural research refers to clinical biomedical research that involves subjects and investigators from different cultures. The most typical--and most problematic--type of transcultural research is that in which the investigators come from a developed country and the subjects are located in a developing country. The possibility of dissonance between the ethical expectations of the researchers and the subjects from different cultural backgrounds raises the following fundamental practical question: Is it possible to justify ethical rules to govern the conduct of investigators from one cultural background who are performing research on subjects from another? This question has been raised most commonly in the setting of AIDS research, but it is not limited to it.[1] Current debate about this question typically construes it within the frameworks of ethical universality versus relativity--the belief that the ethical principles governing the conduct of research are the same wherever research is conducted versus the contention that ethical principles vary according to cultural setting.

Because it brings investigator and subject together across a cultural boundary in a real research situation, the conduct of transcultural research gives the theoretical tension between ethical universality and ethical relativity palpable, practical significance. The psychiatrist and anthropologist Arthur Kleinman has argued that:

clinical investigations in developing societies must be understood as taking place within the particular contexts of practical, everyday beliefs, values, and power relationships that constitute local cultural systems and [must be understood] as creating potential conflicts between these non-Western systems and the Western cultural conceptions and norms that are usually an unrecognized part of clinical research projects and the expectations and behaviors of clinical researchers. . . .[2]

There is considerable controversy regarding how such conflict should be resolved and regarding which system of ethics should govern the conduct of multinational, transcultural clinical research. Some contend that all research, wherever it is conducted, should and can be evaluated by universally applicable standards.[3] Others contend that universal standards are possible, but must be flexibly implemented and conceived.[4] Still others contend that, at best, few standards are universal and that ethical rules are and should be culturally relative.

Virtually always, however, solutions to the question are framed within the extremes of universalism and relativism. But there is another framework which provides a more workable solution to the question: ethical pluralism. Ethical pluralism addresses many of the problems inherent in the relativist and universalist positions. Its superiority arises from two attributes: it acknowledges the key position of culture in shaping both the content and form of ethical rules and it includes a mechanism of dispute resolution through mutual evaluation and negotiation.

UNIVERSAL STANDARDS FOR CLINICAL RESEARCH ETHICS ARE PROBLEMATIC

International guidelines regarding clinical research ethics, such as the *Nuremberg Code*,[5] the *Declaration of Helsinki*, 1964 and 1975,[6] and even the *Guidelines of the Council for International Organizations of Medical Sciences* (CIOMS),[7] are problematic on two broad levels.[8] First, by asserting their universality, international guidelines obscure real and legitimate cross-cultural differences in ethical expectations. International guidelines seek to make homogeneous something which is not necessarily so. Second, existing international guidelines are ambiguous about their objectives and purposes. On the one hand, guidelines are structured as a set of goals and are largely aspirational in language and content. But on the other hand, the guidelines assume a normative character, by providing a set of standards to judge and, if appropriate, to sanction investigators' conduct. Consequently, international guidelines and their application may unavoidably and wrongly marginalize alternative visions of what is ethically correct, and they may therefore proscribe or be used to proscribe necessary investigations in certain locales that are conducted by local investigators in good faith and with local community approval. Indeed, there have been several examples of research that both subjects and investigators wished to conduct that were abandoned for nonconformity to international guidelines.[9]

There are two broad ways that a universal system of research ethics might be developed.[10] One way--the only way so far employed—is to use Western research ethics as the international standard. However, this solution does not speak to non-Western ethical expectations. Moreover, such an outright application of Western research ethics is confounded by serious cultural variation in the interpretation of certain essential ideas (such as personhood, disease causation, and randomization). Another way is to abstract a new system of research ethics through cross-cultural examination of systems of medical ethics. But this is complicated by the lack of other research traditions. Where present, other systems of medical ethics are largely professional in nature and, in a fundamental way, do not speak to the concerns of the Western tradition of clinical research. Both ways, in other words, are practically unworkable.[11]

A particularly good illustration of the debate between the positions of relativism and universalism is found in disagreements over the extent to which variability in individual informed consent is permissible. Articulate proponents of the universal nature of informed consent correctly argue that neither the difficulty of achieving informed consent in the developing world nor the urgency of conducting research justify compromising ethical principles.[12] But the argument about the need for individual informed consent is also often extended to include moral justifications for the universality of individual informed consent. Universalists argue that "ethical standards in medicine . . . cannot be relative; they must be judged by their substance. The force of local custom or law cannot justify abuses of certain fundamental rights, and the right of self-determination, on which the doctrine of informed consent is based, is one of them."[13] They argue that individual informed consent "expresses important and basic moral values that are universally applicable, regardless of variations in cultural practice."[14] These arguments reflect the belief that, since one aspect of modern medicine is to prescribe its cure for patients, why not prescribe its morality as well? Arguments for the universalism of Western research ethics often seem to conflate technological superiority with moral superiority.

A further problem with the universalist position is that it does not seem to recognize that the requirement of first person informed consent is deeply imprinted with the emphasis on individualism and individual rights that is paramount in Western culture and that in many ways is peculiar to it. Moreover, the universalist perspective is disrespectful of the more social conceptions of the person that prevail in most regions of the world.

The Western principle of informed consent is predicated upon the notion of respect for persons and upon the notion of individuals as autonomous agents.[15] However, a fundamental problem arises in the application of the respect for persons principle because of cross-cultural variation in the very definition of personhood. Western societies stress the individualistic nature of the person and put much emphasis on the individual's rights, autonomy, self-determination, and privacy. This is at variance with more pluralistic definitions of the person found in other societies which stress the embeddedness of the individual within society and define a person by his relations to others. The Kongo of Lower Zaire, for example, have conceptions of illness and medicine that "consistently [draw] the effective boundary of a person differently, more expansively, than classical Western medicine, philosophy, and religion. The outcome is usually disconcerting or unreal to Western medical observers. . . ."[16] The very definition of "body" by the Kongo embraces "constant reference to social relations."[17]

Anthropologist Clifford Geertz provides another example in his consideration of the nature of personhood in Bali; Geertz notes: "One of these pervasive orientational necessities is surely the characterization of individual human beings. Peoples everywhere have developed symbolic structures in terms of which persons are perceived not baldly as such, as mere unadorned members of the human race, but as representatives of certain distinct categories of persons, specific sorts of individuals."[18]

The teknonymous Balinese system, moreover, leads to ongoing shifts in how members of this society are given names during the individual's lifetime, depending on their social position. In general, the definition of a person and of the self is more fluid, more expansive, and more relational in that it depends on the relatives of a given individual; the definition, that is, depends on *other members of the society*.[19]

Important practical implications arise from this kind of variation in the definition of a person. Since the notion of persons as individuals is undermined, the consent of the individual may not be viewed as essential in certain cultural settings. Indeed, the focus of the consent process may shift from the individual to the family or to the community; for example, in contemporary China, consent for a procedure might be first elicited from relatives who would in turn persuade the individual of the virtue of the proposed intervention.[20] Thus, in the context of research, it may be necessary to secure the consent of a subject's family or social group instead of, or in addition to, the consent of the subject himself.

The question of whether individual informed consent is universal across all cultures is indeed amenable to cross-cultural empirical research. But it seems unlikely--should such research be undertaken--that individual informed consent will prove to be universal across all cultures akin to, say, the incest taboo. On the contrary, much research suggests that conceptions of individual consent and of the "person" are highly variable.[21] If anything, the American view is in the minority.

Indeed, even in our own society, informed consent is not exclusively individualistic. For instance, although the Uniform Anatomical Gift Act has made it legal for individuals to give consent for *post mortem* organ donation, physicians and other healthcare providers almost always request the written consent of the cadaveric donors' families before they harvest organs for this purpose. It would seem that in the face of a surgical act that they still consider extraordinary, however routinized it may have become, health professionals not only feel compelled to acknowledge the importance of the family's connection with the patient-donor, but also to make sure of their consent.[22]

Ethicist Lisa Newton has cogently summarized the problems with the universalist perspective on informed consent by arguing that,

> seeking informed consent to research from individuals [in certain developing world settings] may tend to weaken the social fabric of a non-individualistic society, forcing it to deal with values it does not hold, and possibly sowing disorder that the community will have to reap long after the investigators have gone home. . . . It is questionable that [our vaunted Western individualism] has been an unmitigated good for our own civilization and very questionable that it is up to standard for export. We ought, in truth, to be suitably humble about the worth of procedures [that is, individual consent] developed only to cater to a very Western weakness. . . . How can it be a sign of our respect for people, or of our concern for their welfare, that we are willing to suppress research that is conducted according to the laws and cultures of the countries in which it is being carried out?[23]

The difficulty in achieving consensus on the applicability of individual informed consent is reflective of the difficulty in achieving consensus on a host of other issues related to the conduct of transcultural clinical research. That is, other aspects of clinical research ethics, including the principles of beneficence and justice, are even less likely to be found to be universal than the requirement for individual informed consent.[24]

ETHICAL RELATIVISM

The point of view that is ordinarily placed in opposition to universalism is relativism. The basis for relativistic thinking about ethics is *skepticism* and its corollary, *tolerance*. Skepticism is the contention that nothing is inherently right or wrong, that no moral principles are inherently legitimate. Skepticism supposes that actions are defined as right or wrong by given peoples in specific cultural contexts at specific times and that behavior is culturally relative. As a result, ethical relativity contends that value judgments should be forsworn in assessing foreign systems of belief. Moreover, ethical relativity contends that the impossibility of objectively determining moral action obliges tolerance towards other cultures. Thus, in the conduct of transcultural clinical research, value and prescriptive force are accorded to all systems of ethics, and transcultural research might be required to independently meet the ethical requirements of the two cultures involved (that is, the cultures of the investigator and of the subject).

Several practical problems are raised by this position. If research is designed so that it meets the ethical expectations of both the subjects and the investigators, then the research, it would appear, is perforce ethical and permissible. Yet, it is possible to envision research meeting the ethical criteria of both the investigator and the subjects which, under some third standard, would be considered unethical. Does this mean that all clinical research projects should meet all possible ethical standards for research, or only the two standards of the involved researchers and subjects? What if, to an outsider, the research ethics articulated within a given setting are perceived as reprehensible? The relativist position, it is clear, fundamentally precludes *evaluation* of differing ethical systems.

A further problem with this relativistic model is that it provides no guidance for resolving conflicting ethical expectations: if neither system is superior and the two conflict, to which one should there be recourse? If the resolution of the conflict is in favor of the subject and is antithetical to the investigator, is the investigator relieved of his or her ethical duty? Can the research then proceed? If no resolution between conflicting ethics is possible, what is to be done if both societies perceive the research to be essential? Or, if no resolution between conflicting ethics is possible--and the research is therefore impermissible--may the investigators conduct it elsewhere?

Aside from the foregoing practical problems with the relativism position, there is a major theoretical problem as well. Ethical relativism is *not* value-free, for a value judgment is contained in its call for tolerance: it asserts that we *ought* to respect other value systems. The problem here is that no definitive reason is provided as to why tolerance is desirable. The evidence regarding cross-cultural variation in basic moral beliefs does not in itself justify tolerance. Anthropologist Elvin Hatch has articulated the problem thus:

The factual evidence [regarding the existence of variation in values] is beside the point. The relativists make the error of deriving an 'ought' statement from an 'is' statement. To say that values vary from culture to culture is to describe (accurately or not) an empirical state of affairs in the real world, whereas the call for tolerance is a value judgment of what ought to be, and it is logically impossible to derive the one from the other. The fact of moral diversity no more compels our approval of other ways of life than the existence of cancer compels us to value ill-health.[25]

Though on liberal, humanistic grounds tolerance has some appeal, critics of relativistic thinking, Hatch included, have pointed out that tolerance should not be extended beyond its limits. But there is no uniform way to decide at what point tolerance should stop.

ETHICAL PLURALISM

Most of the problems with both the universalist and relativist positions on clinical research ethics arise from a maladroit handling and incomplete recognition of the influence of culture upon the question at hand. The pluralist position is fundamentally based on the fact that culture shapes (1) the content of ethical precepts, (2) the way ethics as a concept is configured (that is, the form of ethical precepts), and (3) the interaction between conflicting ethical expectations (that is, the way ethical conflict itself is handled).

Addressing the first issue (how culture shapes ethical rules) requires careful analysis of indigenous ethical expectations.[26] It is in many respects the easiest of the three. Addressing the last two issues, however, is more difficult: it requires the development of a special perspective on ethical systems. Orthodox Western bioethical approaches may well be inadequate to deal with not only the manifest variability in the ethical norms of differing cultures, but also the differing ways ethics is understood and ethical conflicts are handled in other cultures.

Medical ethics is not the same kind of thing in all societies. Sociologists Renee Fox and Judith Swazey have argued, for example, that the Chinese "medical morality" is *not* equivalent to Western "bioethics."[27] More generally, ethics do not just regulate behavior, they construe it. Ethics are a form of "local knowledge," which Geertz has described as "local not just as to place, time, class, and variety of issue, but as to accent--vernacular characterizations of what happens connected to vernacular imaginings of what can."[28] As local knowledge, ethical systems are highly variable and situation-specific. Geertz observes that a paradox arises when we conceptualize systems of ideas with the realization that "socio-political thought does not grow out of disembodied reflection but 'it is always bound up with the existing life situation of the thinker.' "[29] The solution to this problem, Geertz argues, lies in a more adroit handling of socio-political thought by conceptualizing it as an ordered system of cultural symbols. That is, it is not the ethical rules themselves which are so important, it is their *meaning* within respective cultures. The rules, in a sense, may be taken to reflect how a given culture perceives that human beings should be treated by others, how investigator and subject should communicate, or how medical knowledge is to be acquired. Medical ethics may also be different in respective cultures in part because of the activities ethics is viewed as appropriately governing. For example, the distribution of resources that maintain or restore health is configured as necessarily a moral problem within contemporary Western medical ethics. Yet, in other societies, the distribution of such resources might not be configured as a moral issue at all.[30]

A culturally sensitive perspective on systems of medical ethics has a further consequence. According to the prevailing view, medical ethics, as part of a positivist tradition in Western philosophy, consists of rules and principles directed at what ought to be the case. An alternative, contextualist, view of medical ethics, however, focuses on accounting for the *phenomena* of medical ethics. It seeks to understand the practice of medical ethics by locating its cultural context.[31] A contextualist perspective on morality offers a way out of the thorny methodological and substantive issues raised by a positivist--and culturally myopic-- perspective on morality, issues brought to the fore by the conduct of transcultural clinical research.

A contextualist approach also contributes to a solution to the problem of determining which ethics should govern transcultural research, because the contextualist approach broadens the philosophical basis of research ethics. Part of the problem with current analysis of the problem--even from a Western point of view--is that the full richness of Western philosophy itself has not been tapped.[32] Bioethics has, until very recently, based itself almost exclusively on Anglo-American analytic philosophical thought and largely ignored other Western philosophical traditions, such as phenomenology, virtues theory, existentialism, communitarianism, social ethics, and the like.

Present American concepts of medical ethics are too detached from the clinical reality in which ethics come into play. A significant source of ethical meaning is the particular situation in which ethical issues are raised. Clinical research ethics have a concrete existence, expressed in each research setting. Ethical rules such as those pertaining to clinical research, like other socio-political and religious thought, are constructed, fashioned, made. And since both the maker and the situation in which they are applied vary, so will the product. In order to resolve the troubling problems raised by the conduct of transcultural clinical research, an ethnography of the practice of morality in medical contexts in general and in transcultural clinical research in particular will be needed.

Indeed, the Western system of research ethics is, itself, a recent creation, largely articulated since World War II. It rests on a medical ethic that was exclusively doctor/patient oriented and which, under pressure of the research endeavor, was expanded to accommodate the investigator/subject relationship. Western medical ethics, that is, were at the outset based on the Hippocratic tradition, and were largely *professional* in nature, meaning that they pertained largely to matters of professional decorum. The concept of essential patient rights, which in themselves create obligations for professionals, is alien to the Hippocratic ethical tradition. This concept found its first important expression in the West in the *Nuremberg Code*. The *Nuremberg Code* abandoned the notion that experimental subjects are protected by professional standards and replaced it with the notion that subjects have intrinsic rights. In short, there has been an evolution in medical ethics--in response to the existence of research and to the abuse of research subjects in certain settings--in the West. The indigenous ethics of non-Western cultures, as they apply to professional etiquette or clinical care, are also capable of evolution. Of course, the form of research ethics that systems of non-Western medical ethics ultimately achieve might be quite different from Western research ethics.[33] But the emergence of non-Western systems of clinical research ethics, such as they might be, must be expected and understood. In view of the importance and proliferation of collaborative research efforts between developed and developing countries, an understanding of the emergence of research ethics in non-Western countries is of enormous practical significance. Moreover, as traditional medical practices converge with Western biomedicine around much of the world, clinical research ethics will be under increasing pressure to adapt to local circumstances and local cultures.[34]

Thus, culture shapes both the content and form of ethical systems. It can also be seen to shape how the existence of conflicting ethical expectations is construed and handled. In the United States in particular, we often seem to expect that a solution to ethical problems is indeed possible, if only we were clever or persuasive or patient enough. The expectation, tempered by our culture, is that ethical dilemmas have a transcendent solution. However, not all conflicts, especially in such a complex area as research ethics, are resolvable. This problem is compounded in the conduct of transcultural clinical research: it is not just ethical principles themselves that might conflict, it is also the interests of varying cultures. Resolving ethical conflict is apt to be especially unlikely when non-casuistic, systematic solutions--those divorced from actual, clinically and culturally specific situations--are applied. American bioethics has an inherent bias in that there is an expectation that final and transcendent resolution of ethical disputes is indeed possible. In the United States, we seem to hesitate to accept inherent ethical irresolvability. Ethical systems, however, do not exist only to eliminate ethical problems. They also exist to provide a framework for such problems--a framework for the confrontation of particular situations that pose ethical dilemmas.

PRACTICAL IMPLICATIONS OF PLURALISM

Such a casuistic, pluralistic view of medical ethics has three major practical implications. The first implication is that an understanding of the *relevant* and *specific* ethical expectations of indigenous peoples will be a prerequisite of transcultural clinical research. It is not, after all, the existence of moral standards that varies cross-culturally, it is their form and content. This pluralistic approach to the problem is different from the approach of ethical relativism in four critical respects: (1) an ongoing *dialogue* between ethical systems is inherent in it; (2) a *negotiation* between ethical systems about *a particular situation* takes place; (3) proponents of both the dissonant ethical systems *assess* the other *and* their own ethical systems; and (4) a rationale for *tolerance* is thus provided, namely, that ethical conflict is sometimes irresolvable but must nevertheless be handled.

These features lead to the second practical implication of ethical pluralism. From a pluralist perspective, the ethical conduct of transcultural research is dependent upon the negotiated settlement of ethical disputes rather than upon the rigid application of previously formed international ethical rules or the lax acquiescence to all systems of clinical research ethics. The kind of negotiation between equals that this approach entails would admittedly be difficult to attain in many settings in the developing world where research is conducted--if, for no other reason, because of tremendous differences in education, wealth, and power between investigators and subjects. A paternalistic feeling on the part of the investigator that the ethical expectations of the subjects have been met is not enough. The difficulty in achieving such a cross-cultural negotiation, however, does not mean that efforts should be abandoned. In such a negotiation, the involved parties must accept the existence of alternative ethical systems, and, while not foreswearing assessment of the other systems, must still negotiate with them. Such negotiation and mutual understanding also provides the practical advantage of providing a mechanism for dispute resolution.[35]

With an eye toward respecting the local ideals of both subject and investigator, I have previously proposed the following protocol.[36] This protocol would encourage a negotiated settlement of ethical differences, so that both parties, researchers and subjects, might be comfortable with the proposed research, ethically and clinically.

1. The host country for the research, or, more specifically, the representatives of research subjects, should have a presumptive claim to ethical guidance. In the event of a conflict, the host country's ethical standards, if they are more restrictive, should always prevail.
2. A researcher retains an allegiance to his or her own community. To the extent a researcher's community views the research as unethical, the researcher should not go forward irrespective of what the host nation says, unless the ethical dispute can be negotiated.
3. To the extent that any nation or institution adopts ethical guidelines, including any internationally promulgated guidelines, it should be bound by those guidelines irrespective of to whom they are being applied within the nation.
4. When research that is considered desirable by either party is proscribed by existing international standards or by either party's own standards, formal negotiations between the parties to understand the source of disagreement and to arrive at a consensus, if possible, should take place. Relevant international standards might here serve as aspirational guides. If a consensus is reached, the research should be viewed as necessarily ethical, its deviation from any international standards notwithstanding. The negotiations, of course, must be fair.

Ideally, negotiation would take place between true representatives of those who wish to conduct the research and those who would be the subjects. Such negotiations would not necessarily be based on national boundaries and could conceivably take place within a given country as well as between two countries. Implicit in this position is support for an ongoing international dialogue that privileges all perspectives on the ethics of clinical research (not just Western perspectives). In this regard, the question of the composition of international bodies and the ability of alternative voices to be heard is critical. To date, international bodies have tended to mirror the distribution of power within the world. The more powerful, principally Western nations have dominated the debate. Although Western representatives are often commendably sensitive to the concerns of the developing world, this is no substitute for actual participation by those nations themselves.

The quintessential dilemmas in such a protocol thus become (1) to discover local ethical expectations, (2) to assess the good faith and legitimacy of the representatives, and (3) to ensure adequate expertise on the part of the subject representatives.

These requirements, finally, lead to the third practical implication of ethical pluralism. Pluralism suggests a shift from current content-based international ethical standards towards procedure-based protocols directed at addressing the above three dilemmas. Such procedural guidelines would specify how transcultural ethical disputes in transcultural research projects, if they arise, might be mediated, rather than specifying *a priori* which ethical rules should be followed. And they would be concerned with the specification of fair procedures for negotiation rather than the articulation of principles of research ethics.

Ideally, such guidelines would encourage a negotiated settlement of ethical differences, so that both parties--researchers and subjects--might be comfortable with the proposed research, ethically and clinically. But a necessary predicate to the fair application of such guidelines is the legitimacy and good faith of local representatives and the integrity and fairness of the dialogue between the parties.[37] Cultural sensitivity and the privileging of local ethics should not be used as a shield to abuse developing world citizens as research subjects. I emphasize that the legitimacy and good faith of local representatives is fundamental to the process. I am not advocating the view that the assertion by a host nation regarding these matters is perforce acceptable. Otherwise, for example, it is easy to envisage the selective abuse of minorities within host nations or bad faith actions by research subject representatives. This type of evaluation is analogous to the inquiry common in human rights investigations. Monitors of international bodies are not ordinarily satisfied by a mere formal adoption of applicable human rights covenants by a given nation.[38]

Indeed, there are many egregious examples of the abuse of research subjects in the developing world, and they are to be strongly condemned. For example, one researcher outlined high risk experiments conducted in Bangladesh that would "not have been passed by ethics committees elsewhere." This research involved cholera patients and included administration of radioactive materials and withholding of proper treatment (leading directly to a death in at least one case).[39] Other cases have emerged during the development of contraceptive medicines; critics argued that coercion to participate in the research was rife and that the Third World poor might become "the guinea pigs or beagle dogs for the world's contraceptive testing."[40]

Yet another, more recent, problematic case is that of an AIDS vaccine trial conducted in Zaire in the late 1980s. Africans were concerned that they were serving as subjects for research deemed too risky to be conducted in the West, with good reason. An unidentified source close to the research group conducting the trial informed a *New York Times* reporter that "It was easier to get official permission here [in Zaire] than in France."[41] It later emerged that the research subjects were mostly minors. African critics were also concerned that Western investigators, unchecked by foreign or local supervision, might conduct "savage experiments" in Africa.[42] There was a feeling that "Western science often comes to Africa with dirty hands."[43]

Such examples warrant caution and safeguards when reviewing the conduct of multinational research. But the history of the abuse of research subjects in the developing world (and in the developed world) does not mean that we necessarily abandon a sociologically informed, pluralistic research ethic, replacing it, presumably, with a narrow, Western-based ethic which is not *necessarily* representative of the wishes of the research subjects it allegedly is protecting. Indeed, it may even be true that it is not ethical codes themselves--even Western or "universal" ones--that truly protect research subjects. It is not, in other words, necessary to adopt a universalist position on transcultural research ethics in order to support high standards of ethics. Ethical behavior and philosophical outlook are distinct. No system of rules alone, no matter how extensive or enlightened, will completely protect subjects from unscrupulous investigators.[44] Instead, research subjects may perhaps best be protected by being involved as equals in the conduct of research. This, of course, is largely equivalent to arguing that local culture should inform the ethics of clinical research trials.

Since systems of ethical rules are socially constructed, they will vary according to the cultural setting in which they are formulated.[45] This fact suggests that *both* cultural analysis and moral analysis should be part of ethical research. Indeed, it is not possible for moral analysis to be totally acultural, even if this were desirable. Pluralism challenges the presumption that cultural analysis is not integrally related to moral analysis.

It has become apparent that existing international standards of research ethics are not a mechanism for the resolution of conflicting ethical expectations under circumstances where the universality of the principles articulated within them is not recognized, where the principles as articulated are insufficiently specific, or where the principles articulated within the standards conflict with each other. Ethical relativism, on the other hand, is essentially nihilistic: it does not provide a solution because it is non-evaluative and because it does not offer a means for the resolution of conflict. Pluralism does away with the most troubling aspect of both universalism and relativism: namely, the lack of critical appraisal of one's own and the other ethical system. Pluralism is an intermediate solution to the problem of which ethics should guide the conduct of transcultural clinical research, a solution that sits between the autocracy of universalism and the anarchy of relativism.

NOTES

1. M. Barry, "Ethical Considerations of Human Investigation in Developing Countries: The AIDS Dilemma," *New England Journal of Medicine* 319 (1988): 1083-86; N.A. Christakis, "The Ethical Design of an AIDS Vaccine Trial in Africa," *Hastings Center Report* 18 (June/July 1988): 31-37.

2. A.M. Kleinman, "Cultural Issues Affecting Clinical Investigation in Developing Societies" (Paper presented at the National Academy of Sciences Institute of Medicine Workshop, Bellagio, Italy) 2-7 October 1979; also available as A.M. Leinman, "Problèmes culturels associés aux recherches cliniques dans les pays en voie de développement," in *Médecine et Expérimentation*, ed. M.A.M. de Wachter (Quebec, P.Q.: Les Presses de l'Université Laval, 1982).

3. B.G. Schoepf, "Ethical, Methodological and Political Issues of AIDS Research in Central Africa," *Social Science and Medicine* 33 (1991): 749-63; M. Angell, "Ethical Imperialism? Ethics in International Collaborative Clinical Research," *New England Journal of Medicine* 319 (1988): 1081-83.

4. R.J. Levine, "Informed Consent: Some Challenges to the Universal Validity of the Western Model," in *Development of International Ethical Guidelines for Epidemiological Research and Practice* (Geneva: CIOMS, 1991).

5. U.S. Department of Defense, "The Nuremberg Code," in *U.S. v. Karl Brandt, Trials of War Criminals before Nuremberg Military Tribunals under Control Law No. 10* (Washington, D.C.: U.S. Government Printing Office), 2: 181-83. This code is replicated in this volume's Appendix A.

6. World Medical Assembly, "Declaration of Helsinki," and revisions, in this volume's Appendix B.

7. CIOMS, *Proposed International Guidelines for Biomedical Research Involving Human Subjects* (Geneva: CIOMS, 1982). The finalized version of the guidelines (1993) are replicated in this book's Appendix F.

8. N.A. Christakis and M.J. Panner, "Existing International Ethical Guidelines for Human Subjects Research: Some Open Questions," *Law, Medicine & Health Care* 19 (1991): 214-21.

9. M. Barry, "Ethical Considerations of Human Investigation in Developing Countries;" N.A. Christakis, L. A. Lynn, and A. Castelo, "Clinical AIDS Research That Evaluates Cost-Effectiveness in the Developing World," *IRB: A Review of Human Subjects Research* 13 (July-August 1991): 4-7. There have also been examples of developing world research where international guidelines have mandated the inclusion of meaningless revisions in the protocol; see, for example, A.J. Hall, "Public Health Trials in West Africa: Logistics and Ethics," *IRB: A Review of Human Subjects Research* 11 (September-October 1989): 8-10.

10. N.A. Christakis, "Ethics Are Local: Engaging Cross-Cultural Variation in the Ethics for Clinical Research," *Social Science and Medicine* 35 (October 1992): 1079-91.

11. *Ibid.*

12. C.B. IJsselmuiden and R.R. Faden, "Medical Research and the Principle of Respect for Persons in Non-Western Cultures," Chapter 12 in this volume.

13. M. Angell, "Ethical Imperialism?" 1082.

14. C.B. IJsselmuiden and R.R. Faden, "Research and Informed Consent in Africa: Another Look," *New England Journal of Medicine* 326 (1992): 830-33.

15. U.S. Department of Health, Education, and Welfare, National Commission for the Protection of Human Subjects of Biomedical and Behavioral Research, *The Belmont Report: Ethical Principles and Guidelines for the Protection of Human Subjects of Research*, DHEW Publication

No. (OS) 79-12065 (Washington, D.C.: U.S. Government Printing Office, 1979), 4; reprinted in this volume's Appendix C.

16. J.M. Janzen, *The Quest for Therapy in Lower Zaire* (Berkeley, Calif.: University of California Press, 1978), 189.

17. *Ibid.*, 169.

18. C. Geertz, "Person, Time, and Conduct in Bali," in *The Interpretation of Cultures* (New York: Basic Books, 1973), 363.

19. The nature of personhood has, among other things, come increasingly to be the focus of "new" ethnography. See G.E. Marcus and M.M.J. Fischer, *Anthropology as Cultural Critique, An Experimental Moment in the Human Sciences* (Chicago: University of Chicago Press, 1986), especially 45-73.

20. For this example and for a description of cultural variation in other ethical issues, see H.T. Engelhardt, "Bioethics in the People's Republic of China," *Hastings Center Report* 10 (April 1980): 7-10.

21. W. DeCraemer, "A Cross-Cultural Perspective on Personhood," *Millbank Memorial Fund Quarterly-Health and Society* 61 (1983): 19-34. Regarding the notion of the person more generally, see R.C. Fox and D.P. Willis, "Personhood, Medicine, and American Society," *Millbank Memorial Fund Quarterly-Health and Society* 61 (1983): 127-47; M. Mauss, "A Category of the Human Spirit," *The Psychoanalytic Review* 55 (1968): 457-81. There is considerable cross-cultural variability in ethical expectations. See, for example: K.N.S. Subramanian, "In India, Nepal, and Sri Lanka, Quality of Life Weighs Heavily," *Hastings Center Report* 16 (August 1986): 20-22; B.W. Levin, "International Perspectives on Treatment Choice in Neonatal Intensive Care Units," *Social Science and Medicine* 30 (1990): 901-12; P. Ratanakul, "Bioethics in Thailand: The Struggle for Buddhist Solutions," *Journal of Medicine and Philosophy* 13 (1988): 301-12; A.A. Nanji, "Medical Ethics and the Islamic Tradition," *Journal of Medicine and Philosophy* 13 (1988): 257-76.

22. R.C. Fox and J.P. Swazey, *Spare Parts: Organ Replacement in American Society* (New York: Oxford University Press, 1992).

23. L.H. Newton, "Ethical Imperialism and Informed Consent," *IRB: A Review of Human Subjects Research* 12 (May-June 1990): 11.

24. N.A. Christakis, "The Ethical Design of an AIDs Vaccine Trial in Africa."

25. E. Hatch, *Culture and Morality, the Relativity of Values in Anthropology* (New York: Columbia University Press, 1983), 66-67.

26. B. Hoffmaster, "Morality and the Social Sciences," in *Social Science Perspectives on Medical Ethics*, ed. G. Weisz (Philadelphia: University of Pennsylvania Press, 1990); R.W. Lieban, "Medical Anthropology and the Comparative Study of Medical Ethics," in *Social Science*

Perspectives on Medical Ethics, ed. G. Weisz (Philadelphia: University of Pennsylvania Press, 1990); Barry, "Ethical Considerations of Human Investigation in Developing Countries"; M. Beiser, "Ethics in Cross-Cultural Research," in *Current Perspectives in Cultural Psychiatry*, eds. E.F. Foulks *et al.* (New York: Spectrum Publications, 1977); M. Abdussalam and B.O. Osuntokun, "Capacity Building for Ethical Considerations of Epidemiological Studies: Perspective of Developing Countries," in *Development of International Ethical Guidelines for Epidemiological Research and Practice* (Geneva: CIOMS, 1991); Christakis, "The Ethical Design of an AIDS Vaccine Trial in Africa; Christakis, Lynn, and Castelo, "Clinical AIDS Research that Evaluates Cost-Effectiveness in the Developing World."

27. R.C. Fox and J.P. Swazey, "Medical Morality Is Not Bioethics--Medical Ethics in China and the United States," *Perspectives in Biology and Medicine* 27 (1984): 336-60.

28. C. Geertz, "Local Knowledge," in *Local Knowledge: Further Essays in Interpretive Anthropology* (New York: Basic Books, 1983), 215.

29. C. Geertz, "Ideology as a Cultural System, " in *The Interpretation of Cultures* (New York: Basic Books, 1973), 194.

30. Lieban, "Medical Anthropology and the Comparative Study of Medical Ethics," 227-28.

31. Hoffmaster, "Morality and the Social Sciences."

32. Fox and Swazey, "Medical Morality Is Not Bioethics," 358.

33. Christakis, "Ethics Are Local."

34. N.A. Christakis, N.C. Ware, and A. Kleinman, "Illness Behavior and the Health Transition in the Developing World," in *Health and Social Change in International Perspective*, eds. L.C. Chen, A. Kleinman, and N.Ware (Cambridge: Harvard University Press, 1993), 233-56.

35. Christakis and Panner, "Existing International Ethical Guidelines."

36. *Ibid.* See also Levine, "Informed Consent: Some Challenges," for another set of procedural guidelines.

37. Many formal methods to ensure fair and open dialogue exist. For example, see B.J. Broome and N.A. Christakis, "A Culturally Sensitive Approach to Tribal Governance Issue Management," *International Journal of Intercultural Relations* 12 (1988): 107-23.

38. D. Orentlicher, "Bearing Witness: The Art and Science of Human Rights Fact Finding," *Harvard Human Rights Journal* 3 (1990): 83-136.

39. See, for example, a series of letters published in *Lancet* in 1978 regarding diarrheal research in Bangladesh: W.H. Mosley *et al.*, "International Research Laboratory in Bangladesh," *Lancet* no. *i*

(1978): 602-3; C. McCord, "International Research Laboratory in Bangladesh," *Lancet* no. *i* (1978): 768 (containing the allegations of ethical misconduct); C. McCord, "Cholera Research in Bangladesh," *Lancet* no. *i* (1978): 1207; D.R. Nalin, "Cholera Research in Bangladesh," *Lancet* no. *ii* (1978): 102-3.

40. D.P. Warwick, "Contraceptives in the Third World," *Hastings Center Report* 5 (August 1975): 9-12; see also, M. Potts and J.M. Paxman, "Depo-Provera: Ethical Issues in Its Testing and Distribution," *Journal of Medical Ethics* 10 (1984): 9-20.

41. "Zaire, Ending Secrecy, Attacks AIDS Openly," *New York Times*, 8 February 1987. The results were published as D. Zagury *et al.*, "Immunization Against AIDS in Humans," *Nature* 326 (1987): 249-50. Prior news reports regarding this vaccine trial had appeared: P. Newmark, "First Human AIDS Vaccine Trial Goes Ahead Without Official OK," *Nature* 325 (1987): 290; and, "AIDS Immunization Tested in Humans," *New York Times*, 17 December 1986.

42. "Special SIDA: Des Millions d'Africains condamnés à mort?" *Jeune Afrique Magazine* (February 1987): 87. See also "Who Will Volunteer for an AIDS Vaccine?" *New York Times*, 15 April 1986.

43. A.J. Fortin, "The Politics of AIDS in Kenya," *Third World Quarterly* 9 (1987): 906-19.

44. Indeed, the doctrine of informed consent does not adequately protect research subjects in American society; moreover, the *practice* of informed consent in American society seems often to be so substandard as to not adequately protect research subjects.

45. P. Kunstadter, "Medical Ethics in Cross-Cultural and Multi-Cultural Perspectives," *Social Science and Medicine* 14 (1980): 289-96.

12

Medical Research and the Principle of Respect for Persons in Non-Western Cultures

Carel B. IJsselmuiden and Ruth R. Faden

INTRODUCTION

Should the principle of respect for persons be viewed as morally relative when Western researchers conduct medical research in another cultural setting, or should this principle be regarded as universally valid? And, if its application is to be modified, how should it be changed and who will decide on these changes?

Limiting this discussion to first-person informed consent in cross-cultural research, this paper examines the arguments favoring substantial modifications to the Western notion of informed consent: the obligation to obtain first-person informed consent from competent adult subjects of research. By demonstrating that these arguments are incomplete and deficient and by placing research back in the context of the overall endeavor to improve the human condition, this paper defends the position that Western first-person informed consent requirements should be adhered to in cross-cultural research. If first-person informed consent cannot be obtained for studies where the "unit of measurement" is the individual, then such research should not be undertaken, except in the case of medical or health emergencies.

The obligation of scientists to obtain first-person informed consent from research subjects, grounded in a general moral principle of respect for persons, has developed through philosophical and religious reflection on the scientist-subject relationship, through the medical research establishment in the pursuit of protecting study subjects and, therefore, in the pursuit of a continued societal license to conduct research, and, more recently, through challenges to research practices in courts of law and through consumer activism.[1] Much of this development is recent, occurring in the West, especially in the United States of America, following the proceedings of the Nuremburg trials in the 1940s and the exposure of unethical research practices in the United States in the 1960s and 1970s. Currently, in the Western world, the principle of respect for persons and the practice of first-person informed consent with its well defined component parts have become virtually institutionalized in research practice and government regulation.[2]

Although earlier debates questioned the wisdom and utility of adhering to first-person informed consent requirements by highlighting the deficiencies in their application and the potentially negative influences on opportunities to conduct research,[3] the current debate in the West and elsewhere is now mostly concerned with finding practical mechanisms to increase the meaningfulness of consent obligations in particular contexts, that is, to apply these obligations in ways that will enhance the autonomy of research subjects.[4] It has now become almost unthinkable that these deliberations will ever result in substantial modifications to the practice of first-person informed consent in biomedical research in the West that will reduce patient autonomy.

THE APPLICATION OF FIRST-PERSON INFORMED CONSENT IN CROSS-CULTURAL RESEARCH

Why is it, then, that substantial changes to first-person informed consent requirements are being proposed when discussing the principle of respect for persons in the context of cross-cultural research?[5] When, and in what respects, is a culture sufficiently different from Western culture to warrant modifications? What is the nature of these changes, and who will decide on them? What alternative mechanisms are available to both protect individuals from exploitation by researchers on the one hand and to empower them to choose the possibility of receiving the potential benefits of research on the other? And, lastly, why is it that of the three basic principles in research ethics, respect for persons is specifically targeted for cultural adaptation, whereas justice and beneficence remain unaffected by cultural analysis? In fact, it is the application of the principle of beneficence that underpins most argumentation for modifying first-person informed consent requirements in cross-cultural research. That is, respecting local culture by modifying requirements for first-person informed consent is ultimately considered more beneficial than maintaining Western interpretations of the principle of autonomy.

It would seem inconceivable, for example, to successfully argue for a culturally sensitive interpretation of the principle of beneficence by suggesting that female circumcision be done in clinics rather than by traditional healers. Similarly, in the context of contemporary South Africa, the argument for a culturally relative application of principles of justice would not stand. Why then is there an argument to effect substantial changes to the operational demands of obligations to respect persons?

The answer relies on an explicit or implicit appeal to either moral relativism[6] or to ethical pluralism.[7] The former emphasizes the equality of moral systems and advocates as a consequence that local ethical standards determine what research practices are ethically acceptable in cross-cultural research. Ethical pluralism, on the other hand, seeks to solve conflicts between ethical systems that may occur in transcultural research, by negotiating an optimal ethical practice intermediate between the two positions in particular situations. It demands a re-examination of moral and cultural values held in one society in terms of their relevance to and consonance with another culture. This may result not only in a different emphasis being placed on various moral values, or in a different application of similar moral values; but it is entirely possible that moral reasoning in a different cultural context might lead to substantially different principles, and therefore, to substantially different practices. Both relativism and pluralism rely on a deep understanding of the culture of the research subjects for purposes of adapting Western ethical principles.

The opposite view, that of moral absolutism, holds that at least certain ethical principles, obligations, and commitments are universal. Moral absolutism refers to ethical principles, indicating that practices based on these principles may vary depending on local cultural and ethical expectations. In this sense, absolutism also requires substantial understanding of the locale in which transcultural research is being conducted.

The historical debate on moral absolutism versus moral relativism, and now also pluralism, eludes resolution, certainly in the context of this paper.[8] Accordingly, this paper will defend obligations to honor first-person informed consent requirements in cross-cultural research in two less foundational ways. First, this paper will examine the factual reasoning used in the moral relativist and pluralist views for its validity in arguing that it is permissible to substantially modify Western informed consent requirements in research in certain non-Western cultures. And, second, by formulating the question of first-person informed consent *within* the context of growth and development in non-Western countries, this paper will attempt to demonstrate that there can be no other conclusion than that the Western interpretation of the principle of respect for persons, and its derivative first-person informed consent, in terms of medical research and care, is as valid in Africa and elsewhere in the world as it is in the West.

CHALLENGES TO FIRST-PERSON INFORMED CONSENT IN CROSS-CULTURAL RESEARCH

The challenge to the informed consent process as the major exponent of the ethical principle of respect for persons in medical research centers on the validity of applying this obligation across cultures. Critics defend a culturally sensitive or culturally relevant application of Western medical ethics to research in non-Western settings; while the absence of such cultural relevance is decried as "medical-ethical imperialism."[9]

Intuitively, this reasoning is attractive. It suggests that the researcher is not ethnocentric, that he or she has an appreciation of the good that can be found in non-Western cultures, and that he or she is aware of the potential for damage that can be done by the unquestioned replication of culturally bound practices and principles in another cultural setting. But, intuition by itself is not sufficient to replace a carefully reasoned moral argument.

Cultural sensitivity in the application of obligations to respect autonomy has two distinct interpretations. The first interpretation concludes that first-person informed consent in cross-cultural research is appropriate. The challenge to the researcher in this view is one of making the Western steps of the informed consent process more culturally appropriate, by using local language or dialect, by using locally understandable symbolism, and by respecting local traditions such as informing the village leader of the impending research and, hopefully, of the outcome as well.[10] Cultural sensitivity understood in this way is crucial to respect for individuals and groups, and often to the quality of cross-cultural research being undertaken. In terms of ethical reasoning, such modifications to the practice of informed consent enhance the understanding and decision making ability of study participants, and hence, their autonomy. There can be no problem with this interpretation of cultural sensitivity. In fact, this interpretation should be a norm for the ethical approval of cross-cultural research projects. Even if the result of this process is that a research subject prefers that someone else--such as a husband, relatives, or village leader--make the final decision, the dignity of that person, as well as her or his authority to decide for her- or himself has been acknowledged in important respects.[11]

This is in contrast to a second interpretation of cultural sensitivity that holds that first-person informed consent is in itself inappropriate in non-Western settings where individuality is experienced differently from that in the West. As an alternative, it is suggested that trusted village leaders or even health and government officials may be asked to consent in addition to or on behalf of otherwise competent adults.[12] Where women are assigned a low social status, it is implicitly argued that husbands can consent on behalf of their partners.

The factual arguments given for such substantial modifications of the first-person informed consent process were discussed at length elsewhere.[13] Broadly speaking, three groups of arguments are used to justify substantial modifications to first-person informed consent in cross-cultural medical research: urgency, competency, and culture and anthropology.

URGENCY
The first group of arguments concern the urgency of health problems in developing countries and parallel arguments in favor

of overriding obligations to respect the autonomy of patients in the medical emergency room. The argument of urgency is currently receiving great emphasis in discussions of AIDS vaccine research, much of which will have to be conducted in Africa and elsewhere in the developing world because of the great numbers of study subjects needed to conduct a successful trial and because of the large numbers of AIDS vaccines that will need to be tested.[14]

However, the power of research to improve health problems in the developing world is grossly overrated. Technical solutions to most health problems in the developing world exist, and yet these problems persist and even worsen. The root problem for their continued existence is not the absence of essential medical knowledge, but a poor managerial, economic, and political infrastructure in many countries[15] and a lack of global solidarity.[16] Medical research can do precious little to alleviate this. For example, in the case of AIDS in Africa, the knowledge to greatly reduce its impact exists, but the resources to implement this knowledge are lacking. And, although the World Health Organization has started a discussion with the world's pharmaceutical industries, up to now there is no mechanism or guarantee that an AIDS vaccine will be made available to Africa, not even to countries that participate in trials.[17]

Furthermore, even if research produces positive results that are eventually implemented in the developing world, the time lag between research and implementation of its results is almost always so long that the time saved by by-passing first-person informed consent is negligible. In almost all cross-cultural medical research the argument of urgency is therefore not a sufficient justification for ethical short cuts.[18] Ethical review of research that uses urgency to argue for modification of informed consent requirements should therefore realistically assess the social, economic, and political ability of the study population to act on research findings,[19] not only in non-Western cultures but also in the West.[20] That would probably be a more appropriate interpretation of the concept of cultural sensitivity than modifying Western obligations to respect the autonomy of research subjects.

COMPETENCY

The second argument consists of a confusing appeal to the competency of research subjects in developing countries. Although the term "incompetence" is not invoked directly when referring to subjects in developing countries, it is clear that there are problems related to lack of education, lack of comprehension, lack of a scientific conception of disease, and difficulty in understanding the technical details of the proposed research.[21] For some, this forms the basis for justifying changes to the practice of first-person informed consent akin to the changes that are acceptable in the case of Western research subjects with reduced cognitive capacity.[22]

While it may take considerably more effort to achieve a substantially autonomous decision from persons with different languages, different educational levels, and different conceptions of disease, this argument is in itself not sufficient to warrant substantial changes to the practice of first-person informed consent.[23] Great differences also exist within Western cultures, even within the United States itself, among social classes, among immigrants, migrant workers, and minority groups on the one hand and medical researchers and culturally dominant groups on the other.[24] Yet, no substantial changes to informed consent practices have been proposed for these situations, indicating that differences in culture, itself, are not sufficient reason for changing commitments to basic ethical requirements.

In addition, the competency argument overstates what is required for persons to have an adequate understanding of the implications of participating in research. Research participants can make informed and valid decisions concerning participation based on balancing benefits and risks, without having knowledge about the pathophysiology of the disease in question, or the physics of the procedure being tested.[25] Surely, it cannot be argued successfully that the same person who decides daily on financial, agricultural, educational, and health matters related to herself or himself and her or his family, is not sufficiently sophisticated to decide whether or not to participate in a research study. Invoking a relative incompetency on the basis of culture is not only insulting, it is also a direct challenge to the foundations of the *Nuremburg Code* and the *Declaration of Helsinki*.

In addition, the principle of respect for persons calls for the special protection of those whose ability to decide autonomously is reduced. Even if one were to successfully argue the case for the relative incompetency of otherwise competent adult subjects of research in developing countries, the suggested alternatives to first-person informed consent do not provide the special protection required by the principle of respect for persons. There is no evidence that the best interests of these "incompetent" potential research subjects would be better served by the decisions of husbands, village leaders, or government officials. Nor is there evidence that their decisions constitute a better means of reducing risks or of accepting potential benefits of research than first-person informed consent. The evidence available suggests the opposite: sexual abuse, wife battering, structural discrimination against women, corruption, and abuse of power in non-Western cultures equal, and sometimes exceed, levels experienced in the West.[26] At the same time, research ethics is low on the list of priorities in academic training even in the United States.[27] Scientific fraud by Western researchers has certainly not been eliminated[28] and may even increase in terms of research in developing countries due to the pressure to develop AIDS vaccines,[29] and Western research priorities are not necessarily the same as those from developing countries.[30] Instead of dispensing with first-person informed consent requirements, therefore, we must ensure that through improved communication any obstacles to autonomous decision making are removed, a process which may include the involvement of culturally significant others.

CULTURAL AND ANTHROPOLOGICAL ARGUMENTS

The third argument used is the most profound, and the most difficult to argue. Reasoning from a morally relativist or pluralist position, this argument invokes cultural and anthropological evidence to indicate that a society may be so differently structured from Western society that the practice of first-person informed consent should be modified substantially.[31] As indicated earlier, the alternatives suggested include recruiting consent from husbands, village leaders, or government officials on behalf of, or in addition to that of the prospective research participant. The phrase "in addition to, or on behalf of" is misleading in that "in addition to" automatically becomes "on behalf of" in case the village leader declines to cooperate with the research or intervention. This question is important especially now that the 1991 International Guidelines for Ethical Review of Epidemiological Studies,[32] the August 1992 draft review of the 1981 International Ethical Guidelines for Biomedical Research Involving Human Subjects of the Council for International Organizations of Medical Sciences,[33] and many other papers[34] place an increasing emphasis on the potential benefits of research rather than on the protective function of research ethics. The core of this position is the observation that in some cultures it is accepted that decisions about certain matters are not taken by the individual affected, who is in all other respects a competent person, but by someone else, and that such traditions should be respected by Western researchers. In other words, this interpretation of cultural relevancy gives more weight to the principle of beneficence than to Western operational demands made by respect for autonomy, in that culturally appropriate modifications to the informed consent process are deemed to be ultimately more beneficial for the research subjects and their community than a Western insistence on respect for autonomy. This view will result in a distinctly sexist bias. In most cultures, Western and non-Western, the persons granted decision-making authority over others are male, and the "others," female.

Elsewhere we have argued that the anthropological evidence in support of this view, at least in terms of Africa, is at best fragmented. Often only small, well-defined groups of people have been studied, and most of these studies were conducted in the early and middle part of this century. In spite of their profound influence, little consideration has been given to the impact of education, industrialization, colonialization, urbanization, the enormous warfare that has left no part of Africa, nor many other parts of the non-Western world, untouched, and more lately, the AIDS epidemic on non-Western cultures across the globe.[35] There also is a major discongruence between the drive to be culturally sensitive in research ethics, while at the same time Western cultural features continue to deeply penetrate and alter virtually all other aspects of life. The pictures of "traditional Africa" used in this reasoning are false: they reflect, as Nauta says, performances enacted during visits of heads of state or printed in tourist brochures more than they reflect the lived experiences of real people.[36] Traditional Africa is rapidly disappearing, as are many traditional cultures elsewhere in the world.

Even within a moral relativist or pluralist framework, an appeal grounded on updated and locally relevant anthropological studies is *a minimum requirement* if one wishes to suspend or substantially modify informed consent requirements. Moreover, we would maintain that the supporting evidence for such an appeal must be reviewed by both a local and Western institutional review board before research is undertaken.

Our position has attracted two major criticisms: first, that it is "typically" an ethical imperialist view. This criticism can, of course, not be answered. The second criticism, is that the assessment of contemporary Africa and other developing countries is too sweeping, too generalizing, in that there are still great numbers of rural people who live a "traditional" life.[37] Although we are certainly not alone in our vision of Africa today, we do in fact provide space for a different view, given a disciplined and independent review.[38] However, the debate on numbers or proportions of people still living traditionally does not address the more fundamental questions raised by the anthropological arguments.

The fact that differences in cultures are observed is not in itself a reason to modify the application of the principle of the respect for persons. What the anthropological argument maintains is that there are differences between Western and non-Western cultures. What it should demonstrate further, but fails to do adequately, is that the extent of these differences is sufficiently important to warrant substantial modifications to first-person informed consent, that the character of these differences determines what modifications should be effected, and that there are reasonable alternatives available. It also does not provide guidance on who should decide about these changes.

The ethical pluralist position does not substantially contribute to the question of the applicability of the principle of respect for persons in non-Western cultures.[39] It argues for a casuistic approach towards ethical principles. In terms of this discussion, the pluralist view entertains in principle the possibility that the principle of respect for persons may not be the ultimate outcome of negotiations. As preconditions for sincere ethical negotiations, however, the pluralist view requires a "detailed understanding of the relevant and specific ethical expectations of indigenous people," and argues that the best protection against abuse is for the researchers and subjects to enter these negotiations as equals. Using an equally casuistic approach, however, this chapter has argued that detailed and recent anthropological information is mostly absent, and that the equality between researchers and subjects is rarely, if ever, achieved in the West, let alone in the typical cross-cultural research context of a developed nation conducting research in a developing nation.

Where the ethical pluralist view proposed by Christakis does contribute to the debate is the emphasis on the culturally relevant interpretation of ethical principles, and in terms of this chapter, specifically in the requirements for valid first-person informed consent. For example, the informed consent process in the West is typically concluded with the signing of a consent form, whereas this end point may be nonsensical in a largely illiterate population. On this point, the pluralist view does not differ necessarily from the absolutist view which considers (some) ethical principles as absolute, but does not regard the means by which they are actualized as absolutes.

In practice, even if non-Western scientists are included, usually as a minority group, in achieving a consensus view such as the documents of the Council of International Organizations of Medical Sciences (CIOMS), the decision to suspend partly or in whole the requirements for first-person informed consent will be taken by scientists on behalf of otherwise competent adults, and this decision will be grounded in arguments of cultural differences.[40] It should be obvious that the same anthropological reasoning has formed the justification for the system of apartheid. The anthropological reason for promoting cultural sensitivity in medical research, if taken to mean a substantial modification of the application of the principle of respect for persons, is akin to South Africa's notion of "different but equal," which may very easily lead to a system of ethical apartheid.

RESEARCH AS AN INTEGRAL PART OF DEVELOPMENT

To a large extent the term "non-Western" cultures applies to developing nations. Defining development is difficult, but if one can bypass the images of the large infrastructural projects and economic restructuring, multilateral aid committees and international development organizations, then one can see the basic "unit of development": the individual person. Whereas these large projects, food and development aid programs, and international organizations serve to change the environment in developing countries, it is ultimately individuals who are empowered by these changes to develop to optimal intellectual, human, and social potential. The individual is, therefore, the ultimate purpose of all development efforts, as well as the essential unit that can make or break development efforts.

To increase literacy, for example, adult education facilities and teachers are a necessary but insufficient condition. What is needed in addition is a willingness to learn--an immediate consequence of the level of self-esteem of individuals throughout the world.[41] Respect for autonomy acknowledges this need for self-esteem, while its absence is the basis for what is called the culture of poverty. Recognition of one's worth and of one's value to others and the confidence in one's ability to deal effectively with life's challenges, these are the cornerstones of individual and societal development. These attributes are also the cornerstones for the emancipation of women across the globe, and they form an essential part of the justification of affirmative action programs in the United States and elsewhere. Viewing research in this context, as part of a total strategy for human development rather than as an isolated medical occurrence, makes it nearly impossible to argue that first-person informed consent can be dispensed with in cross-cultural research. Seen in this light, ethical review cannot limit itself to the narrow confines of the specific research project, but must instead see medicine and medical research as a means to an end, an end which will include the full realization of individual potentials. Only in true emergencies where immediate research results have a good chance of reducing human suffering in the short term in the cultural context in which the research is conducted could the case for modifying informed consent practices substantially be argued.

The new International Ethical Guidelines appear less stringent on maintaining the requirements for first-person informed consent than the position just outlined.[42] This is troublesome in that CIOMS works in close collaboration with the World Health Organization, the very organization that initiated the Declaration of Alma Ata, in which health is seen as a basic human right, and in which healthcare is not aimed just at alleviating disease conditions, but also at enhancing the total physical, mental, and social well-being of individuals and communities.[43] Research efforts should not be exempted from this wider view of the promotion of health.[44]

CONCLUSION

The concept of cultural sensitivity is both useful and attractive. It forces researchers engaging in cross-cultural research, at home or abroad, to question some or all of the cultural and moral values that accompany the research efforts in the field. This questioning, when done sincerely and critically, should lead not only to a more appropriate and respectful relationship with persons in other cultures and to a higher quality of research, but also result in a better understanding of one's own values or those of the general or academic society in which one works and lives. It is, however, not cultural sensitivity *per se* that is the topic of this paper. The question addressed here is whether or not the expression--first-person informed consent--of one particular Western moral value--respect for persons--can be substantially modified on the basis of cultural sensitivity or moral relativity.

In addition to the arguments already presented, one more approach to answering this question must be considered. Anthropological concern with cultural imperialism has shown its value past and present, and is often justified. Concern over this issue has helped Westerners to note and appreciate cultural practices and beliefs and has made individuals and societies want to incorporate some of these practices and beliefs to supplement or complement Western culture. However, in regard to informed consent and the principle of respect for persons, anthropology and anthropological research are fundamentally different from medicine and medical research. Not surprisingly, each of these differing approaches is likely to reach different conclusions about the cross-cultural implementation of the principle of respect for persons. It is this difference that is the major cause of the confusion in ethical debates on whether or not to apply Western obligations in non-Western cultures.

Anthropology is concerned with the study of structures and cultures of human beings, often those in non-Western cultures. The aim of anthropological research is the holistic study of human societies: their origins, their development, their social and political organization, their religions, languages, arts, and artifacts.[45] In essence, therefore, anthropology is a descriptive science. Because the main aim of anthropology is to describe what is or was, the notion of changing, intervening, or experimenting with locally held cultural values, including the value of respect for persons, is antithetical to its very nature. A "cultural imperialist" in the anthropological tradition is, therefore, anyone who changes or attempts to change cultural or moral values of another society, *irrespective of the nature of such values.*

The first purpose of medicine and medical research, on the other hand, is to change and to intervene. Medical and epidemiological research attempt to discover what is wrong in individuals or groups with the intention to correct it or to test new interventions. Scientific process in medicine is aimed at increasing the length or the quality of life, or both, and not at describing the body in health or disease *per se.* Medicine is, therefore, interventionist by its very nature. The tools and interventions used in medical research are often, but not exclusively, initially developed in the West. To argue, then, that we should not impose our cultural values in ethical matters when the prime purpose of the presence of medical research in non-Western cultures is to increase health through biological, psychological, social, economic, and political interventions is very hollow reasoning indeed. If, in addition, it can be shown that changes in some cultural values, especially the enhancement of autonomy of persons where cultural norms allocate power unequally, can and will actually increase both the quality and quantity of life--as witnessed by the numerous studies that show a strong relationship between maternal education and infant mortality worldwide,[46] by the mortality experience in Kerala State in India,[47] and by studies relating increased status of women in Turkey to improved child survival[48] --then this hollow reasoning becomes void altogether at least from the perspective of the ethics of medical research, since enhancing life is what medicine is all about.

The debate on the culturally sensitive application of the ethical principle of respect for persons and of the practice of first-person informed consent is, therefore, misplaced within the context of research ethics. Instead, such discussion should focus on the interventionist nature of medicine, medical research, and international medical aid as social phenomena. While this may lead to valid insights, the fact that virtually all cultures in the world have a place for a healing, interventionist profession seems to indicate that the conclusion of this debate is a foregone one.

NOTES

1. R.R. Faden and T.L. Beauchamp, *A History and Theory of Informed Consent* (New York: Oxford University Press, 1986); T.L. Beauchamp and J.F. Childress, *Principles of Biomedical Ethics*, 3d ed. (New York: Oxford University Press, 1989); H.K. Beecher, "Ethics and Clinical Research," *New England Journal of Medicine* 274 (1966): 1354-60; C. Levine, "Has AIDS Changed the Ethics of Human Subject Research?" *Law, Medicine, & Health Care* 16 (1988): 167-73.

2. Faden and Beauchamp, *History and Theory;* Beauchamp and Childress, *Principles of Biomedical Ethics.*

3. F.J. Ingelfinger, "Informed (But Uneducated) Consent," *New England Journal of Medicine* 287 (1972): 465-66; R.L. Katz, "Informed Consent: Is It Bad Medicine?" *Western Journal of Medicine* 126 (1977): 426-8.

4. Faden and Beauchamp, *History and Theory;* Beauchamp and Childress, *Principles of Biomedical Ethics;* Ingelfinger, "Informed (But Uneducated) Consent"; A. Surbone, "Truth Telling to the Patient," *Journal of the American Medical Association* 268 (1992): 1661-62; E.D. Pellegrino, "Is Truth Telling to the Patient a Cultural Artifact?" *Journal of the American Medical Association* 268 (1992): 1734-35.

5. *International Guidelines for Ethical Review of Epidemiological Studies* (Geneva: CIOMS, 1991); *Proposed International Guidelines for Biomedical Research Involving Human Subjects* (Geneva: World Health Organization and CIOMS, 1982); *International Ethical Guidelines for Biomedical Research Involving Human Subjects,* draft document, (Geneva: CIOMS, August 1992); N.A. Christakis, "The Ethical Design of an AIDS Vaccine Trial in Africa," *Hastings Center Report* 18 (June/July 1988): 31-37; C.E. Taylor, "Clinical Trials and International Health Research," *American Journal of Public Health* 69 (1979): 981-83; M. Barry, "Ethical Considerations of Human Investigation in Developing

Countries: the AIDS Dilemma," *New England Journal of Medicine* 319 (1988): 1083-86; R.J. Levine, "Informed Consent: Some Challenges to the Universal Validity of the Western Model," *Law, Medicine & Health Care* 19 (1991): 207-13; M.O.A. Durojaiye, "Ethics of Cross-Cultural Research Viewed from Third World Perspective," *International Journal of Psychology* 14 (1979): 137-41; O.O. Ajayi, "Taboos and Clinical Research in West Africa," *Journal of Medical Ethics* 6 (1980): 61-63; E.O. Ekunwe and R. Kessel, "Informed Consent in the Developing World: Commentary," *Hastings Center Report* 14 (June 1984): 22-24; J.O. Ndinya-Achola, "A Review of Ethical Issues in AIDS Research," *East African Medical Journal* (1991): 735-40; K.S. Jacob and I. Rajan, "Informed Consent in India," *British Journal of Psychiatry* 158 (1991): 576.

6. Christakis, "Ethical Design of an AIDS Vaccine Trial"; Taylor, "Clinical Trials"; Barry, "Ethical Considerations of Human Investigation"; Levine, "Informed Consent: Some Challenges"; P. Kunstadter, "Medical Ethics in Cross-Cultural and Multi-Cultural Perspectives," *Social Science and Medicine* 14B (1980): 289-96; N.A. Christakis, "Letter to the Editor," *Social Science and Medicine* 34 (1992): 589-90; M. Leininger, "Transcultural Care Principles, Human Rights, and Ethical Considerations," *Journal of Transcultural Nursing* 3 (1991): 21-23.

7. N.A. Christakis, "The Distinction Between Ethical Pluralism and Ethical Relativism: Implications for the Conduct of Transcultural Research," Chapter 11 in this volume.

8. *Ibid.*

9. *International Guidelines for Ethical Review of Epidemiological Studies; Proposed International Guidelines for Biomedical Research Involving Human Subjects; International Ethical Guidelines for Biomedical Research Involving Human Subjects;* Christakis, "Ethical Design of an AIDS Vaccine"; Taylor, "Clinical Trials"; Barry, "Ethical Considerations of Human Investigation"; Levine, "Informed Consent: Some Challenges"; Durojaiye, "Ethics of Cross-Cultural Research"; Ajayi, "Taboos"; Ekunwe and Kessel, "Informed Consent in the Developing World"; Ndinya-Achola, "Review of Ethical Issues in AIDS"; Jacob and Rajan, "Informed Consent in India"; Kunstadter, "Medical Ethics in Cross-Cultural Perspectives"; Christakis, "Letter to the Editor"; Leininger, "Transcultural Care Principles."

10. A. Kleinman, "Anthropology and Psychiatry. The Role of Culture in Cross-Cultural Research on Illness," *British Journal of Psychiatry* 151 (1987): 447-54; J. Cassell, "Ethical Principles for Conducting Fieldwork," *American Anthropologist* 82 (1980): 28-41; R.H.L. Feldman and R.B. Hollander, "Issues in Cross-Cultural and International Health Education Research," *Health Education* (November/December 1983):

11-15; L.H. Rogler, "The Meaning of Culturally Sensitive Research in Mental Health," *American Journal of Psychiatry* 146 (1989): 296-303; M. Barry, "Letter to the Editor," *New England Journal of Medicine* 327 (1992): 1103; C.D. Kleymeyer and W.E. Bertrand, "Towards More Ethical and Effective Carrying Out of Applied Research Across Cultural or Class Lines," *Ethics in Science and Medicine* 7 (1980): 11-25.

11. Surbone, "Truth Telling"; Pellegrino, "A Cultural Artifact?"

12. *International Guidelines for Ethical Review of Epidemiological Studies; Proposed International Guidelines for Biomedical Research Involving Human Subjects; International Ethical Guidelines for Biomedical Research Involving Human Subjects;* Christakis, "Ethical Design of an AIDS Vaccine"; Taylor "Clinical Trials"; Durojaiye, "Ethics of Cross-Cultural Research"; Ajayi, "Taboos"; Ekunwe and Kessel, "Informed Consent in the Developing World"; Nidinya-Achola, "Review of Ethical Issues in AIDS"; Jacob and Rajan, "Informed Consent in India"; D.S. LaVertu and A.M. Linares, "Ethical Principles of Biomedical Research on Human Subjects: Their Application and Limitations in Latin America and the Caribbean," *Bulletin of the Pan American Health Organization* 24 (1990): 469-79; A.J. Hall, "Public Health Trials in West Africa: Logistics and Ethics," *IRB : A Review of Human Subjects Research* 11 (September/ October 1989): 8-10.

13. J.M. Last, "Epidemiology and Ethics," *Law, Medicine & Health Care* 19 (1991): 166-74; L. Gostin, "Ethical Principles for the Conduct of Human Subject Research: Population-Based Research and Ethics," *Law, Medicine & Health Care* 19 (1991): 191-201; C.B. IJsselmuiden and R.R. Faden, "Research and Informed Consent in Africa: Another Look," *New England Journal of Medicine* 326 (1992): 830-34; Dr. Adityanjee, "Informed Consent: Issues Involved for Developing Countries," *Medicine, Science, and the Law* 26 (1986): 305-7; C.F. Gilks and J.B.O. Were, "Letter to the Editor," *New England Journal of Medicine* 322 (1990): 200; F. Cabello, "Letter to the Editor," *New England Journal of Medicine* 322 (1990): 200.

14. *International Guidelines for Ethical Review of Epidemiological Studies;* Christakis, "Ethical Design of an AIDS Vaccine"; Barry, "Ethical Considerations of Human Investigation in Developing Countries"; Ndinya-Achola, "Review of Ethical Issues in AIDS Research"; IJsselmuiden and Faden, "Research and Informed Consent in Africa"; W.K. Mariner, "Why Clinical Trials of AIDS Vaccines Are Premature," *American Journal of Public Health* 79 (1989): 86-91; W.C. Koff and D.F. Hoth, "Development and Testing of AIDS Vaccines," *Science* 241 (1988): 426-32; C.O. Tacket and R. Edelman, "Ethical Issues Involving Volunteers in AIDS Vaccine Trials," *Journal of Infectious Diseases* 161

(1990): 356; D.P. Byar *et al.*, "Design Considerations for AIDS Trials," *New England Journal of Medicine* 323 (1990): 1343-48; C.B. IJsselmuiden, "Ethical Aspects of Preventive AIDS Vaccine Development" (paper presented at the Eighth International Conference on AIDS/Third STD World Congress, Amsterdam, The Netherlands, 19-24 July 1992); Z. Bankowski, "Epidemiology, Ethics and 'Health for All,' " *Law, Medicine & Health Care* 19 (1991): 162-63.

15. LaVertu and Linares, "Ethical Principles of Biomedical Research"; IJsselmuiden and Faden, "Research and Informed Consent in Africa"; S. Naipaul, *North of South: An African Journey* (New York: Penguin Books, 1980); R.H. Henderson, "The Expanded Programme on Immunization of the World Health Organization," *Reviews of Infectious Diseases* 6 supplement 2 (1984): 475-79.

16. J. Mann, D.J. Tarantola, and T.W. Netter, *AIDS in the World* (Cambridge: Harvard University Press, 1992).

17. "WHO, Pharmaceutical Industry Unite against AIDS," *Global AIDS News* no.1 (1992): 7.

18. IJsselmuiden and Faden, "Research and Informed Consent in Africa."

19. K.S. Khan, "Epidemiology and Ethics: The People's Perspective," *Law, Medicine & Health Care* 19 (1991): 202-6; F. Carbello, "Letter to the Editor," *New England Journal of Medicine* 322 (1990): 200.

20. S.B. Thomas and S. Crouse-Quinn, "The Tuskegee Syphilis Study, 1932 to 1972: Implications for HIV Education and AIDS Risk Education Programs in the Black Community," *American Journal of Public Health* 81 (1991): 1498-1505.

21. Christakis, "Ethical Design of an AIDS Vaccine"; Barry, "Ethical Considerations of Human Investigation in Developing Countries"; Ajayi, "Taboos"; Ekunwe and Kessel, "Informed Consent in the Developing World"; Ndinya-Achola, "Review of Ethical Issues in AIDS Research"; LaVertu and Linares, "Ethical Principles of Biomedical Research"; IJsselmuiden and Faden, "Research and Informed Consent in Africa"; E.M. Ankrah, "AIDS: Methodological Problems in Studying Its Prevention and Spread," *Social Science and Medicine* 29 (1989): 265-76.

22. *Proposed International Guidelines for Biomedical Research Involving Human Subjects;* Christakis, "Ethical Design of an AIDS Vaccine"; Ajayi, "Taboos"; Ekunwe and Kessel, "Informed Consent in the Developing World"; Ndinya-Achola, "Review of Ethical Issues in AIDS Research"; Jacob and Rajan, "Informed Consent in India"; LaVertu and Linares, "Ethical Principles of Biomedical Research."

23. Cassel, "Ethical Principles for Conducting Fieldwork"; Feldman and Hollander, "Issues in Cross-Cultural and International Health

Education"; IJsselmuiden and Faden, "Research and Informed Consent in Africa"; M. Angell, "Ethical Imperialism? Ethics in International Collaborative Clinical Research," *New England Journal of Medicine* 319 (1988): 1081-83.

24. IJsselmuiden and Faden, "Research and Informed Consent in Africa"; Thomas and Crouse-Quinn, "The Tuskegee Syphilis Study"; M.R. Gillick, "Common-Sense Models of Health and Disease," *New England Journal of Medicine* 313 (1985): 700-3; M. Susser, W. Watson, and K. Hopper, *Sociology in Medicine*, 3d ed. (New York: Oxford University Press, 1985); A. Dula, "Toward an African-American Perspective on Bioethics," *Journal of Health Care for the Poor and Underserved* 2 (1991): 259-69; W. El-Sadr and L. Capps, "The Challenge of Minority Recruitment in Clinical Trials for AIDS," *Journal of the American Medical Association* 267 (1992): 954-57.

25. Faden and Beauchamp, *History and Theory;* Beauchamp and Childress, *Principles of Biomedical Ethics;* IJsselmuiden and Faden, "Research and Informed Consent in Africa"; D. Brahams, "Randomised Trials and Informed Consent," *Lancet,* no. ii (1988): 1033-34.

26. LaVertu and Linares, "Ethical Principles of Biomedical Research"; Naipaul, *North of South;* A. Gürsoy-Tezcan, "Infant Mortality: A Turkish Puzzle?" *Health Transition Review* 2 (1992): 131-49; M. De Bruyn, "Women and AIDS in Developing Countries," *Social Science and Medicine* 34 (1992): 249-62; E.M. Ankrah, "AIDS and the Social Side of Health," *Social Science and Medicine* 32 (1991): 967-80; A. Raikes, "Women's Health in East Africa," *Social Science and Medicine* 28 (1989): 447-59.

27. P.J. Friedman, "Research Ethics: A Teaching Agenda for Academic Medicine," *Academic Medicine,* 65, no. 1 (1990): 32-33.

28. Christakis, "Letter to the Editor"; Christakis, "The Distinction Between Ethical Pluralism and Ethical Relativism"; Dula, "Toward an African-American Perspective"; M.F. Shapiro and R.P. Charrow, "Scientific Misconduct in Investigational Drug Trials," *New England Journal of Medicine* 312 (1985): 731-36; P. Kiatboonsri and J. Richter, "Letter to the Editor," *Lancet,* no. ii (1988): 1491; T. Greenhalgh, "Drug Marketing in the Third World: Beneath the Cosmetic Reforms," *Lancet,* no. i (1986): 1318-20; G. Gillet, "NZ after Cartwright," *British Medical Journal* 300 (1990): 893-94; D.J. Rothman, "Ethics and Human Experimentation: Henry Beecher Revisited," *New England Journal of Medicine* 317 (1987): 1195-99; C. Joyce, "Congress Slams Misconduct in Medical Research," *New Scientist* (15 September 1990): 21; C. Marwick, "NIH Collaboration with French AIDS Vaccine Researcher Put on Hold Pending Investigation," *Journal of the American Medical Association* 265 (1991): 2648-49.

29. IJsselmuiden, "Ethical Aspects of Preventive AIDS Vaccine Development."

30. D. Serwadda and E. Katongole-Mbidde, "AIDS in Africa: Problems for Research and Researchers," *Lancet* 335 (1990): 842-43.

31. *International Guidelines for Ethical Review of Epidemiological Studies; Proposed International Guidelines for Biomedical Research Involving Human Subjects; International Ethical Guidelines for Biomedical Research Involving Human Subjects;* Christakis, "Ethical Design of an AIDS Vaccine"; Taylor, "Clinical Trials"; Durojaiye, "Ethics of Cross-Cultural Research"; Ajayi, "Taboos"; Ekunwe and Kessel, "Informed Consent in the Developing World"; Ndinya-Achola, "Review of Ethical Issues in AIDS Research"; Jacob and Rajan, "Informed Consent in India"; LaVertu and Linares, "Ethical Principles of Biomedical Research"; Hall, "Public Health Trials"; Last, "Epidemiology and Ethics."

32. *International Guidelines for Ethical Review of Epidemiological Studies.*

33. *International Ethical Guidelines for Biomedical Research Involving Human Subjects.*

34. Last, "Epidemiology and Ethics"; Gostin, "Principles for the Conduct of Human Subject Research."

35. IJsselmuiden and Faden, "Research and Informed Consent in Africa."

36. L. Nauta, "Afrika bestaat niet (Africa does not exist)," *Nieuw Wereld Tijdschrift* no. 1 (1985): 71-80.

37. N.A. Christakis and R.C. Fox, "Informed Consent in Africa," *New England Journal of Medicine* 327 (1992): 1101-2.

38. De Bruyn, "Women and AIDS"; Ankrah, "AIDS and the Social Side of Health"; Raikes, "Women's Health in East Africa"; Nauta, "Afrika bestaat niet"; G. Seidel, "The Competing Discourses of HIV/AIDS in Sub-Saharan Africa: Discourses of Rights and Empowerment Vs Discourses of Control and Exclusion," *Social Science and Medicine* 36 (1993): 175-94; B.G. Schoepf, "Ethical, Methodological and Political Issues of AIDS Research in Central Africa," *Social Science and Medicine* 33 (1991): 749-63.

39. Christakis, "The Distinction Between Ethical Pluralism and Ethical Relativism."

40. *International Guidelines for Ethical Review of Epidemiological Studies; Proposed International Guidelines for Biomedical Research Involving Human Subjects; International Ethical Guidelines for Biomedical Research Involving Human Subjects.*

41. Khan, "Epidemiology and Ethics"; Gursoy-Tezcan, "Infant Morality"; De Bruyn, "Women and AIDS"; Ankrah, "AIDS and the Social

Side of Health"; Raikes, "Women's Health in East Africa"; R. Chambers, *Rural Development: Putting the Last First*, 4th ed. (New York: Longman, 1985); A. Hope and S. Timmel, *Training for Transformation. A Handbook for Community Workers.* Parts 1, 2, 3. (Gweru Zimbabwe: Mambo Press, 1984).

42. *International Guidelines for Ethical Review of Epidemiological Studies; International Ethical Guidelines for Biomedical Research Involving Human Subjects.*

43. Alma-Ata. *Primary Health Care* (Geneva: World Health Organization, 1978).

44. IJsselmuiden and Faden, "Research and Informed Consent in Africa"; Khan, "Epidemiology and Ethics"; Carbello, "Ethical Imperialism"; Schoepf, "Methodological and Political Issues."

45. D. Jary and J. Jary, eds. *Collins Dictionary of Sociology* (Glasgow: Harper Collins, 1991), 24; C.G. Helman, *Culture, Health and Illness,* 2d ed. (Oxford: Butterworth-Heinemann, 1990), 1-10.

46. De Bruyn, "Women and AIDS"; Ankrah, "AIDS and the Social Side of Health"; Raikes, "Women's Health in East Africa"; *Strategies for Children in the 1990's* (New York: UNICEF, 1989); "Infant Mortality," *Lancet,* no. ii (1988): 1117-18; J. DaVanzo, "Infant Mortality and Socioeconomic Development: Evidence from Malaysian Household Data," *Demography* 25 (1988): 581-95; J.G. Cleland and J.K. Van Ginneken, "Maternal Education and Child Survival in Developing Countries: The Search for Pathways of Influence," *Social Science and Medicine* 27 (1988): 1357-68; O.B. Ahmad, I.W. Eberstein, and D.F. Sly, "Proximate Determinants of Child Mortality in Liberia," *Journal of Biosocial Science* 23 (1991): 313-26; G.A. Oni, "Child Mortality in a Nigerian City: Its Levels and Socioeconomic Differentials," *Social Science and Medicine* 27 (1988): 607-14; P. Dev Pant, "Effect of Education and Household Characteristics in Urban Nepal," *Journal of Biosocial Science* 23 (1991): 437-43; A. Stein, *et al.,* "Social Adversity, Low Birth Weight, and Preterm Delivery," *British Medical Journal* 295 (1987): 291-93; *Rural Women's Participation in Development, Evaluation Study No. 3* (New York: United Nations Development Programme, 1980), paragraph 609.

47. J. Ratcliffe, "Social Justice and the Demographic Transition: Lessons from India's Kerala State," in *Practising Health for All,* ed. D. Morley, J.E. Rohde and G. Williams (Oxford: Oxford University Press, 1983), 64-82.

48. Gursoy-Tezcan, "Infant Mortality"; B. Aksit and B. Aksit, "Sociocultural Determinants of Infant and Child Mortality in Turkey," *Social Science and Medicine* 28 (1989): 571-76.

PART IV

Critical Issues in Specialized Areas

Introduction to Part IV

Harold Y. Vanderpool

Each of the authors in this section explores ethical issues pertaining to a specialized arena of clinical research. A number of these issues have been debated extensively, yet remain controversial. Some of them represent critical items on an agenda of concerns that await thorough-going analysis, resolution, and policy formation.

In Chapters 13 and 14, Benjamin Freedman and William G. Bartholome critically examine the ethics of cancer and pediatric research respectively. Their probing analyses focus on how the ethical principles discussed in *The Belmont Report* should be understood and put into practice.[1] Freedman refutes the assumption that the influence and applicability of *Belmont's* principles are already realized. Bartholome shows why the work of the National Commission and existing U.S. federal regulations are "nothing more than a good beginning" for exploring the ethics of research with children.[2]

In Chapters 15 and 16, Constance M. Pechura and Eric T. Juengst identify dimensions of philosophical and ethical inquiry that are not addressed in *The Belmont Report* nor in international codes and guidelines. The ethical issues inherent to research involving fetal tissue, fetuses, and embryos discussed by Pechura include questions about the nature and value of human personhood, as well as foreboding questions about the boundaries between humans and other animals. The issues surrounding genome research discussed by Juengst raise knotty questions about how researchers should respect, protect, and benefit families and communities, not just individuals. Whether and when these issues will become settled enough to be framed as general ethical guidelines remain open questions.[3]

Altogether, these authors display the value of exploring the ethics of human subjects' research in light of a thorough understanding of the science and technological capabilities of medical specializations.[4] The principles of research ethics and the powers invested in IRBs call for public scrutiny of and levels of compliance from clinical researchers. At times, researchers have viewed this scrutiny and required compliance as burdensome interferences to therapeutic advancements within their specializations.[5] In the face of criticisms from researcher colleagues, some IRBs have shirked their responsibilities or become overly authoritarian in relation to their investigator colleagues.[6] To exercise their roles and responsibilities effectively, ethicists and IRBs must both thoroughly understand research ethics and regulations and intimately understand the practices and goals of clinical specializations.[7] This section's authors display how these bodies of knowledge must be symbiotically related.

LESSONS FROM CANCER RESEARCH

Freedman's closely-argued essay contains valuable insights and challenges for ethicists and members of IRBs. Viewing cancer research as a model for understanding the ethics of clinical trials generally, Freedman explores several crucial topics: how cancer research led to the development of many of the standard features of contemporary clinical trials; how present-day cancer trials are predictive of many of the changes that are and will be occurring in other fields of research; what contemporary, *Belmont*-based ethical and regulatory oversight usually consists of; and how the ethical principles of *The Belmont Report* call for a far more extensive set of concerns than is presently realized.

Historically, many discussions of research ethics were, in fact, centered on cancer research.[8] Discussions included debates over randomized trials versus nonrandomized studies, the nature of informed consent when diagnosis is disturbing, researchers' conflicts of interest, research with children, and extensive discussions of the ethics of Phase I cancer trials.[9] Still unsettled, the ethics of Phase I cancer trials is discussed by Freedman, who suggests how truly informed consent for these trials should be worded on consent forms.

Freedman's discussion of the normal research ethics of contemporary IRBs succinctly portrays how many review committees conceive their roles and functions. His discussion highlights the virtues and limits of these roles and indicates how they have been shaped and delimited by *The Belmont Report's* legacy of crafting research ethics in response to historic abuses of research subjects.[10]

The final section of Freedman's essay outlines a provocative vision of an innovative and comprehensive approach to the ethics of clinical research. Freedman's approach is deduced from ethical principles embedded in *The Belmont Report*, but advances beyond the report's focus and delimited applications.[11] The challenge of his analysis does not involve new ethical principles nor a more complete understanding of the aims and practices of clinical oncology. Its challenge emerges from probing questions about matters that are often taken for granted--the design of clinical trials and the assumptions upon which they are predicated.[12]

PEDIATRIC RESEARCH

William G. Bartholome's essay is an enduring contribution to the ethics of research with children. His essay should be read by all who are responsible for reviewing and approving pediatric research, who want to become acquainted with the most recent literature, and who hope to publish in the field. The two decades of debate charted by Bartholome parallel the years of his own training, research, and teaching in medical and pediatric ethics. This background enables him to bring to life the ethical concerns that were first voiced by Paul Ramsey,[13] to display the core problems in pediatric research ethics that have evolved over time,[14] to evaluate contemporary discussions from the vantage point of this in-depth perspective,[15] to illustrate how his ethical principles apply to a controversial research initiative, and to forecast future ethical agendas.

Bartholome critically assesses present U.S. federal regulations as failing to incorporate several of the concerns voiced by members of the National Commission (upon which the regulations were based) and as needing to take into account key developments in the ethics of pediatric research since the regulations were formulated.[16] His probing exploration of the ambiguities and easily misunderstood minimal risk standard stipulated in and invoked throughout the federal regulations is as relevant to human subjects' research generally as it is crucial to the categories of pediatric research delineated in federal regulations.[17] Bartholome uses stories and cases to illustrate why degrees of risk and harm faced in research should be determined according to what children of different ages ordinarily experience--a perspective that Bartholome believes can dramatically change minimal risk assessments in pediatric research.

Bartholome's discussion of assent is critical for pediatric research and highly relevant to other research arenas. For pediatric research, assent became and remains the focal point that links the ethical principles of respecting children as developing moral agents and of not harming them psychologically to new understandings of their cognitive and emotional development. Bartholome's discussion of assent--its four elements, questions researchers should ask, answers suited to the child-subject's perspective, and so on--serves as a model of candor, clarity of communication, and researcher-subject honesty that contributes to discussions of the informed consent process.[18]

FETAL TISSUE, FETAL, AND EMBRYOLOGICAL RESEARCH

The chapter by Constance M. Pechura contains a book-length set of timely and controversial topics. Pechura begins with a historical overview of federal and nongovernmental initiatives since the early 1970s, then surveys the current science, regulations, and ethical issues surrounding research in three specialty areas: human fetal tissue, fetuses, and embryos. Predicated on her insider's understanding of past, present, and expected scientific developments in each of these areas, Pechura identifies the complex ethical questions at stake, shows why they are politically contentious, and indicates how they will demand conceptual attention and organizational leadership in years to come.

Biomedical research in each of these areas occurs on--or perhaps, more accurately, intrudes upon--the turf of long-standing theological and philosophical traditions. Like their counterparts in other parts of the world, Western traditions of Jewish, Christian, and secular thought comprise understandings of the world that include overarching visions of human origins, worth, and destiny, as well as directives regarding human sexuality and procreation. These traditions are perpetuated by historically shaped and like-minded social groups, through which persons secure self-identity and measures of comfort and certitude.[19] To heighten their sense of security and certitude, secular and religious groups vie for social power. Their struggle for public and political influence encompasses at least three major medical ethics issues: euthanasia, abortion, and, most recently, fetal and embryological research.[20]

As Pechura indicates, the ideological and political ferment over abortion adds to the polarization of opinion over the ethics of fetal and embryological research. While some authors regard fetal tissue research as by and large forbidden because it is morally tainted by the evil of abortion,[21] others, who view early stage abortions as morally permissible under various circumstances, regard this research as offering great promise in the human conquest over debilitating disease.[22]

Much of the controversy over abortion and research involving fetuses, fetal tissue, and embryos revolves around assessments of the moral status of the human embryo and fetus. Those who believe that a human being's life begins at conception are ardently opposed to research on embryos that are created for research purposes, to most fetal tissue research, and to any fetal research that is not expressly designed to sustain and improve the life and health of the fetuses involved.[23] Those who assign moral status to the fetus depending upon its stage of development (for example, its brain functions) or its capacity for consciousness and social interaction generally welcome much of the research Pechura explores.[24] Those who welcome such research nevertheless argue that limits should be placed on scientific advancements and techniques that are possible, but ethically and socially problematic--for example, transplanting human embryos into other species or creating embryos from the immature eggs of aborted fetuses, then implanting them in mature women for the purpose of bearing children.[25]

The U.S. federal guidelines for these areas of research are found in Subpart B of the *Code of Federal Regulations*. Pechura charts how, in the absence of an ethical advisory board (which, according to these regulations, should have been convened to approve federally funded research in these areas),[26] nongovernmental organizations set forth guidelines for the conducting of *in vitro* fertilization and embryo research and also fund its major research initiatives. Recent rulings at the federal level now permit IRBs to review and approve human *in vitro* fertilization research without prior review by an ethical advisory board, as well as review and approve federally funded research that uses human fetal tissue derived from induced abortions.[27] Additional discussions of the ways the Department of Health and Human Services' *Code of Federal Regulations* should be understood and applied are provided by Robert J. Levine and the Office for Protection from Research Risks (OPRR).[28] Robert J. Levine and John C. Fletcher have critically examined the views of and exchanges between the members of the National Commission, upon whose recommendations the federal *Code's* regulations were drafted.[29]

GENOME RESEARCH

Eric T. Juengst's analysis of genome research serves as a fitting finale to the discussions of the authors in this volume. Genome research, (1) raises ethical questions that call for creative applications of the ethical principles of *The Belmont Report* and for ethical reflection beyond the limits of *Belmont*; (2) involves research that is increasingly cross-cultural and international; (3) intersects with a number of the ethical and regulatory issues over research with children and with human embryos; and, as evident throughout Juengst's essay; (4) generates an agenda of issues with respect to ethical analysis and policy formation that will require attention well into the 21st century.

Juengst's essay centers around two aspects of genetics research involving human subjects--the identifying and deciphering of genes generated by the Human Genome Project (HGP) and, by extension, a second and older tradition of studying the natural history of inherited diseases or conditions--commonly called pedigree research. Two additional areas of genetics research with human subjects include research on genetic testing and gene therapy research. While all four of these areas share a common set of ethical problems and concerns, each also raises a particular set of pressing ethical and policy-related issues.[30]

Having served for a number of years as the Chief of the HGP's Ethical, Legal and Social Implications (ELSI) Branch, Juengst is uniquely equipped to propose a policy agenda for the ethics and regulation of human genetics linkage studies. Established in the late 1980s, the Genome Project will likely alter human self-understanding, as well as give rise to diagnostic and treatment modalities for numerous diseases and disorders--conditions that are both "gene caused" and that, as multifactorial maladies, include genetic components.[31] At its outset, the HGP was recognized as so laden with worrisome ethical, legal, and social concerns that 5 percent of its budget was targeted towards exploring these concerns.[32]

Juengst displays how the numerous and intersecting ethical issues raised by genome research have not yet been formulated into national regulatory guidelines.[33] His proposed policy-making agenda is set forth in the form of 10 questions extracted from the rapidly-expanding literature, as well as from the practical experiences and policies of major institutional centers conducting human genetics research. Throughout, his essay reflects how the older wineskins of respecting individuals as autonomous agents cannot entirely hold the new wine of family dynamics and family-relatedness harvested from genome research.[34] A second and interrelated issue involves the degrees to which the historically "minimal risk" character of blood drawing and gathering data from patients' medical records are, in the context of genetics research, replete with high risks of psychological and social harm that are only beginning to be fully appreciated.[35]

NOTES

1. *The Belmont Report* is printed as Appendix C of this book, and the meaning and import of its ethical principles are debated throughout Part I of the present volume.

2. An overview of the work of the National Commission for the Protection of Human Subjects of Biomedical and Behavioral Research (1974-1978) is given by Fletcher and Miller in Chapter 7 of the present volume under the subheading, "Government as Proactive Advocate of Public Bioethics (1973-1983)."

3. The background commentary on the 1993 *CIOMS/WHO International Ethical Guidelines* notes that

> Certain areas of research do not receive special mention in these guidelines; they include human genetic research, embryo and fetal research, and fetal tissue research. These represent research areas in rapid evolution and in various respects controversial. The Steering Committee considered that since there is not universal agreement on all the ethical issues raised by these research areas it would be premature to try to cover them in the present guidelines.

Council for International Organizations of Medical Sciences (CIOMS), *International Ethical Guidelines for Biomedical Research Involving Human Subjects* (Geneva: CIOMS, 1993), 7. See Appendix F for *The CIOMS/ WHO International Ethical Guidelines*.

4. A selective number of sociological studies have displayed the intricate, unique, and fascinating dynamics of clinical specialties. See the classic study of surgery by C.L. Bosk, *Forgive and Remember* (Chicago: University of Chicago Press, 1972), and the sobering analysis of Robert Zussman, *Intensive Care: Medical Ethics and the Medical Profession* (Chicago: University of Chicago Press, 1992). Also helpful are inside accounts of medical specialization and training, e.g., D. Light, *Becoming Psychiatrists* (New York: W.W. Norton, 1980). For a discussion of research ethics and the values of oncologists, see H.Y. Vanderpool, "The Ethics of Clinical Experimentation with Anticancer Drugs," in *Cancer Treatment and Research in Humanistic Perspective*, ed. S. C. Gross and S. Garb (New York: Springer, 1985), 16-46.

5. See the early, critical article by V.T. DeVita, "The Evolution of Therapeutic Research in Cancer, *New England Journal of Medicine* 298 (1978): 907-10; and the letter reply by A.R. Jonsen, "Therapeutic Research in Cancer," *New England Journal of Medicine* 299 (1978): 259.

6. For a thoughtful discussion on the images, functions, and status of IRBs in medical centers, see R.J. Levine, *Ethics and Regulation of Clinical Research*, 2nd ed. (Baltimore: Urban and Schwarzenberg, 1986), 341-57.

7. The challenge of fulfilling these tasks is met only in part by a diversity of membership within review committees--as is required by the

U.S. *Code of Federal Regulations* at section 46.107. These regulations are found in Appendix D of this book.

8. A comprehensive and annotated bibliography of cancer research from 1966 to 1983 is found within G.B. Weiss and H.Y. Vanderpool, *Ethics and Cancer: An Annotated Bibliography* (Galveston: University of Texas Medical Branch, 1984). See also the informative historical study by James T. Patterson, *The Dread Disease: Cancer and Modern American Culture* (Cambridge: Harvard University Press, 1987).

9. Freedman argues that cancer research was the forerunner of logical, phase-staging in other areas of research, and he defines these phases. Annex II of the CIOMS/WHO International Ethical Guidelines views these phases as standard for all drug-development trials.

10. Vignettes of notable chapters in this history of abuses are given in Chapter 1, pp. 4-10 of this book. See also Fletcher and Miller, Chapter 7, pp. 159-60 of this book.

11. The third paragraph of Section B (Basic Ethical Principles) part 2 (Beneficence) of *The Belmont Report* voices a number of the ethical concerns of Freedman, but the import of this paragraph vis à vis Freedman's vision is absent from the report's discussion of how beneficence ought to be applied to the design and review of research protocols (section C.2). For additional comments on Freedman's contributions to the debates over the ethics of *The Belmont Report*, see the subsection entitled "The Purview of IRBs" in this volume's "Introduction to Part I."

12. Freedman adds a third dimension to the expertise IRBs need for fully responsible and effective protocol review: (1) an understanding of research ethics and regulations in relation to, (2) understanding the practices and goals of clinical specializations (both discussed above) and (3) expertise in clinical research trial design.

13. P. Ramsey, *The Patient As Person* (New Haven: Yale University Press, 1970), Chapter 1: "Consent as a Canon of Loyalty with Special Reference to Children in Medical Investigations." For perspectives on Ramsey's role in the emergence of medical ethics, see D.J. Rothman, *Strangers at the Bedside* (New York: Basic Books, 1991), 95-100.

14. Bartholome focuses on contributions to the ethics of clinical research with children beginning in the 1970s and especially since 1983 (when the U.S. federal regulations regarding children went into effect). For a historical overview of experiments with children, see S.E. Lederer and M.A. Grodin, "Historical Overview: Pediatric Experimentation," in *Children as Research Subjects: Science, Ethics, and Law*, ed. M.A. Grodin and L.H. Glantz (New York: Oxford University Press, 1994), 3-25.

15. For example, M.A. Grodin and L.H. Glantz, eds., *Children as Research Subjects: Science, Ethics and Law.*

16. These regulations are printed in subpart D of Appendix D of this book. See also the discussion by R.J. Levine, *Ethics and Regulation of Clinical Research,* 2nd ed. (Baltimore: Urban and Schwarzenberg, 1986), 235-56. Levine carefully reviews the recommendations of the National Commission and offers numerous suggestions and examples on how the commission's points can be put into practice. In contrast to Levine, Bartholome accents the degrees to which the commission's recommendations were not enacted into the federal regulations--a loss to IRBs that do not conduct their deliberations with the commission's recommendations in hand.

17. These regulations define "minimal risk" of research conducted with human subjects as meaning that "the probability and magnitude of harm or discomfort anticipated in the research are not greater in and of themselves than those ordinarily encountered in daily life or during the performance of routine physical or psychological examinations or tests." (45 *CFR* 46.102.(i)). In the U.S. federal regulations this standard is used as one of the justifications for expedited review (45 *CFR* 46.110 (b) (1)), the altering or waiving of informed consent (45 *CFR* 46.116 (d) (1)) or a signed consent form (45 *CFR* 46.117 (c) (2)); and it is invoked throughout the regulations regarding research with children subjects-- e.g., 45 *CFR* 46.404, 405, and 406.

18. The ethical principles and virtues of Bartholome's discussion parallel a number of the ideals of Jay Katz, who, in contrast to Bartholome's optimism vis à vis assent, views obtaining "morally valid consent" as "inordinately difficult" and time consuming. J. Katz, "Human Experimentation and Human Rights," *Saint Louis University Law Journal* 38 (Fall, 1993), 7-54, esp. 34-38. Bartholome's understanding of assent is also highly useful for adults with diminished cognitive abilities.

19. For an analysis of these world views in relation to euthanasia and the sustaining of life, see H.Y. Vanderpool, "Death and Dying: Euthanasia and Sustaining Life: Historical Aspects," in *Encyclopedia of Bioethics,* revised ed., (New York: Simon & Schuster Macmillan, 1995), 554-63. Interrelationships between Western and non-Western religious traditions and medical theory and practice are explored in R.L. Numbers and D.W. Amundsen, eds. *Caring and Curing: Health and Medicine in the Western Religious Traditions* (New York: Macmillan, 1986); and L.E. Sullivan, ed. *Healing and Restoring: Health and Medicine in the World's Religious Traditions* (New York: Macmillan, 1989). Each of the authors in these volumes deals with a specific religious tradition and often discusses the tradition's view(s) of human sexuality and the beginnings of life.

20. For political controversies over research ethics and the influence of abortion in these controversies, see the discussion of Fletcher and Miller in Chapter 7 of this book. A succinct discussion of abortion "as a graphic cultural symbol" in group struggles over social hegemony is in H.Y. Vanderpool, "Abortion in Texas: Legal Enactments, Religious Traditions, and Social Hegemony," in *Personal Choices and Public Commitments: Perspectives on the Medical Humanities,* ed. W.J. Winslade (Galveston: Institute for the Medical Humanities, 1988), 129-47. The news media often hypes and polarizes intercultural controversy over abortion, euthanasia, and fetal/embryological research. For an aspect of embryological research, see, for example, P. Elmer-Dewitt, "Cloning: Where Do We Draw the Line?" *Time,* 8 November 1993, 1, 3, and 64-70.

21. J.T. Burtchaell, "Case Study: University Policy on Experimental Use of Aborted Fetal Tissue," *IRB: A Review of Human Subjects Research* 10 (July/August 1988): 7-11; and J.T. Burtchaell, "The Use of Aborted Fetal Tissue in Research: A Rebuttal," *IRB: A Review of Human Subjects Research* 10 (March/April 1989): 9-12.

22. J.A. Robertson, "Fetal Tissue Transplant Research is Ethical," *IRB: A Review of Human Subjects Research* 10 (November/December 1988): 5-8; and J.C. Fletcher, "Human Fetal and Embryo Research: Lysenkoism in Reverse--How and Why?" in *Emerging Issues in Biomedical Policy,* ed. R.H. Blank and A.L. Bonnicksen (New York: Columbia University Press, 1993), 200-31.

23. The historical and theological underpinnings for this perspective are charted by J.T. Noonan, Jr., "An Almost Absolute Value in History," in *The Morality of Abortion,* ed. J.T. Noonan, Jr. (Cambridge: Harvard University Press, 1970), 1-59. Examples of popular opinion and rhetoric are referenced in note 20 above.

24. See note 22 above and the discussions of J. Areen, "Limiting Procreation," and L. Walters, "Genetics and Reproductive Technologies," in *Medical Ethics,* ed. R.M. Veatch (Boston: Jones and Bartlett, 1989), 93-124 and 201-28. Walters briefly explores the varying assumptions regarding either the naturalness or artificiality of recently emerging scientific technologies. He indicates how various authors and schools of opinion associate human dignity with an anti-technological point of view, a pro-technological point of view, or a view that mediates between the two. See also the article by Julian N. Hartt, "Images of Man," in *Encyclopedia of Bioethics,* ed. W.T. Reich (New York: Free Press, 1978), 851-57.

25. A compendium of viewpoints on these and other matters is found in "United States and Canada Decide to Slow Down Human

Reproduction Research," *Hospital Ethics* (January/February 1994), 10-12.

26. See Appendix D of this book at 45 *CFR* 46.204 (d) for this provision, and note 27 for its nullification. See also the discussion of Fletcher and Miller, Chapter 7, pp. 161-66 of this book.

27. Section 204 (d) of 46 *CFR* 45 (that required human *in vitro* research to be reviewed by a federally constituted ethical advisory board) was nullified 1 June, 1994--as specified by a ruling published in the *Federal Register* 59 (1 June 1994): 28276. Provisions that allow for human fetal tissue transplantation research (following the ending of a five-year moratorium of such research by a directive from President Clinton on 22 January 1993) were published in the *Federal Register* 58 (30 August 1993): 45495-96.

28. R.J. Levine, *Ethics and Regulation of Clinical Research*, 297-320; OPRR, *Protecting Human Research Subjects* (Washington, D.C.: U.S. Government Printing Office, 1993), 6-2 to 6-10.

29. Levine, *Ethics and Regulation of Clinical Research*, 297-308; and Fletcher, "Human Fetal and Embryo Research," 204-12.

30. These four areas or stages of genetics research are delineated in OPRR, *Protecting Human Research Subjects*, section H: Human Genetic Research," 5-42 through 5-63, which discusses the ethical problems they raise and contains recommendations for IRB review. This discussion was added as a new section to the OPRR's 1993 *Guidebook*.

31. E.P. Hoffman, "The Evolving Genome Project: Current and Future Impact," *American Journal of Human Genetics* 54 (1994): 129-36; and the Office of Technology Assessment, *Mapping Our Genes* (Washington, DC: Congress of the United States, 1988), esp. 55-78, ("Applications to Research in Biology and Medicine"). An overview of changing concepts of disease from the 1820s to the present is provided by H.Y. Vanderpool, "Changing Concepts of Disease and the Shaping of Contemporary Preventive Medicine," in *Preventive Medicine and Community Health*, ed. A.W. Domeck (Galveston: University of Texas Medical Branch, 1983), 7-34. For discussions of disease and health as value-laden human constructs, see *Concepts of Health and Disease: Interdisciplinary Perspectives*, ed. A.L. Caplan *et al.* (Reading, Mass.: Addison-Wesley, 1981).

32. Office of Technology Assessment, *Mapping Our Genes*, 79-89; D.J. Kevles and L. Hood, eds., *The Code of Codes: Scientific and Social Issues in the Human Genome Project* (Cambridge: Harvard University Press, 1992).

33. See the brief discussion of the interplay between ethics and regulations under the last heading, entitled "Ethics and Regulation," of this text's introduction to Part I. OPRR's guidebook on human genetics

research says that for some of the areas it discusses, "no clear guidance can be given at this point [to IRBs], either because not enough is known about the risks presented by the research, or because no consensus on the appropriate resolution of the problem yet exists." OPRR, *Protecting Human Research Subjects*, 5-42.

34. See also the helpful discussions of L. Walters, "Genetics and Reproductive Technologies," and C.R. MacKay, "Discussion Points to Consider in Research Related to the Human Genome," *Human Gene Therapy* 4 (1993), 477-95, esp. 482-88.

35. Genetic research raises questions about the impact of research on subjects, subjects' families, and their future progeny that exceed the levels of concern over these questions in all, or almost all, other areas of research with human subjects. This raises critical issues regarding the nature of informed consent for subjects of genetic research. See "Institutional Review Boards Can Comment on Proposal Consent Changes," *Human Research Report* 9 (April 1994) 1-2; T.H. Murray, "The Human Genome Project and Genetic Testing: Ethical Implications," in a report of a Conference on the Ethical and Legal Implications of Genetic Testing, *The Genome, Ethics and the Law* (Washington, D.C.: American Association for the Advancement of Science, 1992), 49-78; MacKay, "Discussion Points to Consider in Research Related to the Human Genome;" and E.A. Wulfsberg *et al.*, "Alpha-one Antitrypsin Deficiency: Impact of Genetic Discovery on Medicine and Society," *Journal of the American Medical Association* 271 (1994): 217-22.

13

The Ethical Analysis of Clinical Trials: New Lessons for and from Cancer Research

Benjamin Freedman

INTRODUCTION

It was some 10 years ago or more that I had the following dream:

I am walking down the hall, and as the director of transplant services is bustling by, he invites me to their party. I ask him what they are celebrating, and he tells me they have just performed a medical breakthrough: They have successfully completed the first appendix transplant in history. I argue with him: "But what's the point of transplanting an appendix? We take out an appendix, we don't put one back! That's not ethical!" He responds: "What do you mean, 'it's not ethical'? We had the patient's consent!"

I have chosen to take this dream as saying something about the pathology of ethical analysis of clinical research (rather than as speaking to the psychopathology of one particular analyst of clinical research). In theory, we have a rich language and manifold concepts to deploy in considering whether a research proposal satisfies ethical norms. And we do deploy them--in theory. In practice, however--if we consider only the changes to research proposals actually required for ethical approval--research ethics committees such as (in the United States) institutional review boards (IRBs) tend to concentrate on a very few areas: disproportionately, on informed consent.[1]

In this paper I will describe in broad strokes an alternative approach to reviewing the ethics of clinical trials: the ways in which a fundamental re-examination of the ethics of clinical research can be effected; the problems it might reveal; the methods it might use; the results for which it gropes. This approach, which underlies the work of our research team investigating ethical issues in cancer trials at McGill University, takes seriously the idea that each aspect of every planned experimental intervention upon human subjects can be the focus of ethical attention--and may need to be modified to satisfy ethical concerns.

CLINICAL CANCER RESEARCH AS A MODEL: ETHICAL PROBLEMS PAST AND FUTURE

Cancer trials overall--and, to the extent that they can be distinguished, trials on advanced cancer patients in particular--seem to our research group a useful model to employ in considering the ethics of clinical trials generally. The characteristics that make clinical trials ethically important, and problematic, exist in cancer trials in exaggerated form. The issues that will preoccupy ethical analysts of trials for years to come, therefore, often first become clear when considering cancer trials.

One important way in which cancer trials presaged what was to come elsewhere in medicine was in showing us how research and treatment can be connected. In many areas of medicine, historically, research and treatment were only loosely connected. These two endeavors proceeded most of the time side by side, as though they were parallel, only incidentally connected, enterprises. This peaceful coexistence is, however, occasionally disrupted when a research breakthrough occurs. Change in clinical practice occurred in a punctuated equilibrium form: Long stretches in which practice is stable while medical research putters along, short stretches in which major advances in research motivate clinical practice to quickly catch up. In cancer, by contrast, there has been a tight connection between research and treatment. Changes in clinical approaches to cancer have been frequent and incremental, commonly based upon the evidence of incremental benefit provided by the large, often multicenter, controlled clinical trials.

Cancer was also a forerunner for other areas of medical research in establishing the concept of a logical staging of investigation of treatments. The unfolding of research can be thought of in two ways: as the stages in which a new treatment is studied and evaluated, or, as the stages in which progress is achieved in the treatment of a given disease process.

The first process of development is illustrated by the long-established distinction between Phase I, II, and III trials. Phase I trials in cancer are done on small numbers of subjects--often 30 or fewer--to find the maximum tolerated dose (MTD) of a newly developed drug. Phase II trials, that may involve a few hundred subjects, are done to gain experience with the drug at the MTD level and to begin to assess its efficacy. Phase III trials are done to establish a drug's therapeutic benefits when tried on a large population suffering from the disease.

The second is illustrated by the evolution of studies of disease done over many years; our group has called these evolving studies intellectual traditions. For example, one such tradition comprises a dozen trials stretching over 20 years (and continuing), in which the National Surgical Adjuvant Breast and Bowel Cancer Project (NSABP) has studied the value of various forms of treatment in women with stage II breast cancer with limited nodal involvement. While simultaneously or in series trying out varying forms and combinations of surgery, chemotherapy, and radiation, the NSABP has studied breast cancer's treatment by asking increasingly refined questions of an increasingly defined disease population.

Most significantly, perhaps, from an ethical point of view, cancer research has been the paradigm of trials entailing not simply uncertainty but very serious risk on the part of subject participants. Cancer trials use toxic treatments--"slash, burn, and poison"--on persons suffering from this dread and lethal disease. The debate over the propriety of placebo controls was resolved by consensus early on in cancer study, thereby helping other areas of research see the way on this still contentious issue.[2] All areas of clinical research can profit, too, from recognizing the phenomenon long apparent in cancer research: the misconception on the part of patients enrolling in a study that they will be the recipients of effective treatments not otherwise available.[3]

Cancer trials have, therefore, in times past often presaged new ethical issues. Our research group believes cancer research will continue to play this same role of early-warning system in times to come. Prospectively, current experience in cancer research suggests that we can look forward to some of the following new problems:

1. *The medicalization of everyday life*: I am probably not alone in thinking that for cancer researchers, there are only two kinds of people: those who have cancer and those who do not yet have cancer. The recent initiation on the part of NSABP and others of a trial investigating whether tamoxifen can prevent the development of breast cancer is one indication that the second group--persons disease free but at some future risk of developing disease--will increasingly be the objects of study in the future. Interventional trials for primary prevention are certain to become more common as genome research succeeds in identifying subpopulations with specific disease susceptibilities.

2. *The specific ethical dilemmas associated with big clinical science:* Some tasks--like digging a ditch--can be split up among many, so that they are easier as more people participate. For other tasks, like reaching a decision, the more people involved, the more complex and intractable the problem becomes. The ethical analysis of research is, unfortunately, not like digging. Large multicenter cancer trials have begun to illustrate some of the associated problems--for example, confusions over responsibilities of investigators, trial centers, local investigators and their centers, research overseers (like the National Institutes of Health), and the research ethics committees attached to all of the above. Large trials often are long trials as well, and the growing attention to early termination of trials and stopping rules, as well as to early publication of trial results, are similarly issues associated with the structure of big clinical science.

3. *The economic and social fallout of trials*: Cancer research and its fruits have been at the forefront of those posing ethical puzzles associated with the economic implications of medical progress. Anticancer agents in themselves are increasingly expensive, and they bring in their aggressive wake new and expensive anti-anticancer agents, introduced to deal with the biological havoc

which we call side effects: expensive biological products like G-CSF (granulocyte colony stimulating factor) and EPO (erythro-poietin), expensive anti-emetic drugs like ondansetron, expensive interventions like autologous bone marrow transplantation. There is no natural end to this kind of positive feedback loop: Anti-anticancer agents will themselves be shown to have side effects, necessitating the development of new anti-anti-anticancer drugs. At the same time, cancer researchers are increasingly now begin-ning to ask what these increasingly interventional approaches cash out to in the quality of life of patients. Clinical research in cancer is engendering quality of life research and evaluation, a de-velopment which will over time be revealed to be equally neces-sary in other realms of medical treatment.

4. *And every other question of or approach to ethical research known:* As with Rome, all roads lead to cancer--sooner or later, but more often sooner. In bioethics gene therapy is an outstanding example of a realm of research posing its own, new, unique ethical problems. But the first clinical applications of gene treatment were not for genetic disease, but for cancer. New approaches to the ethics of research, such as regulations allowing patients off trial to have access to study medication, may be developed for another disease--in this case, HIV/AIDS--but find early and vigorous application to cancer patients.

To know cancer trials is, then, to know the ethics of clinical research. This leads, naturally enough, to the question: What is the ethics of clinical research?

CLINICAL RESEARCH ETHICS: NORMAL ANALYSIS AND ITS LIMITS

Ethical analysis of clinical trials, in the United States of America and those many other jurisdictions influenced by the American approach as developed in *The Belmont Report*, employs three distinct but interacting moral principles: respect for per-sons, beneficence, and justice.[4] As philosophical constructs, these three principles can be construed broadly enough to encompass all ethical questions that a research proposal may pose. Respect for persons may be taken as that category dealing with all questions arising from concern for a subject's *rights;* beneficence, as covering issues of a subject's *welfare;* justice, as a grab bag of all other ethical issues, and especially those concerning a trial's implications for and impact upon those not participating in a trial, indeed, society generally.

Although these principles are theoretically omnicompetent, in the practice of research committees, no such broad reading of them will be found. Rather, the principles are used to map a much narrower realm. Respect for persons has largely been used in grounding the required norms and practices of informed consent for competent patients, protective practices for those subjects who are incompetent to consent, and confidentiality. Interest in beneficence is largely exhausted in discussions of the risk-benefit (or, harm-benefit; or, risk-hope) ratio associated with enrolling in a trial. Justice, finally, in principle such a broad category, has largely been appealed to when considering discrimination in the selection of subjects for research.

The above, necessarily anecdotal, assertion about the practice of research committees is to an extent supported by examination of the literature on research ethics. In examining the 1979-1990 subject index to the sole journal dedicated to the field, *IRB: A Review of Human Subjects Research,* it appears that outside of certain issues unclassifiable by the above (notably, regulations and law on research and research upon specific diseases), the big-ticket items are roughly as described. Subject consent together with proxy consent for incompetent subjects account for 99 entries; confidentiality, 43; risk-benefit ratio and research design, 60; subject selection and recruitment of disadvantaged subjects, 22.

What accounts for this concentration of effort upon such a small range of ethical issues posed in research? A philosophic apologia might be developed, but I believe the answer is to be sought in history rather than philosophy. The *Belmont* principles were crafted in response to crises caused by specific abuses of research ethics, and so their application has naturally been shaped along the same lines. Respect for persons was adopted in the shadow of Nuremberg, of the Jewish Chronic Disease Hospital, and of the Willowbrook studies developing hepatitis vaccine. In all these cases, the perceived problem was a lack of consent and of protection of incompetent subjects; the perceived remedy, a principle of respect for persons. The principle of beneficence reacted to Beecher's and Pappworth's descriptions of dangerous research, studies posing to their subjects a drastically unfavorable risk-benefit ratio.[5] Finally, the principle of justice responded to racism and exploitation in the conduct of clinical research, as seen in the Tuskegee episode and in prison research, for example, the studies of behavioral treatment in Vacaville.[6]

Two points are suggested: First, that The *Belmont* principles are broad enough to accommodate virtually any imaginable ethical concern; second, that they are not in fact so mobilized except in reaction to outside pressure, especially allegations of abuse. Both points are supported by our contemporary experience. In reaction to pressure from such sources as AIDS activism and the women's movement, room is being found for new issues encompassed under respect for persons (for example, the right to enroll on a trial), beneficence (for example, an increased insistence upon active control arms in trials and the availability of experimental treatments off or following trial), and justice (for example, the systematic exclusion of women from the subject population).

The reading of The *Belmont* principles as suggested by these public forces establishes the kinds of problems with which research ethics in fact deals. This is not to say that those problems have no validity on their own merit, without the benefit of outside pressure; nor is it to say that once the pressure is off these problems vanish from the view of analysts of research ethics. Once recognized, a problem in research ethics remains as a puzzle for analysts.

Borrowing a concept from Thomas Kuhn, I will call puzzle-solving activity addressed to recognized problems "normal research ethics."[7] Let me give an illustration of the puzzle-solving activity normal research ethics provides, drawn from the most dominant such puzzle analysts of research ethics face, informed consent.

The main response to the puzzle of informed consent adopted by research ethics committees is the familiar, never-ending refinement--tweaking--of consent forms. This kind of activity should not, I think, be denigrated. It is ultimately addressed, after all, to the problem of how to fairly, honestly, and comprehensively inform an individual or proxy of what research participation will mean to his or her life. Requiring that subjects be specifically informed of the proportion of subjects to be enrolled in each arm of a trial--the establishment of unequal trial arms, for example, 25 percent to placebo, 75 percent to the experimental arm, seems to be increasingly common research practice--is a small detail, a tweak. It is also nothing more than simple honesty, about a fact that a subject may want to know and is always entitled to know. Yet it is still far from uniformly required. Another tweak: Prospective subjects are, in my experience, usually told about concurrent medications prohibited during the course of the trial. They are almost never told the reason for this requirement. Were I a subject in a cancer trial, I would want to know: Are steroids that I may require for comfort excluded because of their confounding neoplastic effect or because they may render the experimental drug useless or dangerous? If the latter, I would agree to partici-pate, for the drug exclusion is in my interest; if the former, perhaps not. More tweaking is required.

In some cases, indeed, the deficiency in information provided to research subjects is still great. Such was my impression several years ago when, for the first time, the research committee on which I serve reviewed protocols for Phase I cancer trials. The purpose of these studies of untried anticancer drugs is to explore the drug's toxicity. Indeed, the endpoint for these studies is not cure, remission, or prolongation of life, but rather the discovery of the maximum tolerable side effects to the drug under investiga-tion.

In inquiring of the investigator and others how subjects to Phase I dose-escalating, toxicity-limited studies are recruited, I found they are not simply inadequately informed, but often misinformed. For example, a Phase I study of drug x is often said to be a study of x's safety and efficacy. Calling a toxicity study a study of safety is harmless, and perhaps even reflects a laudably optimistic view of the world. Calling it a study of efficacy is, however, simply false; although, to be sure, were there no hope of this new drug's working it would not be tested.

The assumption underlying dose-escalating trials to the point of the maximum tolerated dose (MTD) is that an anticancer drug's chance of benefit, chance of inducing harmful side effects, and dose, are all positively correlated: the higher the dose, the higher the chance of harm and of benefit. In order to honestly present a prospective subject with the relevant information, therefore, two barriers had to be hurdled: First, the structure of this kind of study had to be clearly explained. Second, a subject had to be told where he or she fit into that structure--specifically, into which cohort he or she would be enrolled. Truly informed consent to a dose-varying trial has to be as variant as the doses employed.

Cohort-Varying Information Insert for Consent Form to Participation in Phase I Study

Insert in section on Purpose and Design of Study

In testing new drugs and combinations of drugs for cancer treatment, the first study is designed to establish the highest dose that may safely be given. This is such a study. Underlying this trial is our understanding that, most commonly, drugs to treat cancer are most effective when given at the highest safe dose. The highest safe dose is the dose just smaller than that which produces unacceptable reactions.

A group of subjects is enrolled, and given a very small dose. Their progress is followed, and if those patients do not develop unacceptable reactions to that dose a new group of patients is enrolled at a higher dose. This process continues until a dose is reached that commonly produces an unacceptable reaction. [For cohort at highest dose substitute for last sentence: This process continues until a dose is reached that produces an unacceptable reaction in two subjects of the three enrolled at level. If this unacceptable toxicity is repeated in one person from a further group of three subjects, at] [A]t that point the study is complete. It has shown us what the maximum tolerated dose of the drug or combination is.

In this trial, up to nine groups of subjects will be enrolled, at gradually increasing doses of [drug A]. The earliest group of subjects (Group 1) will be [was] given the lowest dose, at a level that should not produce unacceptable toxicity but may also not be sufficiently potent against the cancer. The later the group into which a subject is enrolled, the higher the dose given. It is often, but not always, true that the higher the dose, the more powerful are the effects against cancer, but also the more likely to produce unacceptable side effects.

If I agree to participate in this trial, I will be in the [nth] group of nine planned groups.[8]

Tweaking--of a consent form, or indeed any other ethically relevant aspect of a study--continues to be necessary; but tweaking is not enough. Each of the above suggestions, for example, follows from a particular view of how respect for persons, undergirding informed consent, requires that a clinical investigator disclose to a prospective subject how participation in research will affect him or her. The underlying view, that clinical research primarily concerns a subject's interests, leaves us with no hook for dealing with other problems that can arise predicated upon a different (or, complementary) understanding of research as a social enterprise. For example, many have asked whether an investigator needs to reveal the sponsorship of a study and his/her financial stake in it. After all, in a strict view of consent as based upon subject autonomy, this information is irrelevant. The subject would only be entitled to self-regarding information, and have no claim to information regarding others. Whatever the investigator's stake in the research, that stake will not *per se* affect the subject. Normal research ethics, engaged in working out the implications of accepted moral principles, does not itself provide any handle for problems that step outside the ordinary presuppositions: in this case, that research is a private transaction between investigator and subject, and that the subject has no legitimate interest in being informed about the social aspects of a trial.

In principle, it is true, our moral principles can be expanded to cover this, or any other, ethical concern. It is possible, for example, to argue on the basis of the principle of justice that information regarding the sponsorship of a trial be accessible to prospective subjects in common with any other interested party in society. This may indeed be or become the current trend, under the impetus of rising interest on the part of politicians and academic medicine in the conduct of drug companies. But it is our contention that we need not wait for outside forces to raise questions before we begin to follow our moral principles to the limits of their concern; that it is indeed preferable that clinical trials be subjected to a comprehensive ethical analysis, not dependent upon the specific problems raised by groups outside the clinical trial community.

TOWARD A COMPREHENSIVE APPROACH

Two examples--one brief, one less so--will help illustrate the alternative approach to the ethical analysis of clinical trials we are pursuing: the manner in which a Phase I trial establishes the dose of a drug which will be pursued in following trials and the manner in which a trial's eligible population is established. Both will be illustrated by instances from the field of cancer research, but both teach lessons that go beyond cancer. Neither has been a traditional target of ethical interest in the past; both are becoming so, under outside pressure; yet in each case, we contend, the focus of concern generated by outside interest would not be sufficiently broad.

As explained above, Phase I trials of new anticancer agents are structured to establish the maximum tolerated dose of the agent. Protocol descriptions of how the MTD will be established seem dry and narrowly technical, speaking as they do of preestablished thresholds for blood values indicating neutropenia or granulocytopenia, of scores on nausea scales, or those measuring peripheral neuropathy. As such, the means for establishing an MTD typically escape ethical attention, on the part of IRBs or commentators. Two questions are thereby begged: MTD for *what*? and, MTD for *whom*?

Simply to ask these questions is to reveal the value-underpinnings involved in defining an MTD. The MTD for an anticancer drug is obviously not the same as the MTD for an antihistamine. When we ask whether the side effects of a drug are tolerable, clearly, we need a frame of reference: "Tolerable compared to what?" Equally clearly, that frame of reference will ultimately need to be supplied by patients themselves, rather than by either trialists or clinicians; for it is patients who are the ones who will be undergoing those side effects. Operationally, if not intrinsically, the definition of a maximum tolerated dose is: the highest dose which patients will accept in their search for a cure or surcease.

To choose an MTD is to declare a preference for one point on the curve representing a trade-off between benefits (drug efficacy) and harm (drug toxicity). Any centralized mechanism for deciding that trade-off will recreate all of the inconsistencies associated with a command-and-control economy. (In the cognate problem of governmentally imposed consumer safety legislation, for example, it is common to find imputed values for safety ranging across an order of magnitude. The cost of safety regulation of some products or activities might be $200,000 per life saved; for others, $2,000,000 or more.)[9] To this problem, the present method of defining *a priori* an MTD by discussion among investigators adds another: a problem essentially involving a prediction of patient preference is tackled without patient representation. And, because this aspect of the trial is treated as a technical measure, that form of patient representation and advocacy that research review by IRB is supposed to provide is commonly lacking as well.

Is it at all likely that a process of MTD definition that attempts to incorporate patient input would yield results systematically different from at present? The short answer is, of course, that we won't know until we have tried. Until then, we can certainly imagine how such a difference might have developed. Ever since *primum non nocere* was first articulated, the medical profession has systematically treated risks of treatment versus those of non-treatment in a biased manner, weighting the first more heavily than the second. When a surgeon declares that a patient with advanced terminal disease is "inoperable," that surgeon declares a bias: better that the patient die of disease than of the scalpel. Some models of rationality would judge this an irrational bias, for example, the classical model of economic rationality that weights foregone benefits exactly equally with costs. Yet even if one, in agreement with me, resists the straitened economic model of rationality, it would surely not be irrational for the patient to fail to share this bias, to prefer to undergo the risks and hope of treatment over the *status quo* of hopeless disease. I personally believe that this difference may in part underlie the high proportion of patients who agree to, and even seek out, participation in Phase I trials.

AIDS activists have sought to be included in the planning of clinical trials. They claim the right, for example, to contribute to discussion of what aspects of disease should be studied, arguing that too much research has been done on antiviral medication and too little on treatments for opportunistic infections. These activists are, in a sense, too moderate in their specific demands; as the seemingly technical problem of defining an MTD demonstrates, no aspect of a trial is immune from ethical interest. IRBs, and scholars interested in the ethical analysis of research, are not doing their job if they wait for others to discern ethical issues before responding.

Another main interest of AIDS activists has been in reforming the recruitment process of subjects for clinical trials, so that such populations as women, intravenous drug abusers, and those in late stages of disease, are no longer routinely excluded. Eligibility criteria--criteria of inclusion and of exclusion--have been a major focus of interest of the McGill research group. Here again, it seems to us that even more fundamental questions should be raised by those comprehensively concerned with the ethics of clinical trials than those now being raised by AIDS activists. To examine this, let us return to cancer research.

A theme recurring often in the cancer literature is the very small proportion (approximately 3 percent) of cancer patients who are studied on protocol.[10] Why, at a time of so much ferment in cancer treatment and research, are so few patients enrolled in studies, even in those areas where appropriate cancer trials are open for enrollment? One familiar with the ethics literature might believe that the biggest single factor is patient resistance. Following Charles Fried, one might believe that patients are unwilling to forego the benefit of personal care necessitated by randomization.[11] One would be wrong. The biggest single barrier to increased patient accrual, as demonstrated in a series of large studies of cancer populations in North America, are the exclusion criteria adopted by trialists themselves.[12] (The next largest factor is the refusal by physicians to enroll their patients or to recommend to their patients that they enroll.)

Eligibility criteria have been singled out for attention before. Begg, and Engstrom for example, reviewing a series of breast cancer studies done by various groups in North America, noted the very large number of criteria employed, disparities between criteria employed by different groups, and the fact that some criteria have little scientific or clinical justification.[13]

Underlying the proliferation of eligibility criteria is the desire of a trial group to restrict its study to a "tight," homogeneous population that has the best chance of responding to the new treatment under investigation. If that could be accomplished, trials would be smaller, shorter, and less expensive. Yet for this to be so, two conditions would have to be fulfilled: First, there would have to exist a real and substantial difference in treatment response across subgroups suffering from the disease under investigation; second, there would have to be a reliable way of determining in advance whether a given individual falls into the group with a good treatment prognosis rather than those with a poor prognosis.

Both points have recently been called into question. For example, Yusuf and colleagues performed meta-analyses of a number of trials with the aim of discerning whether those who were excluded from a trial derive less benefit from the treatment under investigation than those who are eligible.[14] In fact, the prognoses of these groups are broadly similar. Treatment factors--whether or not a treatment works--seems a much more powerful determinant of trial outcome than has the selection of a tight population of responders. Formally, too, as Buyse has shown, the damage created by mistakenly selecting a homogeneous group can be much greater than that caused by the opposite error, failing to select out a group of good responders.[15] Yet trialists, through a consistent preference for tight trials, consistently seem to prefer risking the first type of error. Indeed, these various cautionary results have attracted little attention on the part of trialists, or, to our knowledge, on the part of ethics review committees.[16]

There remain a number of questions about eligibility criteria that need to be answered in connection with the ethical analysis of research. Are eligibility criteria, and particularly exclusion criteria, continuing to increase? If yes, what impact does that have on the cost of trials, on their length, and most importantly, on the proportion of patients with the disease who are eligible for the study? Can results from tight studies be generalized to treatment recommendations for the general patient population? In announcing results, are trial groups careful in pointing out any limitations upon generalizability caused by the trial's criteria of exclusion? Are clinicians scrupulously heeding such warnings, or are they rather applying the results established in a carefully limited population of patients to the patient population at large?

The ethical justification of a controlled trial carries with it certain commitments as well as cautions. For a trial to be ethical, it must be do-able and, other things being equal, aspects of trials that make it less likely that they will be completed require rigorous justification. This is one reason why we have been interested in the apparent proliferation of criteria of eligibility. (This concern in part underlies the call of AIDS activists to open up trial eligibility, but adds to the individual patient's interest in trial participation the scientific and social interest in efficient completion of trials undertaken.) In addition, the second requirement of clinical equipoise requires that clinical trials must be designed in such a way as to potentially support changes in clinical practice upon their successful completion. If trials are done on too small a population to rationally support changes in treatment preference; if they will not be communicated in ways yielding that result; if such communications are routinely misconstrued by clinicians who don't have the trialist's luxury of choosing a patient population; or if, in spite of clinicians' qualms, patient demands for new forms of treatment will result in the application of the trial's results beyond what its methods support; the ethical justification of the trial's very design is itself questionable.

Our group has begun the important, but lengthy process of tackling these questions, including filling in some of the information missing from the literature. We have, for example, been looking at eligibility criteria in cancer trials over time, examining in the first instance the criteria established by NSABP in their 12 trials of treatment modalities for stage II breast cancer (years 1972 through 1992). These criteria have approximately doubled over this period. The pattern of growth of criteria is particularly suggestive. By distinguishing between different categories of, or motivations underlying, eligibility criteria (as shown below) and by using this system to classify the NSABP criteria, it is apparent that the classes of criteria we call definition of disease, exigencies of science, and toxicity, are the most important source of growth. In the NSABP trial, they account together for 95 percent of the increase observed. Unlike adding criteria from the other categories--procedural, and legal/regulatory--which would not affect the external validity (generalizability) of a trial, the criteria in which growth was in fact observed are precisely those with that potential. To complicate matters yet further, there remains the possibility that the exclusion criteria imposed upon a trial may not be attended to at the point of research communications and clinical practice.

CATEGORIES OF ELIGIBILITY CRITERIA

DEFINITION OF DISEASE

The purpose of definitional criteria is to set a defined study population of disease.

[Exclude] Patients with tumors greater than 5 cm in size at the largest dimension on clinical examination.

EXIGENCIES OF SCIENCE (including other patient characteristics)

These criteria, unique to research protocols, are concerned with the scientific validity of the research study. The patient population may be restricted by criteria to render it more homogenous and thus to reduce variability.

[Exclude] Patients who have had prior therapy for their breast cancer, including irradiation and chemotherapy.

TOXICITY

Criteria in this category serve the purpose of protecting the vulnerable patient from the risks of treatment in general or from the risks of specific treatments in the particular research protocol.

There must be evidence postoperatively of adequate hepatic functions (bilirubin within normal limits, SGOT or SGPT within normal limits).

REGULATORY AND LEGAL LIABILITY

Criteria in this category ensure the compliance of the protocol with the regulatory (MRC Guidelines; DHHS Regulations) and/or legal requirements for human experimentation.

Patients must consent to be in the study. The informed consent must be signed, witnessed, and dated prior to randomization.

PROCEDURAL

Procedural criteria set out to ensure the smooth functioning of the mechanics of the clinical trial.

Patients must be geographically accessible for followup.

MISCELLANEOUS

We are continuing research in the questions posed here, as well as other areas related to eligibility criteria. Investigating these questions requires expertise in clinical research and trial design as well as ethics, and applying the results from such studies to the ethical evaluation of protocols will similarly call for a considerable degree of sophisticated interdisciplinary expertise.

Can we expect, let alone demand, this degree of sophistication from research committees? Investigating these questions requires coordinated expertise in clinical research and trial design as well as ethics. Yet it is arguable that law, as well as ethics, demands no less. In the first reported case in North America in which a research ethics committee was found negligent in approving a research protocol, the court based its finding both upon inadequacy in informed consent and in the failure of the research committee to alter the trial's eligibility criteria, by requiring the exclusion of subjects with a history of hypertrophic cardiomyopathy.[17]

It may be argued that in this instance the court was only enforcing the IRB's traditional role of protecting human subjects. From this point of view, research committees might only be bound to add exclusion criteria, rather than, as we are suggesting, consider requiring in some cases that trial eligibility be broadened. Yet even without appealing to the ill-defined "right to be a research subject," it seems that our more comprehensive demand is at least grounded in the research committee's other traditional role, protecting the integrity and clinical relevance of experimentation upon human subjects.

CONCLUSION

That research review should be comprehensive, that it should potentially question any aspect of a protocol, is required by the expectations of others who act in reasonable reliance upon the committee's doing its job. Those "others" include government or professional regulators, trial sponsors, the institution hosting the research and, above all, research subjects themselves. It is true that in principle a local research committee might choose to rely upon the judgment of, for example, the trial designers, having satisfied itself that all concerns raised have been fairly addressed. This does not seem to us at present to be the case. Research protocols at present rarely attempt to provide a rationale for eligibility criteria, for example; without such information, it is impossible for a local committee to judge the quality of judgment that went into the selection of these criteria. Moreover, it seems to us that a very plausible route for reform of the research process might arise through the rigorous work of local research committees themselves.

Such comprehensive evaluation is also grounded in the reality of research. Ethics, after all, dealing with the evaluation of choice, requires first a recognition of choices made and their background, and only then may proceed to the process of normative appraisal. Ethical analysis, properly viewed, includes both text (the choices) and commentary. As in most realms of applied ethics, therefore, the ethical issues of research are a superset, rather than a subset, of other scientific or clinical issues arising in the design, management, interpretation, and application of clinical trials.

ACKNOWLEDGMENT

The ideas presented in this chapter are in the process of development in our research group on ethical issues in the design, management, and interpretation of multicenter cancer trials. The author gratefully acknowledges support provided in preparing this chapter by grant #806-91-0031, awarded from the Social Sciences and Humanities Research Council of Canada's program in applied ethics; and the intellectual stimulation and research support provided by colleagues on this grant, including Myriam Skrutkowski, B.Sc.N.; Amina Riaz; and Jim Robbins, Ph.D. Much of the work reported upon here has been initiated and intellectually directed by the project's postdoctoral fellow, Charles Weijer, M.D., by Stanley Shapiro, Ph.D., and by my co-principal investigator, Abe Fuks, M.D., C.M. The author is also grateful to several audience members at the UTMB conference for their useful comments and questions and to Harold Vanderpool, Ph.D., for arranging the conference and inviting me to present this work.

NOTES

1. B.H. Gray, R.A. Cook, and A.S. Tannenbaum, "Research Involving Human Subjects," *Science* 201 (1978): 1094-1101.

2. B. Freedman, "Placebo-Controlled Trials and the Logic of Clinical Purpose," *IRB: A Review of Human Subjects Research* 12 (November-December 1990): 1-6.

3. P.S. Appelbaum, L.H. Roth, and C. Lidz, "The Therapeutic Misconception: Informed Consent in Psychiatric Research," *International Journal of Law and Psychiatry* 5 (1982): 319-29.

4. Department of Health, Education, and Welfare, The National Commission for the Protection of Human Subjects of Biomedical and Behavioral Research, *The Belmont Report: Ethical Principles and Guidelines for the Protection of Human Subjects of Research*, DEW Publication (OS) 78-0013 (Washington, D.C.: U.S. Government Printing Office, 1978). Reprinted in this volume's Appendix C.

5. H. Beecher, "Ethics and Clinical Research," *New England Journal of Medicine* 274 (1966): 1354-60; M.H. Pappworth, *Human Guinea Pigs* (London: Routledge and Kegan Paul, 1967).

6. On all of these, see J. Katz, *Experimentation with Human Beings* (New York: Russel Sage Foundation, 1972). This volume in itself powerfully helped to shape discourse on research ethics during a crucial period of formation of American policy.

7. T.S. Kuhn, *The Structure of Scientific Revolutions*, 2d ed. (Chicago: University of Chicago Press, 1970).

8. B. Freedman, "Cohort-Specific Consent: An Honest Approach to Phase I Clinical Cancer Studies," *IRB: A Review of Human Subjects Research*, 12, (January/February 1990) 5-7.

9. M. Baram, "Cost-Benefit Analysis: An Inadequate Basis for Health, Safety and Environmental Regulatory Decision Making," *Ecology Law Quarterly* 8 (1980): 485; compare W. K. Viscusi, *Risk by Choice: Regulating Health and Safety in the Workplace* (Cambridge: Harvard University Press, 1983). See generally B. Freedman, *Consensuality, Regulation and Social Risk*, Report for the Law Reform Commission of Canada Project on Protection of Life, Health, and the Environment (1984).

10. A.B. Benson *et al.*, "Oncologist's Reluctance to Accrue Patients onto Clinical Trials: An Illinois Cancer Center Study," *Journal of Clinical Oncology* 9 (1991): 2067-75. Compare K. Antman *et al.*, "Selection Bias in Clinical Trials," *Journal of Clinical Oncology* 3 (1985): 1142-47; J.Y. Lee and S.R. Breaux, "Accrual of Radiotherapy Patients to Clinical Trials," *Cancer* 52 (1983): 1014-16; E. Quoix *et al.*, "Treatment of Small-Cell Lung Cancer on Protocol: Potential Bias of Results," *Journal of Clinical Oncology* 4 (1986): 1314-20.

11. C. Fried, *Medical Experimentation: Personal Integrity and Social Policy* (New York: Elsevier, 1974).

12. C. Begg *et al.*, "Accrual of Patients into a Multihospital Cancer Clinical Trial and Its Implications on Planning Future Studies," *American Journal of Clinical Oncology* 7 (1984): 173-82; C. Hunter *et al.*, "Selection Factors in Clinical Trials: Results from the Community Clinical Oncology Program Physician's Patient Log," *Cancer Treatment Reports* 71 (1987): 559-65.

13. C.B. Begg and P.F. Engstrom, "Eligibility and Extrapolation in Cancer Clinical Trials," *Journal of Clinical Oncology* 5 (1987): 962-68.

14. S. Yusuf *et al.*, "Selection of Patients for Randomized Controlled Trials: Implications of Wide or Narrow Eligibility Criteria," *Statistics in Medicine* 9 (1990): 73-86.

15. M.E. Buyse, "The Case for Loose Inclusion Criteria in Clinical Trials," *Acta Chirurgica Belgica* 90 (1990): 129-31.

16. Colin Begg, personal communication.

17. *Rapports Judiciares* (1989): 731; B. Freedman and K. Glass, "Weiss V. Solomon: A Case Study in Institutional Responsibility for Clinical Research," *Law, Medicine and Health Care* 18 (1990): 395-403.

14

Ethical Issues in Pediatric Research

William G. Bartholome

I began my "hybrid-career" as pediatrician and ethicist by submitting two papers I was completing for my work as a Joseph P. Kennedy, Jr. Fellow in Medical Ethics at Harvard University to the National Commission for the Protection of Human Subjects of Biomedical and Behavioral Research. When these papers were subsequently published in the Commission's *Appendix to Report and Recommendations: Research Involving Children,* they represented my first published work in a new field that a handful of us were calling pediatric ethics.[1] Although this represented an important step in my career in academic medicine, this work also brought me squarely into the middle of one of the most important early debates in the young field of bioethics: the Ramsey-McCormick debate on research involving children.[2] This long exchange between two of the founding fathers of American bioethics set the terms not only for the work of the National Commission on research involving children, but also for what was to count as ethical argument in bioethics, at least in the early years of its evolution. By forcing the other to defend his position on these questions, Ramsey and McCormick exposed the assumptions and methods each had used, and were to continue to use, in their scholarly work on a wide variety of issues in bioethics.

This classical debate also allowed interested clinicians, particularly those who provided care to infants and children, to come to a greater understanding of the many complex, if not intractable, ethical problems that were largely inchoate in clinical disciplines like pediatrics or pediatric nursing. To those of us who had chosen to work in pediatric ethics, Ramsey and McCormick also served as a sobering reminder of the extent to which basic questions about the ethics of parenting and the ethical standing of children had been largely neglected throughout the history of philosophical ethics.

In "The Ethics of Nontherapeutic Clinical Research on Children," I attempted a critical examination of both sides of the Ramsey-McCormick debate. I assumed that the role of a neophyte in this emerging field was to ascertain and describe the strengths and weaknesses of each position. In the process, I discovered that I had found a way to mediate or resolve some of the conflict over research involving children. With considerable temerity, I proposed that children could ethically participate in "nontherapeutic" clinical research if such participation involved "no risk" and was experienced by them as enhancing moral growth and development. I also proposed a brief list of guidelines for such research on children five to 14 years old.

In this paper I will provide a brief history of the evolution of pediatric research ethics from its roots in the early debates, through the construction of a conceptual framework by the National Commission and the development of a set of federal regulations to govern the conduct of such research, to a consideration of contemporary scholarship on some of the core ethical concepts. I hope to demonstrate that our understanding of the critical ethical issues involved in allowing children to participate in research has significantly evolved over this 25-year period. I also hope to show that much work remains to be done, particularly in terms of how our understanding of basic concepts in pediatric research ethics must reflect a greater awareness of the perspective of the child subject.

THE RAMSEY-MCCORMICK DEBATE

The publication in 1977 of the National Commission's *Report and Recommendations: Research Involving Children* represents a crucial watershed event in the debate about the involvement of children in research.[3] I will examine its recommendations in detail. The debate over involvement of children in research was begun by Curran and Beecher almost a decade earlier in an article that examined the status of what they called legal ethical principles related to research on children, starting with the *Nuremberg Code*.[4] The first fully developed ethical position was set forth in the first chapter of Paul Ramsey's first major work in the field of bioethics, *The Patient as Person*, published in 1970.[5] In this work, Ramsey undertook an analysis of what he called the "canon of loyalty" between physicians and patients and between investigators and subjects, namely the ethics of consent. Ramsey claimed that consent establishes and maintains a bond of fidelity or faithfulness between investigator and subject. From this ethical foundation, Ramsey argued that ". . . children who cannot give a mature and informed consent, or adult incompetents, should not be made the subjects of medical experimentation unless, other remedies having failed to relieve their grave illness, it is reasonable to believe that the administration of a drug as yet untested or insufficiently tested on human beings, or the performance of an untried operation, may further *the patient's own recovery.*"[6]

Ramsey also claimed that "to experiment on children in ways that are not related to them as patients is already a sanitized form of barbarism" and "to attempt to consent for a child to be made an experimental subject is to treat a child as not a child. It is to treat him as if he were an adult person who has consented to become a joint adventurer in the common cause of medical research. If the grounds for this are alleged to be the presumptive or implied consent of the child, that must simply be characterized as a violent and false presumption."[7]

Although Ramsey left open the possibility of involving children in research "in the face of epidemic conditions endangering also each individual child," he rejected even Curran and Beecher's suggestion that children could be involved in nontherapeutic research in which there was "no discernible risk."[8] For Ramsey, such activities would still involve "using" children. The final section of Ramsey's chapter critically examines published accounts of the studies on infectious hepatitis undertaken at the Willowbrook State School in the late 1950s by Saul Krugman and his associates.

As the first attempt to provide a critical ethical analysis of the participation of children in research, Ramsey's position is not merely of historical interest. McCormick's response to Ramsey revealed a radically different ethical analysis. McCormick argued that parental consent is ethically valid in the context of a therapeutic intervention "precisely insofar as it is a reasonable presumption of the child's wishes." Why? Because, said McCormick, "we know that life and health are goods for the child, that he *would* choose because he *ought* to choose the good of life, his own self-preservation."[9] From this, McCormick proceeded to argue that "a certain level of involvement in non-therapeutic experimentation is good for the child and therefore he ought to choose it."[10] McCormick did limit what the child ought to choose to research that is scientifically well designed, that cannot succeed unless children are subjects, and in which there is "no discernible risk or undue discomfort for the child."[11]

The debate was joined. Ramsey responded by claiming that McCormick's position treated the child as only a little adult: "He [McCormick] treats the child as a small adult by asking, what *should* he consent to instead of what *would* he consent to if in *childhood* he could?"[12] Ramsey noted that McCormick did place limits on what we can presume children would do, but Ramsey saw McCormick as arguing that "a minimum sociability may be presumed of unconsenting subjects, and extracted from them through proxies."[13] Ramsey also pointed out that this presumptive consent must hold for other potential involuntary human subjects, including unconscious patients, terminal patients, psychiatric patients, prisoners, conscripts, and others. Ramsey quoted with approval the response to McCormick's position developed by William May, another of the founding fathers of American bioethics, namely that a child is not a moral agent, not a bearer of moral obligations, even presumptive ones.[14] May also argued that what justifies our interventions into the lives of children is not that we know what they would choose if they could, nor that we know what they ought to choose, but rather that these interventions are undertaken in response to some demonstrable need of the child. For May, there must be some necessity that we intervene. The child's health or welfare must be imperiled in some way to justify our interventions, particularly interventions associated with significant risks or burdens. Ramsey then challenged McCormick to clarify the meaning of terms like no discernible risk, no realistic risk, and minimum risk. This challenge is one that to this day infects the debate about the appropriate level of risk or harm or inconvenience to which child subjects may be exposed.

McCormick's reply was published four months later in the same journal.[15] It should be noted that, at that time, the *Hastings Center Report* was what might be called *the journal* in the emerging field of bioethics. McCormick argued that his talk of infants and children having an "ought" in terms of participating in no discernible risk research was merely "a device, a construction . . . to get at the reasonableness of our expectations and interventions." He argued that such "oughts" are not rooted in the idea that children are moral agents with duties to others, but rather are rooted in the idea that children, like adults, are social human beings. He pointed out, " . . . we introduce the infant not to the world of adults, but to the world of social human beings, to the world of human beings, not the adults' world."[16] In response to Ramsey's argument that this minimum sociability would extend beyond childhood, McCormick stated that he strongly supported the idea that all members of the community should bear the burden of participation in human experimentation if we are to enjoy the fruits of medical progress. In response to Ramsey's challenge to clarify the meaning of "no discernible risk" or "insignificant risk," McCormick argued that his example of a buccal smear (a procedure in which the inside of the mouth is gently scraped with a wooden spatula to remove superficial cells for use in research) was meant to be used as something of a benchmark against which to compare other interventions. He implied that he would draw the line in terms of risk to child subjects at the level of risk or discomfort involved in obtaining a buccal smear. As I will argue later, most members of the scientific community have interpreted the term "minimal risk" as allowing procedures involving a great deal more discomfort and risk than a buccal smear. This supports Ramsey's original concern about the accordion nature of the minimal risk standard.

Four months later, Ramsey's final reply was published. In it, Ramsey argued that "sociality" and its implications in terms of duties and obligations such as the obligation to participate in research must be "in some measure *actualized* before there can be any meaningful talk about . . . 'participation' in research."[17] He again challenged McCormick to be clear about the extent to which his (McCormick's) position rests on an acceptance of the research imperative. Ramsey argued that the duty to refrain from injuring must be understood as having priority over the duty to help and the good that can come from doing research in terms of being better able to help in the future. As Ramsey noted, the idea that it is *also* immoral *not* to experiment on children was being claimed again and again in the scientific literature. For Ramsey, this claim rests on a clear failure to understand what might be called the gratuitous nature of the research enterprise. To the extent that great good can be achieved through medical research, it should be regarded as valuable and good. However, at least in this society, medical research has *not* been regarded as something so essential that we are willing to conscript unwilling subjects into its pursuit. It is an enterprise not unlike that of organ donation and transplantation in that it is totally dependent on the willingness of persons to volunteer to become partners in the pursuit of medical progress. In a later publication Ramsey noted:

> We are to do all the good we morally can, not simply all the good we can. We are to do all the good we can without doing wrong. To do no harm is a universal prescription in medical ethics; to bring aid is medicine's constant task.
>
> Under the spell of promising research benefits, the disparity between these two principles becomes obscure. By verbal slight of hand, we turn failure to bring aid (or having no aid to bring) into doing harm.[18]

In this same text--which was originally presented at a 1977 symposium in Houston on research on children--Ramsey responded to my suggestion that children may be invited to participate in no-risk clinical research if such participation might be said to be an ingredient in their moral development or education. Although Ramsey challenged me to be clear about the level of risk involved in such activities, he agreed that my proposal might be a way of allowing a shift from debates ". . . about quantification of risks in parent-child relations, and placed on the meaning of parenthood, on what parents mean to do with their child. Parents hope to further their child's moral education in joint research ventures, just as they hope to further his or her physical or social education by entering him or her into little league baseball."[19]

In an important sense, the Ramsey-McCormick debate served to define the ethical tensions involved in research on children.

Since children are unable to be true volunteers as adults can, involving children in research requires ethical justification that reaches beyond the primary criterion identified at Nuremberg: the free and informed consent of the research subject. To what extent can "using" infants and children as research subjects be justified on the basis of its potential benefits to future children, to children as a class? Is there an "imperative" or "duty" to conduct research involving children? If children are to be "conscripted" into research (something that has not been done with adults), under what circumstances can that be done ethically? To what level of risk (if any), to what level of burden can children be exposed, particularly when the research activity is not intended to benefit them directly? If parents cannot "volunteer" their children as research subjects, under what circumstances can they allow their children to become research subjects? What I (and others) brought to this early phase of the debate was the perspective and experience of the child subject and what we felt was the critical issue of the role of children in making their own decisions about their participation in research.[20] As will become obvious, that continues to be one of my major concerns about the ethics of research on children.

THE RECOMMENDATIONS OF THE NATIONAL COMMISSION

The National Commission was established in 1974 under Public Law 93-348 to develop ethical guidelines for the conduct of research involving human subjects and to make recommendations for the application of such guidelines to research conducted or supported by the, then, Department of Health, Education and Welfare (DHEW). In 20 pages, the commission set out its 10 recommendations.[21] Although the basic framework proposed by the commission was incorporated into federal regulations some six years later, there are many important ethical issues raised by the commission that were dropped when these recommendations were transformed into regulations. In recommendation 2, for example, the commission had asked that Institutional Review Boards (IRBs) determine that "where appropriate, studies have been conducted first on animals and adult humans, then on older children, prior to involving infants;" that "risks be minimized by using procedures consistent with sound research design and by using procedures performed for diagnostic or treatment purposes whenever feasible;" that "adequate provisions are made to protect the privacy of children and their parents, and to maintain confidentiality of data;" and, finally, that "subjects be selected in an equitable manner."[22] None of these recommendations was incorporated into the regulatory language.

Following the set of general requirements set out in its second recommendation, the commission developed recommendations concerning what it believed were four separate categories of research. Recommendation 3 dealt with "research that does not involve greater than minimal risk"; recommendation 4 with "research in which more than minimal risk to children is presented by an intervention that holds out the prospect of direct benefit for the individual subjects." For this so-called therapeutic research, the commission also required that the risk to the child "is justified by the anticipated benefit," and that "the relation of the anticipated benefit to such risk is at least as favorable to the subjects as that presented by available alternative treatments." Recommendation 5 dealt with "research in which more than minimal risk to children is presented by an intervention that does not hold out the prospect of direct benefit to the individual subjects." Two of the 11 commissioners dissented from approval of this category of research. The commission attempted to limit the involvement of children in this category of research by insisting that "such risk represents a minor increase over minimal risk"; that the intervention "presents experiences to subjects that are reasonably commensurate with those inherent in their actual or expected . . . situations, and is likely to yield generalizable knowledge about the subject's disorder or condition"; and, "the anticipated knowledge is of vital importance for understanding or amelioration of the subject's disorder or condition."

In recommendation 6, the commission left open the possibility that research that did not fall into one of these three categories might be conducted if "the research presents an opportunity to understand, prevent or alleviate a serious problem affecting the health or welfare of children."[23] Research in this last category would require review and approval at the federal level. The commission originally proposed that projects in this category be reviewed by a national ethical advisory board. In the federal regulations this was changed to the approval of the Secretary of the DHEW--called the Department of Health and Human Services (DHHS) beginning in 1980--following consultations with "panels of experts" and following opportunity for public review and comment. These four categories of research involving children were incorporated with minor modifications into 45 *CFR* 46 subpart D, entitled "Additional DHHS Protections for Children Involved as Subjects in Research." (See this volume's Appendix D, 46.404 to 46.407.)

The commission also broke new ground in its seventh and eighth recommendations, which dealt with what had traditionally been called parental or proxy consent. The commission explicitly rejected the concept of consent in this context. "The commission uses the term parental or guardian permission rather than 'consent,' in order to distinguish what a person may do autonomously (consent) from what one may do on behalf of another (grant permission)."[24] In addition, the commission proposed that investigators be obligated to solicit the assent of children and proposed that this be required when children are seven years of age or older. The commission also recommended that at least one parent or guardian be involved in the conduct of the research (by being present during some or all of the conduct of the research); and, that "a child's [of any age] objection to participation in research should be binding unless the intervention holds out a prospect of direct benefit that is important to the health or well-being of the child and is available only in the context of research."

Unfortunately--from this author's perspective--neither of these latter recommendations were incorporated into the regulations. (See Appendix D of this book, 46.408.) In fact, even the commission's recommendation that the age of seven be used as an "age of assent" was not incorporated into the regulations. IRBs were given the task of determining, presumably on a protocol-by-protocol basis, which children should be treated as having the capacity to assent. As I will argue later, this decision has thwarted the evolution of the concept of child assent.

The commission's eighth recommendation dealt with research in which the requirement to obtain parental permission might be waived. Its ninth dealt with research involving children who are wards of the state. Both of these recommendations were incorporated into the regulations. The tenth recommendation dealt with institutionalized children. It was not incorporated into the regulations.

Before leaving this discussion of the recommendations of the commission, I will briefly examine the basis for the dissents of commissioners Cooke and Turtle to research activity which fell under the commission's fifth recommendation. Cooke argued that only subjects who were truly able to volunteer should be involved in research involving greater than minimal risks which does not offer the prospect of benefit to the subject. He observed that the ethical justification for allowing research in this category could be based merely on the "principle of utility," which he felt "indicate[s] the perilous nature of the recommendation and the ethical uncertainty of the commission."[25] Commissioner Turtle was even more scathing in his dissent: "I believe that the substantial majority of the commission has committed a clear error in approving Recommendation (5), potentially subjecting sick children to greater risks than other children without regard to foreseeable benefit." He found the arguments of the majority to be "shams" and argued that "there is no legal, ethical, or social basis for subjecting sick children to more than minimal risks merely because a foreseeable benefit might accrue to an identifiable class of children in the future."[26]

Clearly a major problem for both Cooke and Turtle was that recommendation 5 allowed research involving "a minor increase over minimal risk" to the child subject. Yet the commission's own definition of "minimal risk" was so unclear that the meaning of a "minor increase" over "minimal" was even less clear. The commission had defined minimal risk as "the probability and magnitude of physical or psychological harm that is normally encountered in the daily lives, or in the routine medical or psychological examination, of healthy children."[27] As will become obvious, vigorous debate continues over the meaning of this elusive phrase.

The report and recommendations of the National Commission were published in the *Federal Register* on 13 January 1978.

The secretary of DHEW published a notice of proposed rulemaking on 21 July 1978. Yet, it was not until 8 March 1983 that the "final rule" was published for the regulations, which went into effect on 6 June 1983. Why it took the secretary five years to respond to the 127 comments that were received in response to the original proposal has never been satisfactorily explained. The entire text of the regulations is included in Appendix D of this book.

In the remainder of this discussion, I will review some of the literature that has been published since the promulgation of the regulations and point out several core ethical issues which are both reflective of the ongoing debate about the involvement of children in research and which have been inadequately examined from the perspective of the child subject.

ONGOING DEBATE ABOUT RISKS

As noted above, the National Commission proposed and the federal regulations adopted the standard of minimal risk. The definition--which is now used in all federally sponsored or funded research--is that the risks anticipated in the proposed research are not greater, considering probability and magnitude, than those ordinarily encountered in daily life or during the performance of routine physical or psychological examinations or tests. Obviously, this standard is crucial in the analysis of projects under all four of the categories of research on children in the regulations.

One of the more systematic critiques of this definition is undertaken by Kopelman in an article in an important pediatric ethics text.[28] Kopelman points out that both parts of this definition are problematic. The idea that minimal risk can be defined in terms of those ordinarily encountered in daily life can be interpreted as "all the risks ordinary people encounter; the risks all people ordinarily encounter; or the minimal risks all ordinary people ordinarily encounter."[29] Kopelman demonstrates that each of these interpretations yields unsatisfactory results. She then turns to the second half of the definition--the risks encountered during the performance of routine physical and psychological examinations or tests--and points out that it leaves IRBs with the almost impossible task of figuring out which interventions are ordinarily encountered or routine for a wide variety of health care professionals in an equally wide variety of clinical settings. Kopelman refers to the often-cited survey of Janofsy and Starfield in which pediatric departmental chairs and directors of pediatric research programs were asked to select from a wide range of possible interventions those that would fulfill the criteria of minimal risk.[30] This survey documented that a substantial minority of its respondents regarded interventions such as arterial puncture, placement of a naso-gastric tube, and typmanocentesis (aspirating fluid from the middle ear with a needle placed through the ear drum) to be minimal risk interventions.

A recent Canadian text devotes an entire section to risk-benefit assessment in which authors attempt both philosophical and practical analyses of the problem of risk assessment.[31] In his chapter on philosophical considerations, Meslin not only notes the objections of Kopelman, but also provides a detailed analysis of the risk-assessment process. Using data from a wide range of sources, Meslin argues that risk assessment involves both objective and subjective aspects in the identification of risk, in the estimation of risk, and in the evaluation of risk by both experts and lay persons. Meslin argues that "the way risk information is generated and interpreted is due in large part to the way risk is perceived and framed."[32] He also argues that the process of risk assessment must be combined with the complex task of judging the acceptability of risk. He proposes that the standard approach, in which experts undertake the identification and estimation of risk followed by judgments about acceptability by those who will bear the risks of harm, may be flawed. It is not clear that risk identification and estimation can be done in a manner that is free of subjective bias. It is also not clear that information about these objectively defined risks can be disclosed to potential subjects in a manner they can understand without framing effects.

In concluding his philosophical analysis, Meslin points to recent work by Shrader-Frechette which suggests that the entire risk-assessment process is influenced by subjective preferences and values. For Meslin, these findings suggest that the accepted model may have to be adapted to allow subjects (or in our case both children and their parents) to be involved in the entire risk-assessment process, not merely the limited role of judging the acceptability of risk. Following Meslin's chapter, Koren--who chairs the Research Ethics Committee at the Hospital for Sick Children in Toronto--attempts to provide a practical approach.[33] Unfortunately, the data he provides and the studies he cites do little more than support Kopelman's observations and Meslin's analysis of the problematic nature of the minimal risk standard.

Brock, in an essay in a newly published American textbook observes: "The procedures now used to determine the level of research risk to which children can be exposed are complex and involve different assessments, at several different points, by different persons in different institutional roles with different institutional responsibilities."[34] Brock notes that the first assessment is made by the principal investigator(s) and his or her research associates. He notes, however, that there is empirical and historical confirmation that this is not sufficient. He then points out that externally funded research is often reviewed by committees of peers in study sections where "flagrant abuses would likely be identified." Depending on one's interpretation of the word "flagrant," I am not sure this is the case. The number of research projects reviewed by IRBs that have received prior review by study sections or the like has been shrinking dramatically in recent years. The majority of externally funded projects reviewed by most IRBs today are those funded by drug or device manufacturers, not those sponsored by federal agencies or programs. Brock argues

this mix of communal and individual evaluations [including review by individual researchers, the peer reviewers, the funding agency, and the IRB] employ[ing] shared, communal standards of risks and benefits, [followed by the evaluation of the parents and the child is] well suited to combine judgments about what research risks a community will tolerate with what risks are reasonable from the perspective of the child and those responsible for his or her welfare.[35]

Unfortunately, this argument relies on the highly controversial claim that something called shared, communal standards of risks and benefits exists.

Grodin and Glantz's textbook contains a more helpful (and comprehensively referenced) analysis of risk assessment by

Wender, who argues that the primary issues in risk assessment involving research in children concern psychological rather than physical risks.[36] A similar, but even more helpful, analysis is provided by Thompson. Thompson offers a set of nine guidelines that are framed as general propositions (or, at times, working hypotheses). Rather than reviewing each of these complex guidelines here, I will list the following as examples: His first guideline is "in general, the younger the child the greater the possibility of general behavioral and socioemotional disorganization accompanying stressful experiences; with increasing age, the child's growing repertoire of coping skills permits greater adaptive functioning in the face of stress;" his fourth, "The capacity to make sophisticated psychological inferences of others' motives, attitudes, and feelings increases with age;" his fifth, "Self-conscious emotional reactions--like shame, guilt, embarrassment, and pride--emerge later in development than do the primary emotions. But once they are acquired, young children may be more vulnerable to their arousal because of their limited understanding of these emotions;" and his sixth, "Young children's understanding of authority renders them more vulnerable to coercive manipulations than older children, for whom authority relations are better balanced by an understanding of individual rights."[37]

What is helpful about the analysis of Wender, Thompson and others is the focus on the experience of the child subject in discussions of risk assessment, rather than a focus on attempting to develop objective measures of physical harm.[38] For an example that totally neglects the first of these perspectives, I invite you to read Gaylin's description of a scene involving a physician-investigator, a father, and his nine- or 10-year old son. Following a routine physical examination, the physician asked the boy if he could take a small sample of blood from his arm. The boy asked, "Will it hurt?" Hearing the doctor's affirmative response, the boy replied, "I don't want it." According to Gaylin, the father then said, "Listen, young man, you just get your hand up on that table and let the doctor take the blood." Gaylin quotes the father as adding:

This is my child. I was less concerned with the research involved than with the kind of boy I was raising. I'll be damned if I was going to allow my child, because of some idiotic concept of children's rights, to assume he was entitled to be a selfish, narcissistic little bastard.[39]

When this story was first recounted as a shorter, excerpted version in the *Hastings Center Report,* I was outraged enough to write to the editor.[40] I pointed out that the concept of assent was not even mentioned in Gaylin's article. I wrote: "Assent of the child is indeed an idea before its time. It is a fragile idea that can easily be crushed amidst the boulders of consent, autonomy, rights, and competence. It's an idea that is so foreign to adult reality that its central thrust is missed even by astute minds like Gaylin's."

I then asked:

What value was instilled here? What did the boy learn? It is virtually impossible for me to believe that he learned about the virtue of love, of selflessness, of concern for other children. Clearly he learned a lesson that children learn over and over and over--do what they say; obey the grown ups; listen to the authoritative tone in their voices, or pay the consequences."[41]

In a recent article, Freedman, Fuks, and Weijer attempt to push the analysis of "minimal risk" beyond the analysis of Kopelman. In the process they provide--I believe--a linkage to the analysis of Wender and Thompson regarding the psychological and developmental aspects of the determination of risk.[42] They argue that the term minimal risk seems to raise more problems than it solves since it is being used to attempt to make quantitative judgments rather than what they call categorical judgments. They suggest that the concept of minimal risk is not governed by its link to the risks of everyday life, but is anchored to that idea. It is a concept that functions primarily by

defining the terms of the argument, the kinds of questions that will need to be posed in the committee's (IRB's) deliberations. The arguments will parallel those familiar to any parent considering allowing a child to undergo a new experience. The committee, acting *in loco parentis,* will need to debate whether the demarcated research intervention is similar to a common experience of this child and whether the incremental research risks are similar to the risks this child or others like him runs on a routine basis.[43]

What members of IRBs are asked to do is to imagine what the child will experience in undergoing the research-related intervention. Obviously, the younger the child, the more difficult it is to imagine what the child will experience and to relate this proposed new experience to those already encountered by the child in his or her life up to that point. However, I think the evidence is clear that the major burdens and risks associated with most research involving children can only be understood if the research intervention is seen *from the child's point of view.* What will the child see, hear, and feel? How will the child experience the grown ups who are undertaking the activity? What will the child take them to be doing? What will the child understand the intervention to be about? What will it mean to the child? Will the child feel comfortable and in control during the process?

Take a simple example--that of the physical examination of the child. If the child is a two-month-old baby girl whose daily experience includes being laid on her back, being stripped naked from the waist down, and having her bottom and genitalia systematically examined and methodically rubbed with a wet cloth, a research project involving careful examination and measurement of the size of the clitoris and characteristics of the hymen in infants will likely not expose the infant to any experience that is radically new. It involves experiences that do not depart significantly from those of her daily life. She is likely to experience the research intervention as a diaper change that involved her parent and someone else who touched her in ways not dissimilar from those involved in the diaper change. Yet, if the same research project is proposed for a population of 13-year-old girls, the IRB might well see such examination and measurement as involving an experience that significantly departs from these young women's daily lives. If the investigator proposed to undertake a speculum examination of the vagina in addition to the inspection and measurements, one would hope that the IRB would limit participation to girls who had previous experience with pelvic examination (including speculum) or to girls who had a medical need for such an examination , that is, a prospect of direct medical benefit to the subject. The IRB might even approve such a study on girls who had no previous experience with pelvic examination and did not need one if the examination were to be performed as gently and respectfully as possible by an adolescent medicine specialist who was motivated both by her desire to do research on normal pelvic anatomy and by a desire to provide young women with an education in how a good pelvic examination should be conducted by ensuring that their first examination was as minimally stressful and as maximally educational as possible.

What if the investigator proposed not only to perform a pelvic examination, but also an endometrial biopsy involving dilation of the cervix and insertion of a suction catheter into the uterus to remove a small sample of the lining tissue? One would hope that the committee would regard this minimally risky, but painful procedure, as one that was too large a step beyond the experience of most 13-year-old girls. Yet, even this degree of burden and risk might be undertaken on a special population of 13-year-old girls, girls who had previously experienced the vaginal birth of a child. In such a population of young women, the cervix would be much easier to dilate (dilation might not even be necessary) and they would be in a much better position to understand what the experience of having an endometrial biopsy involves in terms of the instruments to be used, the discomfort involved, how to deal with post-biopsy bleeding, and the like.

Shifting the focus of the assessment from the nature of the intervention and measurable harms that may result to that of assessment of the experience of the child subject can dramatically change the assessment of what constitutes minimal risk. For example, one of the most commonly performed invasive research interventions in children involves venipuncture. If the focus is on the nature of the intervention and measurable harms, this seems like an intervention that clearly fits into the category of minimal risk. However, many studies--including a recent study from The Netherlands--document that the distress a child experiences in undergoing this procedure varies dramatically by age.[44] In 12- to 18-year-old subjects with previous experience of more than five venipunctures, severe distress with loss of control was experienced by only 5 percent of subjects, and none of them experienced "panic" reactions. Yet, 34 percent of subjects who were 30 months to six years of age experienced severe distress and loss of control, and 13 percent of this group developed frank panic reactions. Panic reactions were also observed in 2 percent of subjects from seven to 11 years. Thus, an IRB undertaking review of a study involving five venipunctures to be conducted over a period of a week might well approve the study if it was to be conducted on 12 year olds and disapprove the project if it was to be conducted on 12-month-old subjects. In fact, the number of blood samples required for drug studies in infants was a central question in an analysis of rejected protocols in a study reported by Koren from the University of Toronto.[45] One children's hospital has recently proposed that studies involving venipuncture in healthy children can only be approved for subjects over age eight.[46]

THE MEANING OF ASSENT

In addition to this description of the complex debate over risk assessment in research on children, I will briefly analyze work published since the National Commission's original recommendations dealing with the concept of assent. Again, I will argue that a failure to examine this concept from the *child's point of view* has thwarted the evolution of this important concept. The National Commission provided a bare-bones definition of assent, which was then incorporated into the federal regulations: "Assent means a child's affirmative agreement to participate in research. Mere failure to object should not, absent affirmative agreement, be construed as assent." (See Appendix D, 46.402.) The National Commission provided a slightly more expanded description of assent in its *Research Involving Those Institutionalized as Mentally Infirm:*

The commission has chosen the term assent to describe authorization by a person whose capacity to understand and judge is somewhat impaired by illness or institutionalization, but who remains functional. The standard for "assent" requires that the subject know that procedures will be performed in the research, choose freely to undergo those procedures, communicate this choice unambiguously, and be aware that subjects may withdraw from participation. This standard for assent is intended to require a lesser degree of comprehension of the subject than would generally support informed consent and is not related to judicial determination of incompetency or commitment status.[47]

Unfortunately, this set of regulations were never incorporated into federal regulations.

One of the first scholars to incorporate the concept of assent into his work was Leiken from Children's Hospital National Medical Center. In an important 1983 article, Leiken noted the work of the National Commission and its use of the term "assent" in the research context. He then undertook an "ethical analysis of the assent or dissent by minors for medical therapy."[48] Leiken compares information available from studies of child development to the basic elements of informed consent. Unfortunately, this analysis fails to set out the basic elements of the concept of assent. However, in a recent article, Leiken does undertake an examination of assent "with particular attention to when it is appropriate to seek minors' assent, and what it means to them when it is sought."[49] Leiken argues that consideration must be given to information we now have about cognitive development, to children's understanding of the nature and purpose of medical research, and to the capacity of the child subject to "reason about research." His analysis includes references to the critically important studies undertaken by Weithorn and her associates on the developing capacity of children to participate in decision-making in both the clinical and research contexts.[50] Leiken also argues that for assent to be meaningful, child subjects must have a basic understanding of the concept of rights, particularly the right to refuse to participate and the right to withdraw from a research activity.

Although I find much that is helpful in Leiken's analysis, I find his recommendations regarding assent to be misleading because of an excessive emphasis on the ability to reason. His analysis leads him to imply that it does not make sense to solicit assent below age nine.

Studies of young people's reasoning, described here, indicate that older children and adolescents (that is, individuals over nine years of age) generally have sufficient cognitive capacity to be involved in decision making concerning participation in research. Thus individuals of this age should be considered candidates for assent.[51]

An interesting way to examine how distorting an emphasis on children's reasoning skills can be is provided by Koren in a recent article which examines the practice of babysitting and proposes that we use a "babysitter test" as a way to determine when children are mature enough to consent to participate in research.[52] Note that I did not say merely assent to participate.

I propose that the concept of assent be understood as applying to minors who have not yet achieved the capacities needed to make autonomous choices, that is, provide or refuse consent. These minors have what might best be called a developing capacity to participate in decision making. Respect for a child as a moral agent requires respect for the developing capacity of the child for autonomy. The growth and development of a child are thwarted and undermined by failure to respect this developing autonomy. The self-image and self-esteem of children are not well established. They are fragile, insecure, and vulnerable aspects of the developing child. The child's evolving self is in need of regular reinforcement through multiple acts of respect by parents and other adults involved in the child's life. This is why I was so disappointed when the National Commission's recommendations regarding respecting the objections of the child subject were not incorporated into federal regulations.

Assent is, most fundamentally, about respect. As a father and as a pediatrician, I have learned that--from their perspective--my daughters and my patients value my respect more than my love. Particularly in times of stress or crisis, it is more important to accept and respect our children and our patients as developing children than to care about or care for them. The use of force, coercion and manipulation in dealings with children are destructive of the child's sense of predictability and control over her life. Failure to respect a child's persistent objection to participating in a research project undermines that child's sense of mastery and the child's sense of adults as trustworthy. To be used as a research subject may or may not involve a risk of harm to the child. For a child to be used as a research subject against her will, against her expressed persistent objection *does* involve doing her predictable harm.[53] It is impossible for me to imagine how one would justify--to the child--using her as a subject over her persistent objection to non-therapeutic research. The Committee on Drugs of the American Academy of Pediatrics has strongly supported the idea that children over age seven must be seen in the research context as having "the right to say no."[54]

In addition, resort to force or coercion in dealing with children undermines the relationship between the child and healthcare providers, the essential nature of which we are just beginning to acknowledge. We are learning the hard lesson that the development and maintenance of a functional patient-provider relationship is an indispensable aspect of healthcare, particularly when patients are experiencing chronic illness. Even in the therapeutic, as opposed to research context, any last resort utilization of force or coercion in dealing with a child should be acknowledged to the child as unjustifiable from the child's perspective. Adults in such situations should always see themselves as owing children an apology for undertaking acts which from the child's perspective are seen as arbitrary, imposed, and harmful. Failing to respect the objection of a child of any age involves--*from the perspective of the developing person*--doing harm to the child. Few of us as parents allow ourselves to realize how often we fail to honor our children when we inflict harm on them "for their own good." The use of force or coercion in the name of discipline may be justifiable. In some situations it may even be necessary to prevent a grave harm from befalling the child. However, we should always honor the fragile developing persons children are by acknowledging to them that--from their perspective--our justifiable actions are experienced as disrespectful and, often, very hurtful.

Thus, I would argue that subjects with developing autonomy may be invited to participate in research activities. Such activities may well provide opportunities for the exercise of autonomy and support the child's evolving sense of self and self-worth. They may, in short, contribute to the psychological and moral growth of a child. However, in order for such opportunities to be present in these activities, the child subject must be informed that she is considering a completely voluntary activity, one she understands she may refuse to participate in or withdraw from even if parental permission has been obtained or her parents object to her decision to withdraw. The dissent of the child subject should be binding in all but the most exceptional circumstances. There are few, if any, clinical situations in which a child's participation in research is *the only* means of responding to the child's healthcare needs. I would also argue that formal review procedures by an IRB or an institutional ethics committee should be required and utilized in the rare situation in which a provider or parent feels that the dissent of a child subject or the child's decision to withdraw from participation should not be respected.

What are the elements of assent understood from the perspective of the child subject? First, the child must be assisted to develop an awareness of the nature of her condition that is developmentally appropriate. What is it about her that makes her an appropriate candidate for participation in this project? Why is she, rather than some other child, being invited to participate?

Second, the investigator must disclose to the child subject the nature of the proposed intervention and what she is likely to experience in undergoing it. From the child's perspective this means answering questions like: What is going to happen to me? What am I being asked to do? What will it be like? What will it feel like? Will I be scared? Will it hurt?

The third element involves the assessment by the investigator of the child's understanding of the information provided and the factors influencing how she is evaluating the situation (with particular emphasis on the presence of undue internal or external pressures). It is clear that children are extremely vulnerable to coercion. It is this extreme vulnerability that led Ackerman to wonder if we shouldn't abandon the entire assent process as proposed by the National Commission.[55] It is also helpful to remember that it may well be the case that parents who volunteer their children to participate in medical research may themselves be very vulnerable to undue external pressures.[56] Investigators must be extremely sensitive to this element with both parents and potential child subjects. Parental permission/child assent forms should clearly document that the parents and the child subjects understand that both parental permission and child assent are necessary for a child to participate in research. Parental permission forms should include a statement such as: "I understand that the assent (statement of willingness) of my child will be solicited by the investigator. I understand that my child is free to refuse to participate in this research and to withdraw from participation in this research even if I have given permission or wish him/her to continue in the project." Assent language might include: "I understand that I do not have to be part of this research even if my parents give permission for me to do it. I also know that I can stop being part of this research at any time even if my parents want me to stay in the research." Obviously, the spirit of this language must also permeate the permission/assent process and the conduct of the research.

The fourth element of assent is the solicitation of the child's expression of willingness to accept the proposed intervention. From the child's perspective, this necessitates an affirmative answer to the question: Will you do it?

It is important to note that nothing in these four elements of assent requires a sophisticated ability to reason or a sophisticated understanding of the risks and benefits of participation in the project or alternatives to participation. Nothing in these four elements requires that a child understand the nature and purpose of medical research in general or the purpose of the proposed research project in particular. Nothing requires that the child subject understand the nature of basic human rights or even that she is a rights-bearing subject. (Although, I would be prepared to argue that most children seven years and older have a good basic understanding of how rights work. For example, one six-year-old in a focus group on children's rights told us, "To have rights is to be treated like a grown up.") The only right that is assumed by the concept of assent is one that children learn very early in life, namely, the right to say no. Assent is a concept that is best understood from the standpoint of the child's reality, the child's perspective, the child's experience.

APPLICATION OF THE CONCEPTS OF EXPERIENCED RISK AND CHILD ASSENT

In this concluding section, I invite the reader to examine an ongoing controversy in pediatric research ethics in light of the idea that risk and assent need to be understood from the child's point of view. In 1989 the NIH began clinical trials (originally submitted to the National Institute of Child Health and Development [NICHD] in 1984) of the use of biosynthetic growth hormone in "extremely short" children. A suit was filed in 1990 by the Foundation on Economic Trends directed by Jeremy Rifkin to put a halt to these studies. In response to the suit, the NIH conducted an internal review of the short-stature studies which resulted in a report in 1992 supporting the trials. In May of 1993 the NIH resumed recruiting for the studies. And, in June of 1993, the Foundation for Economic Trends and the Physicians Committee for Responsible Medicine headed by Neal Barnard again filed suit to stop the trials. The joint plaintiffs claimed that the study posed risks to the children that were clearly more than minimal, failed to hold out the prospect of direct benefit to the subjects, and was studying a condition that was not clearly a disease, that is, short stature. There is no question that the information that could be produced by these randomized, prospective, placebo-controlled trials may be very valuable. There is mounting evidence that growth hormone is being administered to ever increasing numbers of short children who do not have evidence of a deficiency of growth hormone. In fact, there is evidence to suggest that growth hormone is being given to some short children who do not have clearly documented growth failure.

The findings of the NIH review panel have been systematically analyzed by White and by Tauer, who conclude that serious questions remain about these trials. White argues:

It is imperative that value assessments about whether physical stature alone constitutes a physical impairment that should be remedied by medical intervention be made *before* a clinical trial is constructed. Neither the fact that the biotechnology industry is poised to market synthetic hGH to a wider audience nor that physicians may be pressured to prescribe it by parents of non-hGH-deficient, short children is, in and of itself, a good reason for conducting a clinical trial in which children are exposed to more than minimal risk and may not benefit.[57]

Tauer finds reason for concern in the fact that the NIH study panel seems to have created a dangerous precedent by "bending" federal regulations to allow for these projects:

Such an application of 46.406 [see Appendix D of this book] creates a precedent for approving greater than minimal risk research with healthy children in order to study any condition researchers or clinicians would like to be able to modify. If there are people who regard the condition as disadvantaging and who seek "treatment" for it, then that condition would seem to qualify for studies under 46.406.[58]

Tauer supports the recurrent recommendation of Jay Katz that Congress establish a permanent, national human investigation board to respond to studies like these, rather than to find creative ways to interpret the regulations to cover them.[59]

Although I support the critical analysis of these trials offered by White and Tauer, I use these trials as examples of challenges involved in understanding the concepts of risk and assent from the perspective of the child. Although there may well be significant risks for the short children in these studies who are randomly assigned to the growth hormone arm, it might be argued that these risks could be balanced by the possibility that taking growth hormone injections three times a week for 18 to 24 months may result in a significant increase in their ultimate adult height. (It should be pointed out that most of these subjects would need to continue to take growth hormone injections for an extended period after completion of the study for these potential benefits to be realized.) However, when one examines the issue of risk to the children in the placebo arm, things get very muddy. These children are being asked to take injections three times a week for at least 18 months (more than 200 injections), to have radiological monitoring by a series of wrist x-rays, to undergo bone-density measurements, multiple venipunctures, multiple urinalyses, nude photography against a height grid, and extensive psychological testing. Since they are in the placebo arm, they will not experience any of the potential direct benefits of participation. The NIH study panel argued that there were potential benefits to members of their class, that is, to nongrowth hormone deficient, short children, and that there were potential benefits to the research subjects' possible future children who might also be significantly short. One of these two studies involves girls with Turner's syndrome. The other involves normal children who have growth rates at or below the first or second percentile and predicted adult heights that are two standard deviations below normal. It should also be noted that there is no lower age limit for enrollment of children in either trial. Thus, children below the standard age of assent of seven years are allowed to enroll.

To enroll children too young to assent to involvement in such an activity raises serious ethical questions. There can be no question but that participation in this study would be experienced by these very young subjects as extremely burdensome. It is impossible to imagine that the world of a child who is three or four years old would not be disturbed in significant ways when that child has to incorporate into her reality injections three times a week from her mother or father.

Assuming, however, that the study were limited to children who were willing to become research subjects and to give their assent, what should be written in the child assent section of the consent instrument to be used in these studies? First, the child would have to be told why she is being asked to become a research subject, namely that she is excessively short and growing poorly. Meanwhile, the parents of this child would also be doing everything in their power to help her understand that even though she is very short, she is still a perfectly acceptable little girl. What would a child of eight believe about her body, her self? On the one hand, the people who are important to her would be telling her that being short does not mean that there is anything wrong with her. At the same time, she would be told that she is being invited to participate in research on the treatment of this very same condition.

What should she be told about the experience of being a research subject? It would be necessary to tell her that only half of the children in the study would be getting growth hormone injections, and that neither she nor her parents would know whether or not her injections contained the hormone. She would clearly need to be told that she would have to be given or take shots three times a week for at least 18 months in addition to the other multiple experiences called for by the protocol. What would she make of being asked to do all this? Clearly, she would secretly hope and pray that she was one of the lucky children that had been assigned to the growth hormone arm. On the other hand, she may very well feel intense guilt about these same feelings, since that would mean that some other child was getting placebo injections.

Is it possible for a child of this age to see herself as free to join or not join this adventure in spite of her parents' obvious deep concern over her growth and ultimate adult height? Recruitment of subjects into this study has been slow and difficult since few parents are willing to subject their children to the 50:50 chance of being assigned to the placebo group. They would much rather simply have their short child treated with growth hormone even though there is little available data on the efficacy of growth hormone in significantly increasing ultimate adult height. One recent uncontrolled study from Israel found a "modest" increase in final heights of 5.4 cm (a little over two inches), following an average of almost four years of growth hormone injections.[60] An Italian study published in the same journal found that "growth hormone treatment did not generally increase final height over target height in short non-growth-hormone-deficient children."[61] The fact that large numbers of parents are willing to give their children three times weekly injections of growth hormone in the face of such unimpressive results should give one pause in assessing the voluntary nature of assent in these circumstances.

Finally, what of the child's willingness to participate? In particular, what about the monitoring of her willingness to continue to be a subject of this level of intervention? The injections which are clearly the major burden from the child's perspective are being administered by the parent, not by the investigator. They are being administered in a very private setting, namely the child's home. Will a parent whose child objects to continued participation be willing to respect the child's decision to withdraw from the study? What will happen on one of those days which we have all experienced as parents when everything is going wrong and the child objects to having her injection? How many times will the child have to object before she is finally heard as wanting to withdraw from the study? Is it fair to place a child in this kind of situation for periods as long as two years?

CONCLUSION

I have attempted to share with the reader a glimpse into the evolution of pediatric research ethics. We began with an historic ethical debate between two of the founding fathers of American bioethics, Paul Ramsey and Richard McCormick. I described in considerable detail the work and recommendations of the National Commission, which were subsequently incorporated into federal regulations governing research on children. A review of scholarly work and critical examination of two aspects of these regulations--assessment of risk and the concept of assent--constitutes the contribution attempted here. Finally, we examined the value of this analysis by application of an understanding of risk and assent *from the child's perspective* to the ongoing controversy involving research on the use of biosynthetic growth hormone in children who are excessively short.

In conclusion, addressing the many ethical challenges involved in allowing children to participate in research remains very much work-in-progress. I hope that we can come to see that the conceptual framework constructed by the National Commission on the basis of our understanding of pediatric research ethics in the 1970s and incorporated into federal regulations in the 1980s is nothing more than a good beginning of our exploration of these issues. We have developed a reasonably functional conceptual framework and a language that allows adult investigators, members of IRBs, federal investigators, and others to communicate with one another and to make ethical judgments concerning when it appears to be justifiable for adults to undertake research involving children. It is essential that we continue to respond to the many ethical challenges involved in pediatric research ethics in a manner that is more sensitive to the experience of the child subject, a manner that reflects an awareness of both child subjects' vulnerability and developing capacities, as well as honors the "second-mile behavior" of the young heros and heroines who willingly place themselves in harm's way so that the next generation of children may benefit from biomedical and behavioral research.

NOTES

1. W.G. Bartholome, "The Ethics of Nontherapeutic Clinical Research on Children and Proxy Consent in the Medical Context: The Infant as Person," in The National Commission for the Protection of Human Subjects of Biomedical and Behavioral Research, *Appendix to Report and Recommendations: Research Involving Children* (Washington, D.C.: DHEW Publication No. (OS) 77-0005), 3-1 to 3-54; W.G. Bartholome, "Parents, Children and the Moral Benefits of Research," *Hastings Center Report* 6 (December 1976): 44-45.

2. P. Ramsey, "Consent as a Canon of Loyalty with Special Reference to Children in Medical Investigations," in *The Patient as Person* (New Haven: Yale University Press, 1970), 1-58; P. Ramsey, "The Enforcement of Morals: Nontherapeutic Research on Children," *Hastings Center Report* 6 (August 1976): 21-30; R.A. McCormick, "Experimentation in Children: Sharing in Sociability," *Hastings Center Report* 6 (De-

cember 1976): 41-46; P. Ramsey, "Children as Research Subjects: A Reply" *Hastings Center Report* 7 (April 1977): 40-41.

3. National Commission for the Protection of Human Subjects of Biomedical and Behavioral Research, *Report and Recommendations: Research Involving Children* (Washington, D.C.: DHEW Publication No. (OS) 77-0004, 1977).

4. W.J. Curran and H.K. Beecher, "Experimentation in Children: A Reexamination of Legal Ethical Principles," *Journal of the American Medical Association* 210 (1969): 77-83.

5. Ramsey, "Consent as a Canon of Loyalty."

6. *Ibid.*, 11-12.

7. *Ibid.*, 12-14.

8. *Ibid.*, 16.

9. McCormick, "Proxy Consent in the Experimentation Situation," 11.

10. *Ibid.*, 13.

11. *Ibid.*, 14.

12. Ramsey, "The Enforcement of Morals," 22.

13. *Ibid.*, 24.

14. W.E. May, "Experimenting on Human Subjects," *Linacre Quarterly* 41 (1974): 238-52.

15. McCormick, "Experimentation in Children: Sharing in Sociability."

16. *Ibid.*, 42.

17. P. Ramsey, "Children as Research Subjects: A Reply," 40.

18. P. Ramsey, "Ethical Dimensions of Experimental Research on Children," in *Research on Children: Medical Imperatives, Ethical Quandaries, and Legal Constraints*, ed. J. van Eys (Baltimore, Md.: University Park Press, 1978), 57-67.

19. *Ibid.*, 66.

20. L. R. Ferguson, "The Competence and Freedom of Children to Make Choices Regarding Participation in Research," *Journal of Social Issues* 34 (1978): 114-21; P. Keith-Spiegel, "Children's Rights as Participants in Research," in *Children's Rights and the Mental Health Professions*, ed. G.P. Koocher (New York: Wiley, 1976).

21. National Commission, *Report and Recommendations: Research Involving Children*, 1-20.

22. *Ibid.*, 2-3.

23. *Ibid.*, 5-12.

24. *Ibid.*, 13.

25. *Ibid.*, 146.

26. *Ibid.*, 146-7.

27. *Ibid.*, xx.

28. L.M. Kopelman, "When is the Risk Minimal Enough for Children to be Research Subjects?" in *Children and Health Care: Moral and Social Issues*, eds. L.M. Kopelman and J.C. Moskop (Boston: Kluwer Academic, 1989), 89-99.

29. *Ibid.*, 95.

30. J. Janofsy and B. Starfield, "Assessment of Risk in Research on Children," *Journal of Pediatrics* 98 (1981): 842-46.

31. G. Koren, ed., *Textbook of Ethics in Pediatric Research* (Malabar, Fla.: Krieger, 1993), 25-76.

32. *Ibid.*, 48.

33. G.A. Koren, "A Practical Approach to Risk-Benefit Estimation in Pediatric Research," in *Textbook of Ethics in Pediatric Research*, 57-62.

34. D. Brock, "Ethical Issues in Exposing Children to Risks in Research," in *Children as Research Subjects: Science, Ethics & Law*, ed. M.A. Grodin and L.H. Glantz (New York: Oxford University Press, 1994), 97.

35. *Ibid.*, 98-99.

36. E.H. Wender, "Assessment of Risk to Children" in *Children as Research Subjects: Science, Ethics and Law*, 182-92.

37. R.A. Thompson, "Behavioral Research Involving Children: A Developmental Perspective on Risk," *IRB: A Review of Human Subjects Research* 12 (March-April 1990): 1-6.

38. See N. Garmezy and M. Rutter, eds., *Stress, Coping, and Development in Children* (New York: McGraw-Hill, 1983).

39. W. Gaylin, "Competence: No Longer All or None," in *Who Speaks for the Child: The Problems of Proxy Consent*, ed. W. Gaylin and R. Macklin (New York: Plenum Press, 1982), 27-54.

40. W. Gaylin, "The Competence of Children: No longer All or None," *Hastings Center Report* 12 (April 1982): 33-39.

41. W.G. Bartholome, "In Defense of a Child's Right to Assent," *Hastings Center Report* 12 (October 1982): 44-45.

42. B. Freedman, A. Fuks, and C. Weijer, "*In Loco Parentis*: Minimal Risk as an Ethical Threshold for Research Upon Children," *Hastings Center Report* 23 (March-April 1993): 13-19.

43. *Ibid.*, 18.

44. G. B. Humphrey *et al.*, "The Occurrence of High Levels of Acute Behavioral Distress in Children and Adolescents Undergoing Routine Venipunctures," *Pediatrics* 90 (1992): 87-91.

45. G. Koren, "Ethical Boundaries of Medical Research in Infants and Children in the 80's: Analysis of Rejected Protocols and a New Solution for Drug Studies," *Developmental Pharmacology and Therapeutics* 15 (1990): 130-41.

46. S.S. Gidding *et al.*, "A Policy Regarding Research in Healthy Children," *Journal of Pediatrics* 123 (1993): 852-55.

47. National Commission for the Protection of Human Subjects of Biomedical and Behavioral Research, *Research Involving Those Institutionalized as Mentally Infirm* (Washington, D.C.: DHEW publ. no. (OS) 78-0006, 1978).

48. S.L. Leiken, "Minors' Assent or Dissent to Medical Treatment," *Journal of Pediatrics* 102 (1983): 169-76.

49. S.L. Leiken, "Minors' Assent, Consent, or Dissent to Medical Research," *IRB: A Review of Human Subjects Research* 15 (March-April 1993): 1-7.

50. L.A. Weithorn and S.B. Campbell, "The Competency of Children and Adolescents To Make Informed Treatment Decisions," *Child Development* 53 (1982): 1589-98; L.A. Weithorn, "Children's Capacities to Decide About Participation in Research," *IRB: A Review of Human Subjects Research* 5 (March-April 1983): 1-5; L.A. Weithorn, "Involving Children in Decisions Affecting Their Own Welfare: Guidelines for Professionals," in *Children's Competence to Consent,* ed. G.B. Melton, G.P. Koocher, and M.J. Saks (New York: Plenum Press, 1983).

51. Leiken, "Minors' Assent, Consent, or Dissent to Medical Research," 4.

52. G. Koren, "Maturity of Children to Consent to Medical Research: The Babysitter Test," *Journal of Medical Ethics* 19 (1993): 142-47.

53. R.B. Redmon, "How Children Can Be Respected as 'Ends' Yet Still Be Used as Subjects in Nontherapeutic Research," *Journal of Medical Ethics* 12 (1986): 77-82.

54. R.E. Kauffman, "Drug Trials in Children: Ethical, Legal and Practical Issues," *Journal of Clinical Pharmacology* 34 (1994): 296-99.

55. T.F. Ackerman, "Fooling Ourselves with Child Autonomy and Assent in Nontherapeutic Clinical Research," *Clinical Research* 27 (1979): 345-48.

56. S.C. Harth, R.R. Johnstone, and Y.H. Thong, "The Psychological Profile of Parents who Volunteer their Children for Clinical Research: A Controlled Study," *Journal of Medical Ethics* 18 (1992): 86-93; Y.H. Thong and S.C. Harth, "The Social Filter Effect of Informed Consent in Clinical Research," *Pediatrics* 87 (1991): 568-69.

57. G.B. White, "Human Growth Hormone: The Dilemma of Expanded Use in Children," *Kennedy Institute of Ethics Journal* 3 (1993): 401-9.

58. C.A. Tauer, "The NIH Trials of Growth Hormone for Short Stature," *IRB: A Review of Human Subjects Research* 16 (May-June 1994): 1-9.

59. J. Katz, "Ethics and Clinical Research Revisited: A Tribute to Henry K. Beecher," *Hastings Center Report* 23 (September-October 1993): 31-39.

60. Z. Zadik *et al.*, "Effect of Long-Term Growth Hormone Therapy on Bone Age and Pubertal Maturation in Boys with and without Classic Growth Hormone Deficiency," *Journal of Pediatrics* 125 (1994): 189-95.

61. S. Loche *et al.*, "Final Height after Growth Hormone Therapy in Non-Growth-Hormone-Deficient Children with Short Stature," *Journal of Pediatrics* 125 (1994): 196-200.

15

Fetal and Embryo Research: A Changing Scientific, Political, and Ethical Landscape

Constance M. Pechura

This chapter presents an overview of the scientific and ethical issues pertaining to three of the most controversial areas of human experimentation--research involving fetal tissue, fetuses, and embryos. Over the past two decades, the questions regarding research ethics in these areas have continuously evolved. This now richly textured canvas has been created from science, politics, and the growth of bioethics as an academic field. Fundamental and important scientific discoveries regarding in vitro fertilization (IVF), fetal surgery and diagnostics, and the use of human fetal cells to ameliorate adult disease, have raised increasingly complex ethical questions. Likewise, the legalization of abortion in 1973 has fueled political controversies and pressures, which have had an enormous influence on both science and research ethics in the United States. In many instances throughout these decades, scientific and technological advances and political struggles have preceded ethical debate, and hard-won resolution of ethical questions has not always been able to wrest political change. What about the future?

The major conclusion of this chapter is that each of the three research areas will continue to pose new ethical questions and that mechanisms in the United States for ongoing consideration of these questions must be in place on a national level. Such a conclusion is not unique. Indeed, a variety of proposals for national mechanisms to address bioethical issues have been put forward, and new federal efforts are being implemented. This chapter, however, addresses some of these efforts with specific reference to the potential scientific advances in research with fetuses and embryos.

The chapter begins with a historical overview of the bioethics initiatives regarding fetal and embryo research over the past two decades. Following this overview, the state of the science and current regulations applicable to each research area are summarized, followed by an overview of potential future advances and their ethical implications. This chapter is not meant to be a complete review of the scientific and ethical literature. Rather, it is intended to present selected issues to give the reader a sense of these research areas and the ethical dilemmas they engender. Finally, although the chapter focuses primarily on the ethical guidelines and policies that govern these types of research in the United States, key developments and documents from other countries are also discussed.

HISTORICAL OVERVIEW

FEDERAL BIOETHICS INITIATIVES

There has been a long and tortuous history of federal regulatory efforts in the area of fetal and embryo research. This history was described by the Association of American Medical Colleges in 1988 and examined in the broader context of biomedical ethics in a recent report by the Office of Technology Assessment of the U.S. Congress.[1] Additional historical and analytic perspectives regarding publicly constituted bioethics bodies can be found in Chapter 7 of this book. Presented here is a brief distillation of past and very recent federal efforts specific to the research areas considered in this chapter, along with a description of activities of nongovernmental groups.

The development of federal regulations to govern fetal research began with the 1973 Supreme Court decision in *Roe v. Wade* that legalized abortion and overturned the many state laws that banned or indirectly regulated research on fetuses. Also in 1973, all states ratified the Uniform Anatomical Gift Act that prohibited the for-profit sale of human organs and tissues (including fetal tissue) and regulated their use for research or therapeutic purposes. In 1974, the National Research Act (Public Law 93-348) set up the National Commission for the Protection of Human

Subjects in Biomedical and Behavioral Research. As part of this act, all research on fetuses was prohibited pending a report from the commission. The National Commission issued its report in May 1975, recommending that fetal research following an abortion be permitted, but that all research, including that following abortion, either involve no more than minimal risk or be undertaken for a therapeutic purpose.[2]

However, a waiver from these restrictions could be obtained on a project-by-project basis by application to an Ethics Advisory Board, whose establishment was recommended in the commission's report. It was not until 1978 that the first Ethics Advisory Board (EAB) was convened. The EAB issued only one waiver, for a project to use fetal blood samples for prenatal diagnosis of sickle cell anemia, before its charter expired in 1980. The EAB also produced four reports. These included one on human IVF and embryo transfer, one on fetoscopy, and two others unrelated to its charge to address research issues involving the fetus, pregnant women, and IVF.[3] The President's Commission for the Study of Ethical Problems in Medicine and Biomedical Research was created by Congress in 1978 (Public Law 95-622). This body operated from January 1980 to March 1983 and produced reports on a wide range of topics, none of which directly addressed issues of fetal or embryo research.[4]

In 1985, the Health Research Extension Act (Public Law 99-158) imposed a three-year moratorium on the issuance of any waivers for fetal research beyond that involving minimal risk. The act also established a Congressional Biomedical Ethics Board to appoint and oversee a Biomedical Ethics Advisory Committee (BEAC). The first meeting of BEAC did not take place until September 1988 and, as a result of political wrangling among the members of its congressional oversight board, the committee expired in 1989 having issued no reports.[5]

An important development pertaining to fetal tissue transplantation also occurred in 1988. The trigger was a request from the National Institute of Neurological and Communicative Disorders and Stroke to study human fetal brain cells as transplant material for patients with Parkinson's disease. Assistant Secretary for Health, Robert Windom, issued a memorandum in March placing a moratorium on such research until the National Institutes of Health (NIH) could convene an outside advisory group to consider 10 specific questions. His questions mostly focused on the implications of fetal tissue transplantation research for elective abortions. The resulting Human Fetal Tissue Transplantation Research Panel issued its report in December 1988, with the majority of panel members recommending lifting the moratorium.[6] NIH did not forward the panel's report to the Department of Health and Human Services (DHHS) until January 1989, the last days of the Reagan presidency. Following additional months of consideration at DHHS, the secretary, Louis Sullivan, sided with the minority opinion in November 1989 and extended the moratorium. This moratorium remained in effect until January 1993, when it was lifted by President Clinton in a memorandum (58 FR 7468) that also directed NIH to establish guidelines for fetal tissue transplantation and fetal research. The first project in fetal tissue transplantation research following the end of the moratorium was funded by NIH in January 1994.[7]

In June 1993, the Public Health Service Act was amended under the National Institutes of Health Revitalization Act (Public Law 103-43) to provide for the establishment of ethics advisory boards by the secretary of the Department of Health and Human Services. Additional amendments upheld the 1988 NIH panel's findings and set out regulations for publicly funded fetal tissue transplantation research. The regulations prohibit and impose criminal penalties on the sale of fetal tissue or the designation of such tissue to a specific recipient or relative.

As soon as one controversy seemed to end, however, another emerged with the announcement that researchers at The George Washington University Medical School had "cloned" human embryos.[8] Under the revised Public Health Service Act, the NIH convened an ethics advisory panel on human embryo research in February 1994. This panel's report, although still subject to a public hearing and final acceptance by the director of NIH, was released on 27 September 1994.[9]

NONGOVERNMENTAL BIOETHICS INITIATIVES

From 1980 until quite recently, a tremendous vacuum existed in bioethics inquiry at the federal level, which had particularly chilling effects on fetal and embryo research, as well as fetal tissue transplantation research. Federal funding was unavailable for these types of research and funding sources shifted to private foundations and corporate entities. Nevertheless, the clinical practice of IVF expanded greatly during this period, often in the absence of an adequate scientific base.[10] Although other countries were establishing national bioethics bodies, many of which issued reports on ethics of research with the fetus and embryo, the task of grappling with such ethical guidelines in the United States, with one exception, fell to nongovernmental organizations.[11] The exception was the U.S. Congress Office of Technology Assessment (OTA), which under its establishing mandate was charged to evaluate the policy implications of developments in science and technology. As policy and ethics are not easily disentangled, OTA has consistently found itself incorporating bioethics in many of its reports.[12]

In 1984, the American College of Obstetricians and Gynecologists (ACOG) issued a report outlining ethical issues to be considered in the practice of IVF. They later established a Committee on Ethics, which addressed the ethical issues of embryo research. The American Fertility Society also formed an Ethics Committee that reported its guidelines for IVF and embryo research in 1986.[13]

A report on infertility and research in IVF was released by OTA in 1988.[14] The ethical and legal issues of both clinical practice and research were summarized in this report. In addition, policy options relating to the reestablishment of the EAB, implementation and update of the EAB's 1979 recommendations, and the possibility of directing the Congressional Biomedical Ethics Board to address such issues were outlined. In 1989, the Institute of Medicine (IOM) issued a report on medically assisted conception that assessed the scientific base of IVF, outlined a research agenda, and summarized the relevant ethical issues.[15] This report recommended that, in the absence of a reconstituted EAB or some other federal bioethics body, "a nongovernmental organization should be established to develop guidelines for embryo and fetal research." Partly in response to this IOM recommendation, ACOG and the American Fertility Society formed the National Advisory Board for Ethics in Reproduction (NABER) in 1992. This group is now supported by private foundations and operates independently from its founding professional societies.[16]

By the late 1980s, the ethical implications of the use of fetal tissue in transplantation research became an additional area of focus. Again, a vacuum was created by the failure of the HHS secretary to implement the recommendations of the 1988 report by the NIH Human Fetal Tissue Transplantation Panel. In a report assessing the political underpinnings of specific decisions about the funding and applications of advances in biomedicine, the IOM analyzed the deliberations of that NIH panel as one of its case studies. An assessment of the scientific findings of neural grafting and relevant policy options had been completed by OTA in 1990. NABER also considered the ethical issues of fetal tissue transplantation in a paper published in 1993.[17]

In June 1993, before the controversy surrounding human embryo cloning emerged, the IOM sponsored a conference to revisit the scientific advances in embryo and fetal research.[18] Fetal tissue research was also included in this conference, as were presentations and discussions of the ethical and legal issues relevant to research in these areas. A workshop on the ethical issues of embryo cloning was convened by NABER in February 1994 (the same month that the NIH advisory panel on embryo research met for the first time). An excellent summary of this conference and the conclusions of NABER members was published in September, 1994.[19]

FEDERAL INITIATIVES REVISITED: OUTLOOK FOR THE NEAR FUTURE

There is broad and continuing discussion over the best mechanisms by which to address present and future bioethics concerns in the United States. These discussions have been complicated recently by rapid changes in Congress and the Executive Branch. For example, in their 1993 paper, Hanna, Cook-Deegan, and Nishimi called for both a reconstituted EAB to resolve ethical debates generated by research advances and a relatively autonomous body, "such as a President's Bioethics Commission," to handle broad policy issues.[20] Even before their paper was printed, the Public Health Service Act was amended allowing the formation of ethics advisory panels. These panels, however, differ importantly from the previous EAB in that they are to be convened on an ad hoc basis only when the need arises. Nevertheless, a variation of one of the two mechanisms suggested by Hanna and her colleagues is now possible and the second mechanism may be on the horizon.

A National Bioethics Advisory Commission, to be established within the executive branch, has recently been proposed by the Office of Science and Technology Policy.[21] The proposed charter directs this body to two areas of inquiry: "issues in the management and use of genetic information and protection of the rights and welfare of research subjects." However, specific reference to issues relating to fetal and embryo research, which might fall into one of these broad charges, is absent. The final charter of this body may be further revised, following public comment, in the months ahead.

FETAL TISSUE RESEARCH

OVERVIEW OF THE SCIENCE

Fetal tissue research uses cells and tissues from dead fetuses, following induced or spontaneous abortions, to establish cell lines or organ cultures or for transplantation into human beings or animals for therapeutic or research purposes. Although extensive research into its use as transplant material for treatment of human disease is relatively recent, fetal tissue has been used in research for decades because most fetal cells grow and proliferate easily in culture. For example, human fetal cell lines were used in the 1950s to develop polio vaccine and are still used today in research and diagnostic virology, bacteriology, immunology, as well as for research in blood cell differentiation, embryological development, cell physiology, and molecular biology.[22]

There are four major advantages to the use of fetal tissue for transplantation. First, fetal cells lack most of the cell-surface markers that trigger immune responses in transplant recipients. Thus, the chances of graft rejection are greatly reduced. Second, fetal cells from all body areas continue to grow and divide. This capacity is particularly important for application to diseases of the brain, because adult brain cells essentially lose their ability to regenerate. Fetal brain cells, in contrast, grow readily following transplant. Fetal cells also retain their ability to differentiate after transplantation and they continue to produce factors that stimulate growth. The ability of fetal cells to differentiate is crucial to their usefulness in a number of diseases. For example, fetal thymus and liver contain so-called stem or precursor cells, which differentiate into all the various types of blood cells or certain specialized types of immune system cells and are absent or lost in a number of diseases.

Most fetal tissue transplantation research has involved the use of tissue from the pancreas, thymus, liver, or brain. Successful use of fetal thymus transplants was first reported in 1968.[23] In these attempts, fetal thymus was transplanted into two infants born with DiGeorge's syndrome, a congenital birth defect characterized by multiple anomalies, including absence of a specific type of immune cell (T lymphocytes) due to failure of the thymus to develop. In the absence of T cells, the immune system is so compromised that patients usually die within a year. By 1988, fetal thymus transplants were the treatment of choice for DiGeorge's syndrome and it remains today the only condition for which fetal tissue transplantation is not experimental.[24]

Serious efforts to employ human fetal pancreas tissue to correct diabetes emerged in the late 1970s and early 1980s, following experiments in animals showing that islet cells from the fetal pancreas could function to restore normal glucose levels in diabetic adults. Application of fetal pancreas transplants in human diabetes, however, has proven more problematic.[25] Despite more than 1,500 individual human transplant cases reported to the International Islet Transplant Registry, rigorous analysis has revealed problems with successful engraftment of the transplants, immunological problems, and difficulty demonstrating physiological functioning of the transplanted cells.[26] For example, the presence of lymphoid tissue in the fetal pancreas and its capacity to induce an immune reaction in the transplant recipient have necessitated the use of immunosuppressive drugs in these patients. This requirement is undesirable because diabetic patients are already prone to infections, some of which are potentially life-threatening. Continuing research in this area has focused on improving preservation of fetal pancreatic tissue by freezing, to increase the quantity of tissue transplanted and finding ways to isolate the functional pancreatic cells to obtain purified cell fractions and reduce the need for immunosuppressive therapy.

Fetal liver transplants, often in combination with fetal thymus to provide T lymphocytes, have been attempted with mixed success for a number of immunodeficiency diseases and inborn errors of metabolism, as well as for certain blood disorders.[27] In contrast to adults in whom bone marrow is the primary site of blood cell formation (hematopoiesis), the liver is a primary site of hematopoiesis in the fetus. There are also large numbers of stem cells for blood formation in the fetal liver. Although bone marrow transplantation can cure some immunodeficiency diseases and blood disorders, there are stringent requirements for acceptable donor tissue for all bone marrow transplants. All cells have a complement of specific sets of genes (major histocompatibility complex, MHC) that vary from individual to individual. The MHC encode a group of cell-surface molecules, called human leukocyte antigens (HLA) because they were discovered on lymphocytes. When the HLAs of a bone marrow donor do not match the HLAs of the recipient, the T lymphocytes from the donor will eventually mount an immunological attack against the recipient known as graft-versus-host disease. Fetal T lymphocytes are immature and, thus, tolerate the antigens of the recipient.

Severe combined immunodeficiency disease is a rare and lethal congenital disorder that has been successfully treated with fetal liver and thymus transplantation.[28] Inborn errors of metabolism, such as Gaucher's disease and Hurler's syndrome, have also been treated with some success using fetal liver transplants.[29] Touraine has reported three cases of fetus-to-fetus transplant in which cells from fetal liver and thymus were injected into umbilical veins and, thus, transplanted into two fetuses diagnosed with immunodeficiency disease, and one fetus diagnosed with thalassemia.[30] Attempts to treat adult blood disorders, including aplastic anemia and acute myelogenous leukemia, with fetal liver transplants have been disappointing, largely due to insufficient engraftment without prior treatment with immunosuppressive drugs.[31]

The first efforts to transplant fetal brain cells to treat Parkinson's disease brought worldwide publicity to fetal tissue research.[32]

Parkinson's disease is a progressive degenerative condition caused by loss of a specific group of brain cells that contain the neurotransmitter dopamine. Although the drug L-dopa reduces the symptoms of Parkinson's disease, its effectiveness diminishes over time. Until about 10 years ago, animal experiments in neural grafting for a number of neurological diseases, despite many decades of investigation, often did not mirror human diseases precisely enough. For Parkinson's disease, however, a tragic accident allowed the development of a highly reliable model that was directly applicable to humans. A severe form of Parkinson's disease developed in a group of young men who had taken an illegally produced drug that contained a contaminant. Once isolated, this contaminant, 1-methyl-4-phenyl-1,2,3,6-tetrahydropyridine or MPTP, was injected into animals to produce a syndrome that matched human Parkinson's disease quite well. Shortly after fetal brain transplants were shown to work in the animal model, the first attempts in human patients were made in a number of centers around the world, including the United States.[33] By 1992, more than 100 patients had received fetal tissue transplants for Parkinson's disease, and, although many of these patients have shown improvement, key questions await further study.[34]

CURRENT REGULATIONS APPLICABLE TO FETAL TISSUE RESEARCH

In general, fetal tissue research in the United States is regulated under the Uniform Anatomical Gift Act (UAGA), but special regulations apply to fetal tissue transplantation research, many of which derive from the issues and topics assigned to the 1988 NIH Human Fetal Tissue Transplantation Research Panel.[35] Often ignored, however, is the fact that state laws take precedence over federal regulations and guidelines and some states prohibit research with fetal tissues.[36] This precedence is explicit in the UAGA, DHHS regulations on human subjects (45 CFR 46), and the amendments specific to fetal tissue transplantation research in the NIH Revitalization Act of 1993 (Public Law 103-43).

Three prohibitions are outlined in federal regulations concerning fetal tissue research (45 CFR 46) under the principle that the decision to abort should be separate from any research interests. Researchers are prohibited from participating in any decision relating to the timing or method of an abortion; physicians are prohibited from changing the abortion procedure in any way for the sole purpose of research; and, monetary or other inducements to obtain consent from women for use of fetal tissues for research are prohibited. For fetal tissue transplantation research, many other stipulations were added by the amendments contained in Public Law 103-43. These include requiring the following signed statements, which must be available for confidential audit by the Secretary of DHHS:

1. A signed statement by the woman agreeing to donate the fetal tissue for research, specifying that the donation is without any restrictions regarding particular recipients and testifying that the identity of any recipient is unknown.

2. In the case of an induced abortion, the physician must submit a signed statement to guarantee that he or she obtained consent for the abortion before requesting consent for research use of the tissue; that no change in the timing, method, or procedure was made for research purposes; and, that the abortion was in concert with state law. Assurances must be included in the physician's statement that the woman had been fully informed of medical and privacy risks and any interest of the physician in the research to be carried out with the fetal tissue.

3. The researcher must submit a statement certifying appropriate informed consent of the woman; promising to inform fully any recipient of the tissue; and, testifying that the researcher had no part in the decisions about timing, method, or procedures used in the abortion.

In addition, the regulations impose criminal penalties on persons who would sell fetal tissues for transplantation, knowingly donate tissue to a specific individual or relative, or solicit a donation of fetal tissue.

ETHICS AND SCIENCE IN THE FUTURE

It may seem that lifting the moratorium on federal funding of fetal tissue research and establishing regulations for fetal tissue transplantation research mark the end of ethical debate. This could not be farther from the truth for three reasons. First, the politics of the abortion issue will continue to spur reexamination of the moral status of the fetus, and dominance of one view over another in the future may even overshadow the current regulations. Second, there are important ethical questions left unresolved by the establishment of regulations, which even by their establishment raise new questions. Finally, new scientific applications and advances on the horizon will generate yet other, largely unexplored, ethical issues. The latter two reasons are appropriate subjects for this chapter.

The current regulations, as stated above, derive in large measure from issues addressed by the 1988 NIH Human Fetal Tissue Transplantation Research Panel. The deliberations of this panel were analyzed by James Childress in a 1991 report from the Institute of Medicine.[37] A major issue that dominated much of the NIH panel's time was the morality of abortion and whether or not that question could be separated from the morality of fetal tissue transplantation, given that abortion was legal. Related to this were the moral implications for the researchers, who according to two panel members would be participating or cooperating in the moral evil of abortion. In terms of the recent regulations, however, the panel's response to questions about whether fetal tissue transplantation research would increase the number of abortions, proved pivotal.

Childress organized his analysis of this question by describing three scenarios for how women could be motivated to have an abortion in order to donate fetal tissue: general altruism, to donate for the good of others; specific altruism, to donate for the good of a particular individual; and financial incentives. While noting that no evidence existed that abortions were increased by the previous three decades of fetal tissue research, the NIH panel recommended that ways be found to assure that the decision to abort preceded the decision to donate tissue and that women should not be allowed to designate the recipient of donated fetal tissue. This separation of the decision to abort from the decision to donate and the prohibition against designating a specific recipient, are common in regulations developed in other countries, including the United Kingdom and Canada.[38]

That the NIH panel's recommendations are reflected in the current regulations is unmistakable, but the requirements of the 1993 amendments to the Public Health Service Act for signed statements by the woman, the physician, and the researcher, along with the possibility of audit, seem to exceed the intent of the NIH panel. Indeed, when similar legislation was attempted as part of the NIH Revitalization Act of 1991, the House bill called for the woman to certify that her decision to have an abortion was not for the purpose of donating fetal tissue. This version additionally contained no explicit protection of confidentiality. In response to the proposed legislation, Kearney, Vawter, and Gervais argued strongly that certification requirements and the potential for government audit would seriously threaten the right of privacy of women, that it represented an unprecedented intrusion of the government into personal motivations, and that the bill essentially "misread" completely the ethical intent of the NIH panel.[39] Although the current law does not require a woman to certify her motivation for seeking an abortion and protection of confidentiality is included, its requirements for signed statements by all three parties and the potential audit of these statements can be expected in the future to be the subject of serious concerns.

In the broadest context, there are those who argue that any restriction on the motivation of a woman to seek an abortion may be ethically faulty--as long as abortion is legal, that is--and that ethical debate must continue, even about those aspects for which a consensus is apparent. For example, in his recently released book, John Robertson argues that the concept of procreative liberty should be a primary guide for public policy on reproductive technologies, including fetal tissue transplantation. In considering the implications of procreative liberty for a woman contemplating becoming pregnant for the sole purpose of donating fetal tissue, Robertson writes:

In sum, deliberate creation of fetuses to be aborted for tissue procurement is more ethically complex and defensible than its current widespread dismissal would suggest. Such a practice is, of course, not in itself desirable, but in a specific situation of strong personal or familial need may be ethically justified. Persons who rationally compare the competing concerns may well conclude that in some circumstances, with safeguards to protect women from coercion and exploitation, the use of one's reproductive capacity to obtain fetal tissue for transplant should be ethically and legally accepted. When the need for such abortions arises, this should be fully debated and not dismissed out of hand as ethically unacceptable.[40]

This cursory glimpse at some of the implications of current regulations demonstrates that even some of the oldest ethical questions pertaining to fetal tissue research continue to present vexing dilemmas. It will be against this backdrop that advances in science will complicate these questions and create new ones. Although a clear view of the scientific future is daunting, certain directions are already emerging.

Fetal pancreas and fetal brain transplants are still experimental and many knowledge gaps exist that require further study. In trials for diabetes, for example, tissue from 16- to 20-week-old fetuses has been found to be better than tissue from younger gestational ages. It is also not clear what the optimum age is for fetal brain tissue transplanted into patients with Parkinson's disease, or what the best age will be for newer applications for Alzheimer's disease or other neurological diseases. If older fetuses are found to be preferable in these procedures, then the quantity and sources of fetal tissue may be more limited because most elective abortions are legal only up to week 12 of gestation. Investigation into methods of maintaining fetal cell populations in culture are currently under way as a possible solution. Work with brain precursor cells is aimed to determine what conditions favor differentiation of particular types of brain cells and whether, once transplanted, the cells will function properly. Other culture methods may involve immortalization of the cells by altering them in such a way that they continue growing. However, immortalized cells can behave like cancer cells, so ways to prevent overgrowth of such cells will be important to their usefulness as transplant material. Experimentation in this area is now confined to animal work but will pose special ethical questions if, and when, the technology develops sufficiently for human clinical trials.

A federally funded fetal tissue bank was proposed to handle the possible need for older fetal tissue, as well as a way to insure an adequate supply of fetal tissue. Although such a bank was established by President Bush in May 1992, many saw this action as merely a political move to quiet scientists, ethicists, and legislators who were arguing for an end to the moratorium. By 1993, following nullification of the moratorium and despite the funding of five centers for this purpose, NIH cancelled the program. Cohen and Jonsen argued on behalf of NABER that the fetal tissue bank project should be continued because it provided a "barrier between those who undergo and carry out abortions and those who receive and perform fetal tissue transplants."[41] Also cited as reasons to continue the program were the developing knowledge about optimum age of tissue and the amount of tissue needed for successful transplants. NABER also referred to the existence of such a bank in the United Kingdom and made the point that a tissue bank could develop uniform quality standards for fetal tissue, thus helping to ensure their safety.

Another scientific challenge is circumventing the immune system in fetal pancreas and even fetal brain transplants. In both these cases, immunosuppressive drugs are needed and, as more applications of fetal tissue transplant are developed, new methods to reduce the antigenicity of transplanted cells, or their ability to mount an immunological attack against the recipient will be developed. Will these methods require a change in tissue collection techniques? If so, current guidelines may be questioned. Another way to protect cells against immunological attack is to encapsulate them in special material that allows the biochemical products of the cells to exit the capsule, but prevents antibodies or immune-active cells from entering. The potential development of unique methods to culture purified fetal cell populations, cell populations with special properties, or methods to encapsulate such cells for transplant would raise intellectual property and commercial questions not addressed by current regulations and guidelines. Canada's Royal Commission on the New Reproductive Technologies has foreseen this potential, writing: "Commissioners believe strongly that fetuses should never be an appropriate subject for patents. However, if they are intended to benefit human health, and if the safeguards we have recommended for obtaining and using fetal tissues are in place, innovative products and processes using fetal tissue as a source may warrant some limited form of patent protection."[42]

Two additional areas of potential scientific advance deserve mention: the development of methods to expand human stem cells using animals as the culture environment and the potential use of fetal germ cells as transplant material. It is now possible to grow intact human organ pieces in animals and to replace an animal's blood entirely with human blood cells.[43] A particularly useful model for these techniques is the SCID mouse, a mutant strain that lacks T and B lymphocytes and exhibits severe immunodeficiency. Implants of human fetal thymus have been shown to result in production of human T cells tolerant to both the mouse and human donor. Transplanted human fetal bone marrow in these mice reconstitute all the human blood cell types. For this reason, these mice are called SCID-hu mice indicating the presence of functional human cells. Because it is also now possible to isolate human blood stem cells, this work has important implications for a variety of diseases, including diabetes. In addition, SCID-hu mice can be used to study human viral diseases, such as AIDS. The model also suggests that blood stem cells can repopulate the bone marrow of a recipient and correct acquired disease states, such as leukemia, or even genetic disease states, such as severe combined immunodeficiency and thalassemia. The SCID-hu mouse can also potentially be used as a culture environment to expand the sources of human stem cells. These advances raise not only intellectual property and commercial concerns, they also carry with them some of the same ethical questions as do animal-to-human organ transplants (xenografts) and germ-line gene therapy.

Although much of the publicity regarding fetal germ cells has focused on the potential use of fetal oocytes to create embryos (to be discussed below), the potential also exists, and is currently being studied, to use transplants of fetal gonadal tissue to reverse sterility, to restore sex steroid production, or even to circumvent transmission of genetic disease.[44] The advantage, particularly for female sterility, is that ovaries from one aborted fetus contain enough potential oocytes to repopulate the ovaries of many sterile children and women. Obviously the barriers to applying this work to humans are not only technical, but also ethical. The prospect of thousands of genetic half-siblings with unborn biological mothers raises profound ethical and legal implications far beyond what ethics commissions and bodies have grappled with so far. Indeed, the only fully enacted response to date has been an outright ban on the use of fetal oocytes in infertility treatment.[45]

FETAL RESEARCH

OVERVIEW OF THE SCIENCE

Fetal research is conducted on a living fetus inside or outside the uterus, involving both invasive and noninvasive procedures. Fetal research has been extensive and extremely successful in many cases, making fundamental contributions to health for both pregnant women and their children through improved monitoring, early diagnosis of a host of illnesses, and improved or more timely therapeutic intervention. Although some types of fetal research are no longer allowed--such as drug studies to assess the ability of pharmacologic agents to cross the placenta and the effects of these agents on the fetus--it continues to be an active area of research.[46] Noninvasive techniques developed through fetal research, such as ultrasonography, are able to evaluate the age and growth of a fetus, detect malformations, determine sex, and detect multifetal pregnancies. Invasive techniques, such as amniocentesis and chorionic villus sampling, can detect infection, chromosome abnormalities, neural tube defects, and Rh disease, as well as assess the maturity of fetal lungs. Fetoscopy allows direct visualization of the fetus *in utero* and allows the collection of blood samples or biopsy material.

Still experimental, percutaneous umbilical blood sampling (PUBS) permits diagnosis of genetic diseases and fatal hemolytic diseases in the fetus. In addition, the PUBS technique can be used to introduce cells into a fetus, including blood transfusions. By 1991, an international registry recorded more than 7,000 PUBS procedures with a fetal fatality rate of 1 percent; PUBS transfusion of more than 400 fetuses exhibiting severe edema caused by Rh disease resulted in an 82 percent survival rate.[47]

Surgical interventions into fetal diseases have had mixed results.[48] Urinary tract obstructions, for example, have been treated by the surgical placement of shunts. Although the shunts helped to insure survival if no other complication was present, there were a number of undetectable complications resulting in fetal loss, and there was a high risk of severe kidney problems in survivors. Prenatal surgery to correct diaphragmatic hernia resulted in more deaths than postnatal surgery, so this procedure was halted. For hydrocephalus, fetal surgical shunt placement increased the survival rate, but infants were born profoundly brain-damaged and, so, this procedure is no longer performed.[49]

CURRENT REGULATIONS APPLICABLE TO FETAL RESEARCH

DHHS regulations for human experimentation (Section 46.208 (a), Title 45-*Code of Federal Regulations*, Part 46) limit research on the living fetus *in utero*, unless "(1) the purpose of the activity is to meet the health needs of the fetus and the fetus will be placed at risk only to the minimum extent necessary to meet such needs, or (2) the risk to the fetus imposed by the research is minimal and the purpose of the activity is the development of important biomedical knowledge which cannot be obtained by other means."

Further, consent must be obtained from both parents in most cases, although the mother's consent alone is acceptable under certain conditions. The regulations make no distinction between living or dead fetuses *ex utero* except to stipulate certain restrictions on artificial life support and activities that could terminate fetal heart beat or respiration. Before the moratorium, these restrictions came under the waiver provision and, thus, research beyond minimal risk, or that which would not meet the health needs of the fetus, could be allowed after review by an ethical advisory board. In fact, the only waiver ever issued by the former EAB was for the development of fetoscopy to diagnose sickle cell anemia and other blood diseases. The EAB also recommended that, under certain circumstances, similar projects need not be reviewed and could be funded.[50]

ETHICS AND SCIENCE IN THE FUTURE

Ethical questions about fetal research tend to be complex because they involve all of gestational life and issues of personhood become more prominent.[51] In addition, the range of potential interventions is broad, including continued research into PUBS, selective reduction of multifetal pregnancies, treatment of metabolic disturbances and vitamin deficiencies *in utero*, and others. There are no present activities comparable to the new federal guidelines for funding fetal tissue transplantation research or the deliberations of the NIH Embryo Research Panel to address the many unresolved questions for fetal research. For example, in practice and with nonfederal funding, considerable fetal research has been done prior to abortion when it involves more than minimal risk, but when there is a reasonable expectation that the techniques developed will benefit the future generations. Arguments over this issue can also apply to a nonviable fetus *ex utero* and have been summarized by Levine.[52] Thus, one question raised is whether or not future DHHS regulations will change, or waivers will be granted, to distinguish between a viable fetus intended to be carried to term and a nonviable fetus, or a fetus to be aborted. However, in the absence of a standing EAB, it is not clear how such waivers would be issued without convening a special advisory group.

Increased focus on women's health has also raised new questions about the need for research to provide effective medications for serious illnesses affecting pregnant women.[53] Will pharmacological research protocols to test effectiveness of medications for pregnant women or to test the medication's effect on the fetus be approved again if it is conducted prior to an abortion? A recent IOM committee recommended that the automatic exclusion of pregnant women from clinical trials in DHHS regulations be dropped.[54] Although this IOM committee made no recommendations regarding the parts of the DHHS regulations dealing specifically with fetuses, they did ask NIH to "facilitate clinical research to advance the medical management of pre-existing medical conditions in women who become pregnant (for example, lupus); of medical conditions of pregnancy (for example, gestational diabetes); and, of conditions that threaten the successful course of pregnancy (for example, pre-term labor)."

On the scientific frontier, research to develop additional applications for the PUBS technique seems certain. Of particular interest is the ability to transfuse fetuses. As mentioned in the section above, fetal bone marrow has been injected into a few fetuses with immunodeficiencies and thalassemia.[55] PUBS is also being used to collect platelet samples from fetuses in studies of maternal-fetal blood incompatibilities, such as thrombocytopenia, to assess the effectiveness of various maternal therapies.[56] Another technique, called embryoscopy, is in the early stages of development and may allow access to the blood supply of fetuses less than 12 weeks of age.[57] This capability would have implications for very early diagnosis and potential use of interventions, including blood transfusions and genetic therapy. Finally, fetal surgery done outside the uterus, with replacement of the fetus into the uterus following surgery is being attempted.

The scientific developments in the field of fetal research do not seem to elicit the publicity and political pressure that has been targeted to fetal tissue transplantation and embryo research. This may, in part, be due to the fact that much fetal research is for the more socially desirable purpose of enhancing fetal survival and reducing birth defects. Nevertheless, fetal research has greatly increased the ability to diagnose genetic and other diseases and, thus, increased the number of parents faced with the choice to continue or terminate their pregnancies. In this respect and others, then, the ethical issues of fetal research will always be closely tied to the variety of ethical views regarding abortion. Indeed, it can be argued that the current ambiguities in the regulations governing fetal research and the number of unresolved ethical questions, while not the most visible, represent important issues for future ethics bodies to consider.

EMBRYO RESEARCH

OVERVIEW OF THE SCIENCE
In addition to the discovery of basic biological processes of reproduction, embryo research has been crucial to the medical practice of human in vitro fertilization (IVF). It is this biology and the applications of such research that makes the term "embryo research" useful but overly restrictive because it denies the importance of research with male and female gametes--sperm and ova. In addition, the literature is filled with different terms for the embryo. Textbooks of embryology define various stages of the embryonic period of development--zygote, blastomere, blastocyst--depending on the number of cells in the mass. There are also distinctions between preimplantation embryos, also sometimes

called preembryos or early embryos, and postimplantation embryos. In this section, unless otherwise noted, the term embryo denotes a preimplantation embryo.

In 1988, the OTA report on infertility estimated that success rates of IVF, in the hands of the best practitioners, was 15 to 20 percent.[58] In addition to assessing the practice and policy options affecting IVF, the OTA report identified a number of areas requiring further research to improve this success rate, including development of ways to inject a sperm into an ovum and better understanding of the biology of ova. A year later, the IOM assessed the scientific base underlying IVF practice and developed a research agenda to increase understanding of the biology of gamete maturation, fertilization, and embryo development. There has been some progress since 1989, but lack of federal funding for much of the research in the United States has hampered work in this field and, unfortunately, the success rates of IVF have not changed.[59] Clearly, much more research is needed, particularly regarding fertilization and the biology of the embryo.

Research with human oocytes (immature ova) and ova have additionally been hampered by a lack of supply, but important findings have been possible. For example, proteins on the gelatinous coating of the ovum, the *zona pellucida*, have been found to bind sperm to the ovum and facilitate sperm entry. Antibodies to zona proteins are also being investigated as possible contraceptives. Better ways to preserve oocytes have been developed, and it is now possible to mature primitive oocytes in culture.[60] This capability may be applied to the development of methods to culture adult ovarian follicles, which could obviate the need for drugs used in IVF, which overstimulate follicles and have significant side effects. Culture of fetal oocytes can also provide a greatly expanded number of oocytes available for research, but not without significant controversy regarding their use to create embryos.

Much has been learned about the biology of sperm, including the molecular biology of sperm formation and maturation and the role of sperm proteins in fertilization. For example, knowledge about the role of sperm-zona interactions led to attention in IVF clinics to the implantation of only those ova with bound sperm. It has been known for a long time that sperm determine the sex of the offspring by either carrying an X, or a Y, chromosome. However, techniques have been developed recently to separate X- and Y-carrying sperm and so determine the sex of an embryo before fertilization.[61] Because some genetic diseases are sex linked, separation of sperm in this way can, when coupled with IVF, prevent the production of embryos with certain genetic diseases even though the actual gene for that disease may not be identified. The same technique, however, could be used more broadly for sex selection.

Low success rates and technical difficulties have driven the search for more innovative ways to assist fertilization. Application of micromanipulation techniques has permitted holes to be drilled in the zona pellucida so that a sperm can be injected directly into an ovum.[62] These techniques have also been used to help an embryo "hatch" out of the zona, a process necessary for successful implantation, but difficult if the zona is particularly thick. Armed with the powerful methods developed for molecular biology that amplify small amounts of DNA and the identification of genes for a number of human diseases, micromanipulation techniques have enabled researchers to develop preimplantation genetic tests.[63] These tests involve the separation of a single cell (blastomere) from an embryo and have been used to diagnose cystic fibrosis and Lesch-Nyhan disease. In addition, single blastomere biopsy techniques have been used to determine the sex of an embryo for the purpose of detecting sex-linked genetic diseases.[64]

It has been estimated that 30 to 40 percent of IVF-produced embryos have chromosome abnormalities, comparable to rates for natural fertilization.[65] Thus, the ability to perform genetic analysis of embryos and of gametes has another useful application in research, to determine why these abnormalities occur and to improve the success rates of IVF by identifying, but not implanting, embryos with abnormalities.

CURRENT REGULATIONS APPLICABLE TO EMBRYO RESEARCH

Although research is allowed with male and female gametes, all research involving fertilized ova and embryos is prohibited under DHHS regulations unless a protocol is granted a waiver by an ethics advisory board. Section 46.204 (d) of Title 45, *Code of Federal Regulations,* Part 46 states: "No application or proposal involving human in vitro fertilization may be funded by the department or any component thereof until the application or proposal has been reviewed by the ethical advisory board and the board has rendered advice as to its acceptability from an ethical standpoint."

The NIH Embryo Research Panel's recommendations, once formally accepted, will provide such guidance for a number of types of embryo research.[66] However, state laws will apply that may ban or severely restrict certain types of research.[67]

ETHICS AND SCIENCE IN THE FUTURE

Ethical guidelines for embryo research have been put forward by a number of groups within the United States and other countries. The IOM Committee on Medically Assisted Conception summarized 16 extended committee statements on new reproductive technologies published in various countries between 1979 and 1987, including the 1979 EAB report.[68] Among these reports, most found research with human embryos and the use of spare embryos for research acceptable under a variety of circumstances and restrictions. Of the statements that defined acceptable time periods, almost all held that embryos could be kept *in vitro* for up to 14 days. However, much less consensus was found regarding the acceptability of creating embryos for research.

Consideration of more recent guidelines reveals a tremendous increase in the complexity of the issues addressed. The 1993 report from the Royal Commission on the New Reproductive Technologies recommended that research on spare embryos was acceptable, as was the creation of embryos for research and fertilization of spare ova, with permission of the donor and in licensed facilities.[69] However, the commission also considered, and found unacceptable, embryo cloning by nuclear substitution, genetic manipulation of embryos, parthenogenesis, fusion of female gametes, ectogenesis, transfer of embryos to another species, and preimplantation genetic diagnosis for the sole purpose of sex selection.[70] NABER also recently considered embryo cloning by blastomere separation, and, although almost all NABER members agreed that research on split embryos is acceptable if the embryo is not harmed, certain members would allow greater research flexibility, and one found such research totally unacceptable.[71]

As mentioned above, the NIH Embryo Research Panel released its draft report very recently.[72] Their recommendations are similar to the Royal Commission's with some notable exceptions--the NIH panel would allow limited cloning by nuclear substitution and limited creation and study of parthenotes. The NIH panel also would allow creation of embryos for research, but only if the information could not be obtained in other ways and if the research proposed had the potential of being greatly valuable to science or therapy. Like the Royal Commission, the NIH panel recommended that no payments be given to donors, that donors consent to the use of spare embryos for research, and that no embryos should be transferred to another species. In addition, no fertilization or gestation of embryos from fetal oocytes would be allowed by the NIH panel. Research would be allowed in the area of preimplantation genetic diagnosis, but not in the area of sex determination, unless the research in question deals with sex-linked genetic diseases.

Areas of needed and acceptable research in the NIH panel's report included study of the biology of fertilization, effects and methods of embryo freezing, and establishment of stem cell lines. These are interesting developments from a scientific viewpoint, because the panel's report will likely stimulate research in many of the areas that are now emerging in gamete and embryo research. Genetic analysis of embryos and of gametes can be expected to be the subjects of intense investigation in the near future. Also, the possibility of establishing stem cell lines is particularly intriguing, in part due to the concern for adequate and safe sources of transplant material.

What the future will hold for those areas deemed unacceptable today is unclear. The use of fetal oocytes, for example, will likely be discussed and debated over the next few years. Already there is an apparent disparity among the newest guidelines. For example, although banning the use of fetal oocytes to create embryos for IVF, the United Kingdom will allow their use for research--but the United States may not.[73] Canada's Royal

Commission recommended that any fertilization of fetal oocytes be banned under criminal codes.[74] Such disparity underscores the fact that numerous other questions are not fully resolved, despite the recent flurry of ethics panels' activities.

In conclusion, future scientific advances in fetal tissue transplantation and fetal and embryo research will generate increasingly complex ethical questions. In the United States, this research will take place in an environment of strong, and almost certainly changing, political pressures. Such pressures are difficult to predict but will become apparent as the ethics bodies issue their reports. For example, the fate of the NIH Embryo Research Panel's recommendations will be telling, once forged in the fire of public scrutiny and political interest. The nullification of the moratorium that stymied much of fetal and embryo research was cause for celebration for many and disappointment for others. It has also stimulated careful, but varied, thought about how best to structure strong leadership in bioethics at the national level. Whatever structures are established, a proper balance between autonomy from political pressure and self-interest on the part of researchers will be critical to advances in science and to the grounding of science in reasoned ethical principles.

NOTES

1. Association of American Medical Colleges (hereafter, AAMC), *Summary: Fetal Research and Fetal Tissue Research,* 1988; U.S. Congress, Office of Technology Assessment (hereafter OTA), *Biomedical Ethics and U.S. Public Policy--Background Paper,* OTA-BP-BBS-105 (Washington, D.C.: U.S. Government Printing Office, 1993).

2. U.S. Department of Health, Education, and Welfare (hereafter HEW), National Commission for the Protection of Human Subjects in Research, *Research on the Fetus: Report and Recommendations,* DHEW Pub. No. (OS)76-127 (Washington, D.C.: U.S. Government Printing Office, 1975).

3. OTA, *Biomedical Ethics and U.S. Public Policy;* HEW Ethics Advisory Board, *Report and Conclusions: HEW Support of Research Involving Human In Vitro Fertilization and Embryo Transfer* (Washington, D.C.: U.S. Government Printing Office, 1979); HEW Ethics Advisory Board, *Report and Recommendations: Research Involving Fetoscopy* (Washington, D.C.: U.S. Government Printing Office, 1979).

4. OTA, *Biomedical Ethics and U.S. Public Policy.*

5. *Ibid.*

6. U.S. Department of Health and Human Services, National Institutes of Health, Human Fetal Tissue Transplantation Research Panel, *Report of the Human Fetal Tissue Transplantation Research Panel, Volumes I and II* (Bethesda, Md.: National Institutes of Health, 1988).

7. L. Thompson, "Fetal Tissue Research on the Rebound," *Science* 263 (1994): 601.

8. J.L. Hall *et al.*, "Experimental Cloning of Human Polyploid Embryos Using an Artificial Zona Pellucida," The American Fertility Society and The Canadian Fertility and Andrology Society, Program Supplement, *Abstracts of the Scientific Oral and Poster Sessions*, S1:0-001, 1993; G. Kolata, "Researcher Clones Embryos of Human in Fertility Effort: Tough Ethical Challenge," *New York Times*, 24 October 1993, A1, A22.

9. E. Marshall, "Rules on Embryo Research Due Out," *Science* 265 (1994): 1024-26; J.A. Schwartz, "Panel Backs Funding of Embryo Research," *Washington Post*, 28 September 1994, A1.

10. OTA *Infertility: Medical and Social Choices*, OTA-BA-358 (Washington, D.C.: U.S. Government Printing Office, 1988); Institute of Medicine, *Medically Assisted Conception: An Agenda for Research* (Washington, D.C.: National Academy Press, 1989).

11. OTA, *Biomedical Ethics and U.S. Public Policy*; K.E. Hanna, R.M. Cook-Deegan, and R.Y. Nishimi, "Finding a Forum for Bioethics in U.S. Public Policy," *Politics and the Life Sciences* 12 (1993): 205-19. Eleven other opinions on this topic were published in a subsequent issue of this journal (13, no.1, 1994) along with a response by Hanna and her colleagues.

12. Hanna, Cook-Deegan, and Nishimi, "Finding a Forum."

13. American College of Obstetricians and Gynecologists (hereafter ACOG), Committee on Gynecologic Practice, "Human In Vitro Fertilization and Embryo Placement, Committee Statement," Washington, D.C., 1984; American College of Obstetricians and Gynecologists, Committee on Ethics, "Ethical Issues in Human In Vitro Fertilization, and Embryo Placement," ACOG Committee Opinion Number 47, Washington, D.C., 1986; American Fertility Society, Ethics Committee, Ethical Considerations of the New Reproductive Technologies, *Fertility and Sterility* 46, 3 Suppl. (1986): 1S-94S.

14. OTA, *Infertility*.

15. Institute of Medicine, *Medically Assisted Conception*.

16. C.B. Cohen, "Future Directions for Human Cloning by Embryo Splitting: After the Hullabaloo," *Kennedy Institute of Ethics Journal* 4 (1994): 187-92.

17. K.E. Hanna, ed., *Biomedical Politics*, Institute of Medicine (Washington, DC: National Academy Press, 1991); OTA, Neural

Grafting: *Repairing the Brain and Spinal Cord,* OTA-BA-462 (Washington, D.C.: U.S. Government Printing Office, 1990); C.B. Cohen and A.R. Jonsen, "The Future of the Fetal Tissue Bank," *Science* 262 (1993): 1663-65.

18. Institute of Medicine, *Fetal Research and Applications: A Conference Summary* (Washington, D.C.: National Academy Press, 1994).

19. The entire September 1994 issue of the *Kennedy Institute of Ethics Journal* is devoted to a summary of this workshop and recommendations by NABER members.

20. Hanna, Cook-Deegan, and Nishimi, "Finding a Forum."

21. OTA, "National Bioethics Advisory Commission Proposed Charter," *Federal Register* 59 (12 August 1994): 41584-86.

22. Association of American Medical Colleges, *Summary: Fetal Research;* Institute of Medicine, *Fetal Research;* L. Wong, "The Procurement of Human Fetal Tissues for Clinical Transplantation: Practice and Problems," in *Fetal Tissue Transplants in Medicine,* ed. R.G. Edwards (Cambridge: Cambridge University Press, 1992).

23. T. Hansen and J.R. Sladek, Jr., "Fetal Research," *Science* 246 (1989): 775-79; Council on Scientific Affairs and Council on Ethical and Judicial Affairs, American Medical Association, "Council Report: Medical Applications of Fetal Tissue Transplantation," *Journal of the American Medical Association* 263 (1990): 565-70; C.S. August *et al.,* "Implantation of a Foetal Thymus Restoring Immunological Competence in a Patient with Thymic Aplasia," *Lancet* no. *ii* (1968): 1210; W.W. Cleveland *et al.,* "Foetal Thymic Transplant in a Case of DiGeorge's Syndrome," *Lancet* no. *ii* (1968): 1211.

24. R.H. Buckley, "Human Thymus Transplantation for the Correction of Congenital Absence of the Thymus (DiGeorge's Syndrome), Presentation to the Human Fetal Tissue Transplantation Research Panel," in *Report of the Human Fetal Tissue Transplantation Research Panel,* vol.2, (1988), D50-57.

25. Hansen and Sladek, Jr., "Fetal Research"; AMA, "Council Report"; B.E. Tuch, "Clinical Results of Transplanting Fetal Pancreas," in *Fetal Tissue Transplants in Medicine,* 215-37.

26. Tuch, "Clinical Results."

27. Hansen and Sladek, Jr., "Fetal Research"; AMA, "Council Report"; R.P. Gale, J.-L. Touraine, and V. Kochupillai, "Synopsis and Prospectives on Fetal Liver Transplantation," *Thymus* 10 (1987): 13-18; J.-L. Touraine, "Transplantation of Fetal Haemopoietic and Lymphopoietic Cells in Humans, with Special Reference to In Utero Transplantation," in *Fetal Tissue Transplants in Medicine,* 155-75.

28. AMA, "Council Report"; Gale, Touraine, and Kochupillai, "Synopsis"; Touraine, "Transplantation."

29. Gaile, Touraine, and Kochupillai, "Synopsis"; Touraine, "Transplantation."

30. Touraine, "Transplantation."

31. Gale, Touraine, and Kochupillai, "Synopsis."

32. Human Fetal Tissue Transplantation Research Panel, *Report;* J.R. Sladek, Jr. and I. Shoulson, "Neural Transplantation: A Call for Patience Rather Than Patients," *Science* 240 (1988): 1386-88.

33. Hansen and Sladek, Jr., "Fetal Research"; AMA, "Council Report"; Sladek, Jr. and Shoulson, "Neural Transplantation."

34. H. Sauer, S.B. Dunnett, and P. Brundin, "The Biology of Fetal Brain Tissue Grafts: From Mouse to Man," in *Fetal Tissue Transplants in Medicine,* 177-213; L. Thompson, "Fetal Transplants Show Promise," *Science* 257 (1992): 868-70; R. Robbins, "Fetal Tissue Transplantation for Patients with Parkinson's Disease," in *Fetal Research and Applications: A Conference Summary,* 49-51.

35. Human Fetal Tissue Transplantation Panel, *Report.*

36. L.B. Andrews, "Federal and State Regulations of Fetal Research: A Current Perspective," in *Fetal Research and Applications: A Conference Summary,* 11-13; L. B. Andrews, "Regulation of Experimentation on the Unborn," *Journal of Legal Medicine* 14 (1993): 22-56.

37. J.F. Childress, "Deliberations of the Human Fetal Tissue Transplantation Research Panel," in *Biomedical Politics,* 215-48; pages 249-57 contain additional commentaries by Patricia A. King and Walter Harrelson, who were members of the IOM Committee to Study Biomedical Decision Making.

38. J.C. Polkinghorne, "Law and Ethics of Transplanting Fetal Tissue," in *Fetal Tissue Transplants in Medicine,* 323-35; Royal Commission on New Reproductive Technologies, *Proceed with Care: Final Report of the Royal Commission on New Reproductive Technologies* (Ottowa, Ont., Canada: Minister of Government Services, 1993).

39. W. Kearney, D.E. Vawter, and K.G. Gervais, "Fetal Tissue Research and the Misread Compromise," *Hastings Center Report* 21 (September-October 1991): 7-12.

40. J.A. Robertson, *Children of Choice: Freedom and the New Reproductive Technologies* (Princeton, N.J.: Princeton University Press, 1994).

41. Cohen and Jonsen, "The Future."

42. Royal Commission, *Proceed with Care.*

43. I. Weissman, "Isolation of Candidate Human Stem Cells Using SCID-hu Mice Implanted with Human Fetal Tissue," in *Fetal Research and Applications: A Conference Summary,* 55-58; B. Peault *et al.,* "Experimental Human Hematopoiesis in Immunodeficient SCID Mice Engrafted with Fetal Blood-Forming Organs," in *Fetal Tissue Transplants in Medicine,* 77-95.

44. R.G. Edwards, "Overview: Modern Ideas in Embryo Research," in *Fetal Research and Applications: A Conference Summary*, 15-17; C. Holden, "Fetal Egg-Cell Research Scare," *Science* 265 (1994): 608; R.G. Gosden, "Transplantation of Ovaries and Testes," in *Fetal Tissue Transplants in Medicine*, 253-79.

45. Holden, "Fetal Egg-Cell Scare."

46. AAMC, *Summary*; IOM, *Fetal Research*; Hansen and Sladek, Jr., "Fetal Research."

47. K. Moise, Jr., "Percutaneous Umbilical Blood Sampling," in *Fetal Research and Applications: A Conference Summary*, 27-29.

48. Hansen and Sladek, Jr., "Fetal Research"; M. Golbus, "Fetal Therapy," in *Fetal Research and Applications: A Conference Summary*, 37-38.

49. Hansen and Sladek, Jr., "Fetal Research"; R. Berkowitz, "Therapeutic Interventions in Utero," in *Fetal Research and Applications: A Conference Summary*, 35-37.

50. J. Fletcher and J.D. Schulman, "Fetal Research: The State of the Question," *Hastings Center Report* 15 (April 1985): 6-12.

51. R.J. Levine, *Ethics and Regulation of Clinical Research* (New Haven, Conn.: Yale University Press, 1988).

52. *Ibid.*

53. J. Robertson, "Ethical Issues Related to the Inclusion of Pregnant Women in Clinical Trials (I)," in *Women and Health Research, Volume 2, Workshop and Commissioned Papers*, ed. A.C. Mastroianni, R. Faden, and D. Federman (Washington, D.C.: National Academy Press, 1994); B. Steinbok, "Ethical Issues Related to the Inclusion of Pregnant Women in Clinical Trials (II)," in *Women and Health Research, Volume 2, Workshop and Commissioned Papers*, 23-28.

54. A.C. Mastroianni, R. Faden, and D. Federman, eds., *Women and Health Research: Ethical and Legal Issues of Including Women in Clinical Trials, Volume 1* (Washington, D.C.: National Academy Press, 1994).

55. Touraine, "Transplantation"; Moise, Jr., "Percutaneous Umbilical Blood Sampling."

56. R. Berkowitz, "Therapeutic Intervention in Utero," in *Fetal Research and Applications: A Conference Summary*, 35-37.

57. E.R. Reece, "Embryoscopy and New Advances in Fetal Diagnosis and Treatment," in *Fetal Research and Applications: A Conference Summary*, 29-32.

58. OTA, *Infertility*.

59. IOM, *Medically Assisted Conception;* IOM, *Fetal Research.*"; Society for Assisted Reproductive Technology, American Fertility Society, "Assisted Reproductive Technology in the United States and Canada: 1991 Results from the Society for Assisted Reproductive Technology/

American Fertility Society Registry," *Fertility and Sterility* 59 (1993): 956-62.

60. Edwards, "Overview."

61. *Ibid.*; B.L. Gledhill and R.G. Edwards, "Can Spermatozoa Be Typed?" in *Preconception and Preimplantation Diagnosis of Human Genetic Disease,* ed. R.G. Edwards (Cambridge: Cambridge University Press, 1993).

62. J. Cohen *et al., Micromanipulation of Human Gametes and Embryos* (New York: Raven Press, 1992); J. Cohen, "Micromanipulation Research in Clinical Embryology," in *Fetal Research and Applications: A Conference Summary,* 17-19.

63. M. Hughes, "Preimplantation Genetic Analysis of Single Human Blastomeres," in *Fetal Research and Applications: A Conference Summary,* 22-23.

64. A.H. Handyside and J.D.A. Delhanty, "Cleavage Stage Biopsy of Human Embryos and Diagnosis of *X* Chromosome-Linked Recessive Disease," in *Preconception and Preimplantation Diagnosis of Human Genetic Disease,* 239-70.

65. M. Plachot *et al.,* "Are Clinical and Biological IVF Parameters Correlated with Chromosomal Disorders in Early Life: A Multicentric Study," *Human Reproduction* 3 (1988): 627-35.

66. Andrews, "Federal and State Regulations"; Schwartz, "Panel Backs Funding."

67. Andrews, "Federal and State Regulations."

68. HEW, *Report and Conclusions;* IOM, *Medically Assisted Conception.* This summary was based on a presentation by LeRoy Walters.

69. Royal Commission, *Proceed with Care.*

70. *Embryo cloning by nuclear substitution* involves the transfer of a nucleus from one cell into another cell from which the nucleus has been removed. This process differs importantly from *cloning by blastomere separation* in which cells of an embryo are simply divided. For an excellent description of cloning see J. Cohen and G. Tomkin, "The Science, Fiction, and Reality of Embryo Cloning," *Kennedy Institute of Ethics Journal* 4 (1994): 193-203. *Parthenogenesis* refers to the creation of an embryo from only a female gamete. *Ectogenesis* refers to the gestation of an embryo in an artificial womb.

71. National Advisory Board on Ethics in Reproduction, "Report on Human Cloning through Embryo Splitting: An Amber Light," *Kennedy Institute of Ethics Journal* 4 (1994): 251-82.

72. Marshall, "Rules"; Schwartz, "Panel Backs Finding."

73. Marshall, "Rules"; Schwartz, "Panel Backs Finding"; Holden, "Fetal Egg-Cell Search."

74. Royal Commission, *Proceed with Care.*

16

Respecting Human Subjects in Genome Research: A Preliminary Policy Agenda

Eric T. Juengst

INTRODUCTION

The Human Genome Project has been described as "the lightning rod of human genetics."[1] Given the project's goals--to construct fine-grained reference maps of the human chromosomes and to develop more efficient DNA sequencing technologies--some other mechanical metaphor (the "tool box of human genetics"?) might seem to catch the project's purposes better. But in fact, the Human Genome Project represents geneticists' growing ability to explore human heredity. It thus generates a wide range of charged questions about how our society's genetic explorations should proceed and how their results should be used. These questions include a set of unresolved issues regarding the conduct of research involving human subjects. While these issues predate the Human Genome Project and would continue to exist without it, they are becoming increasingly important as genomic tools and genetic strategies become pervasive in biomedical research. In this essay, I will sketch the most prominent of these issues as a proposed agenda for professional ethics and policy development for the future.

BACKGROUND

One of the initial goals of the Human Genome Project is to identify reliable DNA markers--stable molecular features that can be used as landmarks in the DNA--evenly spaced across all 24 human chromosomes.[2] Taken alone, the construction of this "framework map" of the human genome involves no active participation by human research subjects. It is almost entirely a matter of bench molecular biology, using anonymous chromosomes acquired from "immortalized" cell lines long since separated from their varied human sources. While such a genomic marker map will not answer many scientific or medical questions in itself, it will provide a crucial tool for localizing genes on the chromosomes, so that the genes can be identified and decoded. *This* research involves working with human subjects. In fact, human subjects are involved in these studies in a way that was largely unanticipated in our research policies on ethics: they are involved as entire families.

By correlating the inheritance of a given health problem with the inheritance of different DNA markers within a family, geneticists can use "flanking" markers to define the chromosomal region into which the problem's causal gene must fall. Once "mapped" in this way, the causal gene can be isolated by even more fine-grained techniques and deciphered at the molecular level, providing a key clue to the pathogenesis of the clinical problem.[3] If specific molecular mutations can be identified within the gene as necessary and sufficient conditions for the emergence of the clinical disorder, molecular "probes" for these mutations can be quickly developed as powerful prognostic tests for use within at-risk families.[4]

As higher resolution marker maps become available, genetic linkage studies involving large families are becoming increasingly common across the biomedical research landscape. They are already being used in attempts to discover the etiology of health problems as diverse as deafness, heart disease, colon cancer, and schizophrenia.[5] They have become particularly important in the etiology of diseases such as breast cancer, which are understood to be predominantly environmentally caused, but which also seem to run in some families. In these cases, the hope is that if the inherited germ-line mutation can be isolated in families, it may shed light on its somatic counterpart as well.[6]

Like any clinical research, genetic family studies can encounter ethical problems that reflect the unique characteristics and circumstances of the specific diseases and families in question. Family genetic studies also challenge researchers to respect the rights and interests of subjects within the matrix of families. As new research teams take up gene hunting, an increasing number of investigators and institutional review boards (IRBs) find themselves faced with these matters. IRBs quickly discover that both the federal research regulations and the research ethics literature have been virtually silent in this area. If anything, the prevailing standards seem to assume that cohorts of biomedical research subjects usually consist of strangers, rather than people who live with each other as family members.

At the same time, genetic family studies have been conducted for decades, and a variety of home-grown practices and policies have evolved within the human genetics research community to address these challenges.[7] Unfortunately, these precedents can bewilder as easily as they illuminate. While home-grown approaches to specific problems are often defended passionately by their advocates, almost all these approaches have their critics as well. As family-based, gene-hunting protocols multiply within biomedicine, the demand for fuller, more definitive, and more uniform guidance on how best to use our new genomic tools is increasing.

TEN OPEN QUESTIONS

Genetic family studies raise at least 10 questions of research ethics that are incompletely addressed by current rules and practices. Collectively, these questions offer an agenda for research policy making that will become increasingly important as the Human Genome Project's tools become disseminated within biomedicine.

From the outset, it is important to mention a complicating feature of many genetic family studies--the fact that this research is increasingly cross-cultural and international. The large intermarried families and careful record-keeping of culturally insulated populations such as the U.S. Amish and Canadian Hutterite communities make them attractive resources for genetic researchers. The physical isolation of populations like the villagers of Lake Maraciabo in Venezuela also produce useful, high-density pedigrees for study. Even genetic studies that involve mainstream American immigrant families can quickly take investigators all across the globe and across cultures in the Third, as well as the First, World. Large gene-hunting expeditions are increasingly collaborative efforts between scientists in different countries who pool international family resources to expedite their searches. Cultural, linguistic, and socioeconomic factors complicate genetics research, in much the same way they complicate international epidemiological research.[8]

The 10 open questions that geneticists face can be divided into two sets: issues over the recruitment and enrollment of family members as research subjects, and questions about the control and disclosure of research results.

INDIVIDUAL INTERESTS AND FAMILY TIES

Conceptually, genetic linkage studies start with the identification of a person who expresses the inherited trait in question (a *proband*, or *index case*), and then the reconstruction of as much of the trait's pattern of inheritance within the proband's extended family as possible. This genetic pedigree is used to distinguish family members who carry the causal gene from those who do not. For most well-defined genetic conditions, linkage study subjects are recruited from clinical practice settings in which multiple family members have become involved in genetic evaluation and counseling, and the family pedigree for the condition is already at least partially established. Ethical questions arise even in this initial stage. The proband can provide investigators access to his or her own clinical records, which may well include family medical histories compiled for clinical purposes. But the provision of information by the proband about family members for research purposes raises a question: *(1) To what extent can the investigator use the proband or the proband's clinical records as a source of research data about other people, without their permission?*

Appropriating clinical family history information to launch a new genetic family study is a practice so traditional as to be ethically invisible within the community. But as the power of genetic analysis grows, the involvement of family members as research subjects is coming under more scrutiny. At stake is not only the privacy of the genetic information disclosed about other family members, but also the voluntariness of their involvement in the study. Thus, while acknowledging that "no consensus on this issue has yet been reached," the NIH's Office of Protection from Research Risks (OPRR) now suggests that IRB's might

draw a distinction between information about others provided by a subject that is also available to the investigator through public sources (for example, family names and addresses) and other personal information that is not available through public sources (for example, information about medical conditions or adoptions).[9]

IRBs could then allow investigators to collect only the former, public facts about the family from the index case.

RECRUITMENT STRATEGIES

The recruitment strategy that flows most naturally from the OPRR's suggestion is to have the proband provide a bare family tree (one that contains information already publicly available elsewhere), and for the investigators to convert this tree into a genetic pedigree by soliciting relevant health data from each relative directly. In order to pursue the linkage analysis further, investigators must request and collect DNA (usually from a blood sample) from as many members of the extended family as possible. This recruitment approach anticipates the fact that the relatives will all have to be contacted eventually anyway if the study is to proceed to the next stage. If the investigator's solicitation includes an invitation to contribute the preliminary genetic data as well as blood, the subjects' ability to control their own involvement in the study is enhanced.[10]

Other teams of researchers take stronger measures to insulate prospective subjects from premature involvement. Some investigators do not construct family trees immediately, but have the probands carry letters to their relatives explaining the study and inviting them to contact the investigators if they want to become involved.[11] As a result, the researchers only receive pedigree information from those family members who actively volunteer for the study. While this approach does the best job of giving the potential subjects control over the situation, it is important to note its imperfections. If enough family members volunteer for the study, even those who declined to participate may find themselves involved, as information about them is inferred from analyses of their offspring and forbears.

This approach, moreover, highlights a second issue: in some cases it may be the proband's own privacy that the recruitment process puts at risk. *(2) To what extent can the privacy of medical information about an individual subject be protected from other family members recruited into a family study?* This concern arises primarily for genetic studies of socially stigmatizing conditions like psychiatric disorders, the diagnosis of which may not be generally shared within an extended family.[12] To rely on a proband to contact and recruit members of his or her extended family is to assume that the proband's diagnosis is one that can be shared with relatives without prejudice; for this reason most psychiatric geneticists take the responsibility to contact the family themselves. Here, the imposition on the family is justified out of a concern to protect the proband's privacy.

Unless it is handled adeptly, this strategy quickly meets limitations. Without a reference to the proband's diagnosis of, for example, schizophrenia, how do the investigators adequately explain to a proband's cousin why they are interested in her participation in their family linkage study of this disease? Psychiatric geneticists warn,

It should be made clear to psychiatric patients whose relatives will be contacted exactly what information about a subject will be provided to those relatives. This is important because the presence or severity of mental disorders may be considered a secret, and subjects may not want relatives to learn about their diagnoses, prognoses, or past behavior. As part of the "family secrets" concern, when discussing relatives who may be affected by a psychiatric disorder, the pedigree should not be presented to a prospective subject with diagnoses of identified relatives included. Subjects should start with a blank pedigree, rather than being asked to add information to one which reveals sensitive information about other relatives.[13]

Enlisting research subjects to help recruit their relatives has been defended as a means to enhance family members' ability to make voluntary choices regarding participation in genetics research. However, families are not composed of equal peers. In many situations, the subject-recruiter or family facilitator is recruited from the charged atmosphere of the clinic. These subjects, who are motivated by their clinical need to find "their gene," usually proceed as advocates of the research. Thus the pressure of compelling familial relationships may simply replace the researcher's influence in recruiting potential subjects.[14] This problem may be greater for cohesive, hierarchically organized families from cultural groups that have not yet been effected by the 20th century breakdown of the family, families whose size also tends to make them ideal subjects for linkage analysis.

One response to this problem is for researchers to approach families collectively, by presenting their research projects at large gatherings like family reunions, and inviting all interested individuals to contact them to become involved.[15] Some teams of researchers also rely on lay organizations, like genetic disease support groups, to make the initial contact with families in the context of the community support they are providing.[16] However, these approaches also pose risks to the goal of achieving autonomous participation: family members may actually feel less free to demur in large group settings, and lay-led support groups vary in expertise, understanding, and objectivity (particularly when they are helping to fund the research itself). The general policy questions remain: *(3) In seeking to protect the voluntariness of participation in face of the need for the greatest level of participation by families, when should recruiting be done directly by investigators, and when by family members or members of support groups?*

These last two questions regarding recruitment policies raise an important meta-level question for students of research ethics. Do the concerns over privacy and individual autonomy that current research ethics dwell on pose the wrong questions on research that involves the inner workings of family life?

Some argue that because the family is the proper clinical unit of analysis (and allegiance) for geneticists who counsel patients, most questions about the disclosure of intra-familial genetic information should not be regarded as problems about confidentiality in professional practice.[17] If that argument succeeds for genetic counseling, should it not also apply to genetic research? Similarly, others now argue that taking the family seriously means that IRBs or investigators should not attempt to police the inevitable psychosocial forces that come into play in familial decision making, any more than they would second-guess an individual volunteer's internal deliberations. Researchers would do better, they argue, to monitor their own influence and leave the family's internal dynamics intact.[18] Whether the family should be regarded as an entity that can justify these arguments that may discount the privacy and autonomy of individuals is, of course, the question.[19]

MATERIAL RISKS

Questions about the voluntariness of research participation in research and the privacy of participants become more important as the stakes involved in participating in a study increase. Thus another important set of research ethics questions pertains to the levels of risks that linkage studies pose to subjects, and, in turn, the risk-related disclosures that should be made to potential subjects as part of the informed-consent process.

Compared with other, more physically invasive forms of clinical research, the risks of involvement in a linkage study seem minimal: taking a blood sample is usually the only physical contact the research imposes upon a subject. As a result, consent forms for linkage studies, drafted against standard biomedical and bioethical templates, sometimes cite only the minor physical risks of drawing blood, and protocols continue to be expedited through review as minimal risk studies. But the OPRR now admonishes IRBs as follows:

Genetic studies that generate information about subjects' personal health risks can provoke anxiety and confusion, damage familial relationships, and compromise subjects' insurability and employment opportunities. For many genetic research protocols, these psychosocial risks can be significant enough to warrant careful IRB review and discussion. The fact that genetic studies are often limited to the collection of family history information and blood drawing should not, therefore, automatically classify them as "minimal risk" studies qualifying for expedited IRB review.[20]

Supporting this position is the growing body of literature that documents the range of psychological responses,[21] social labeling and stigmatization,[22] and economic discrimination[23] that genetic studies may pose for research subjects.

One of the most controversial forms of risk in genetic research in the United States relates to subjects' ability to retain their insurance and employment. Even if the research results are kept scrupulously confidential, subjects who are at genetic risk for serious illness may be asked to disclose their knowledge when they apply for insurance coverage. To do so places them at the risk of being denied coverage for predisposing medical conditions. But to fail to do so places them at the risk of being charged with fraud and the cancellation of all coverage.[24] Either outcome is a dire consequence of their participation in the research study, albeit not a consequence for which the investigators should be held responsible. Thus, IRBs are now faced with deciding: *(4) To what degree and at what stage should psychosocial risks of participating in genetic studies (like risks to insurability) be included in the informed-consent process?*

Traditionally, investigators and IRBs have been discouraged from over-emphasizing remote or speculative risks of harms that might occur as a consequence of newfound knowledge.[25] But recently the risks of losing insurance coverage have been singled out by several groups as a material element to include in the consent process for clinical genetic testing,[26] and the OPRR now includes the loss of insurance coverage among the social risks that should be disclosed to participants in genetic studies.[27] Critics of this practice point to studies that report there is little evidence of "genetic underwriting" on the basis of research data,[28] while advocates applaud it for its foresight, affirming that "testing of apparently healthy [subjects] for a trait that might stigmatize them for a lifetime requires adequate protections and safeguards, particularly informed consent."[29] Others argue that, given the lack of evidence that economic discrimination is a *bona fide* risk of participating in genetic research, it might be better to simply caution potential subjects that, if the project succeeds, subjects could eventually obtain information about themselves that they might have to divulge voluntarily to others, such as insurance companies. This casts the problem as one of recognizing the limits of investigators' abilities to guarantee the confidentiality of data disclosed by the research, rather than as a risk inherent to the research.[30]

ELIGIBILITY OF SUBJECTS

The concerns over the risks of linkage research are also important in making research policy decisions about who should be considered eligible for enrollment in genetic family studies. The most prominent example is found in the debate over whether to involve children in these studies.[31] The DHHS research regulations allow research that imposes more than minimal risk to be conducted with children only when there is promise of direct benefit to the research subjects. In situations where little can be done to benefit subjects as a result of a positive marker test, the risks of being labelled, stigmatized, or of losing insurance coverage suggest that linkage studies should not involve children. This has been the traditional position on the issue within medical genetics.[32]

Increasingly, however, the case for excluding children from linkage research has become less clear cut.[33] For example, for some, the potential benefits of early warning of cancer risk and the benefits of a negative result clearly justify the inclusion of young children in predictive testing trials, even when the risks are acknowledged to be more than minimal.[34] Since the absence of any efficient monitoring or preventive interventions in this case weakens the clinical value of early warning, the weight of this judgment rests on the weight of the benefit of a negative test: the relief of anxiety it can give to the children who are found to be free of the tested mutations, and to their parents. Others are concerned enough about the psychosocial burden of positive tests results (like the imposition of a "vulnerable child syndrome" on children found to be carriers of a mutation)[35] to strike the balance in favor of excluding minors from studies that are likely to lead to new and effective tests.[36]

A third, moderating response is to approach the involvement of minors in a step-wise fashion, in the tradition of beginning research with the least vulnerable population of subjects.[37] For family studies, this means collecting and analyzing DNA samples only from adult members of the family first, then involving minors only as it becomes scientifically necessary. Some teams now make arrangements in advance to disclose any findings about minors only after pilot clinical testing studies with adults have helped demonstrate the relative medical benefits of presymptomatic testing in that case.[38]

One implication of this third strategy is that a minor subject's parents or guardians--who would ordinarily be expected to give their permission for the subject's participation--are almost always already subjects in the same study. This means that the parents, unlike their counterparts in other pediatric research settings, have had to think through the questions that face the potential subject on a first-person basis, which may enrich their deliberations. But it also may mean that the parents' own decision to enroll will unduly cloud the substituted judgement they must make for their child.[39]

These same concerns about the quality of proxy consent in genetic family studies also surface in research with other subjects who are unable to consent for themselves, such as the mentally incapacitated. In family studies of particularly stigmatizing conditions, researchers are concerned that family guardians may be reluctant to grant permission for research that involves their children or charges. One group advises psychiatric geneticists that, while "conducting a clinical interview and/or drawing blood would not appear to exceed minimal risk as currently defined, . . . Even if a waiver [of consent] is justified, the IRB should consider if permission from the family is appropriate." In this group's view, the answer is not necessarily affirmative.

In family studies, it is important for the IRB to assess whether a family member is the most appropriate person to give permission for another, as there may be a vested interest in the results of the research on the part of the family member giving permission. In cases where obtaining consent is required, but no family member is *ethically available*, then a court appointed representative must be sought.[40]

The familial nature of family studies can thus interfere in different ways with decisions that should be made on behalf of an incompetent research subject: once having weighed the relative risks and benefits of having his or her family studied in a particular way, a guardian's decision on behalf of an incompetent subject should represent the independent interests of the particular family member the guardian represents. Those who design genetic family studies are faced with another general policy question: *(5) Under what circumstances can a research subject serve to grant permission to involve another relative in a study (such as a minor child or an incapacitated adult) of their own family?*

DISCLOSURE AND CONTROL OF
RESEARCH FINDINGS

So far, the questions I have described all arise at the outset of a new genetic family study, during the process of recruiting and enrolling subjects. As genetic family studies progress and begin to yield results, however, a second set of questions emerges. These questions all concern the management of the information that investigators uncover about their subjects.

By comparing the inheritance of a panel of known DNA markers with the familial occurrence of a particular trait, specific markers that have been transmitted through the family in the same pattern as the trait (and therefore its causal gene) can be identified. This is a sign that the DNA markers and the gene reside together on the same portion of a chromosome. The degree of this linkage, or its *lod score*, serves as the measure of the proximity between the marker and the gene.[41] Flanking markers that have lod scores indicating that they are 1,000 times more likely to be physically linked to the gene are considered reliable indicators of the location of the causal gene. This means that they can also be used as clinically detectable surrogates for the gene long before tests can be developed for the gene itself.

For individuals who have a familial risk of carrying recessive genes, or genes for late-onset disorders, the identification of these markers through clinical testing can provide the benefit of increased certainty about their personal genetic status. For those who are found not to carry the genes, this benefit is reassurance and relief. For those who "test positive" for the targeted mutations, the benefit depends on how well they can use the knowledge of their carrier status to prevent or prepare for its ill effects. In either case, as studies acquire the ability to convey clinically relevant findings back to the subjects, a number of questions emerge about how best to do this.

DISCLOSURE OF PRELIMINARY AND
INTERIM RESULTS

(6) When and how should preliminary and interim results be disclosed to subjects? Most genetic family studies begin as basic research projects in molecular and human genetics, and often have relatively indirect connections with the kinds of clinical services

that are relevant to the education and counseling of individuals regarding the results of genetic tests. Thus, one traditional approach to managing findings has been to condition subjects' participation on the understanding that no individual findings will be disclosed to subjects under the auspices of the study. This approach was justified, in part, by the slow pace of research that isolated disease genes, which allowed the clinical community to prepare for the translation of research findings into clinical practice further in advance. Hence, for example, the linkage studies that localized markers for the Huntington's disease gene established the policy of withholding preliminary research results from all subjects until the level of scientific confidence in the reliability of the markers justified the establishment of pilot clinical testing programs.[42]

The pace of research to isolate genes, however, is quickly putting pressure on this approach. Many investigators now find themselves in possession of information that seems to be reliable enough to use clinically in the absence of a developed program for delivering the information. Increasingly, individuals and families request early results directly from the researchers. One group reported that a young woman who participated in a linkage study of familial breast cancer announced her decision to undergo a prophylactic bilateral mastectomy even though the researchers knew that, according to their study, there was little chance that she had a genetic inheritance that placed her at risk.[43] Although the gene in question had not been isolated, the evidence available through flanking markers seemed compelling enough to obligate the team to shift from the research to the clinical mode and disclose their findings to the subject. Their decision was supported by those who argue that subjects should have the right to information about themselves at all stages of the research, particularly when it could have a bearing on clinical decision making.[44] In fact, legal concerns about "look-back liability" on the part of investigators who hold, but do not communicate important findings, have already been raised.[45]

Intermediate approaches to the question of disclosing early results take two forms. One is to establish decision-making guidelines by suggesting the variables that should be considered in each instance. For example, one report recommends that investigators consider the following points:

(1) the magnitude of the threat posed to the subject, (2) the accuracy with which the data predict that the threat will be realized, and (3) the possibility that action can be taken to avoid or ameliorate the potential injury.[46]

The other approach to these issues is procedural: to recommend the creation and use of committees that would be comparable to the "data safety and monitoring committees" used by clinical trials.[47] These committees (usually misnamed as project ethics committees) are charged with deciding when study findings are clinically reliable and useful enough to disclose to the research subjects.[48] To the extent that they involve research subjects or family representatives, these committees may potentially offer a useful middle ground between paternalistic and client-centered views.

All these approaches illustrate the difficulty of establishing firm, substantive standards for the clinical reliability of new, uncertain genetic information. Moreover, as the Human Genome Project progresses and the mapping of linkage markers gives way to direct clinical testing based on DNA sequence information about the mutations in question, the nature of uncertainty concerning clinical reliability will change. Increasingly, as tests for genetic factors in more complex diseases become available, the question will become less whether one has the mutation in question, but what that means for one's future. To be able to use the results of genomic research intelligently, subjects will need to be able to think in terms of shifting ranges of probabilities that are influenced both by genes and environmental factors.[49] As they learn to do this, both subjects of research and investigators will find themselves swimming upstream against our culture's tendency to understand genetic risk factors in a deterministic, even fatalistic fashion.[50]

Even when researchers are confident that the information they have uncovered is reliable, they are often uncertain about their own obligations to provide the clinical services required to convey it back to their subjects. The traditional view has been,

clinical researchers may minimize potential harm to subjects by separating, as thoroughly as possible, their research role from clinical roles. If a genetic test reaches the level of reasonable medical certainty, and a subject wishes presymptomatic testing to learn the risk of carrying a particular defective gene, the subject can be referred to a qualified clinical genetic counselor for provision of such information (rather than obtaining genetic liability test results in the research setting).[51]

Others, however, question whether the traditional separation of research and clinical roles is in the subject/patients' best interest in these situations. Having decided to disclose their interim findings to the families involved in their familial breast cancer study, the team of researchers at the University of Michigan, for example, established a counseling program for the families involved. The Michigan team expressly wanted to keep their genotype records isolated from their subjects' medical files. The argument was that, while the research files enjoyed certain additional privacy protections,[52] information transferred to regular medical records would become more widely accessible to insurance companies and employers, exposing the family members to increased socioeconomic risks as a result of their research participation.[53] Since this approach would clearly add to the cost and complexity of genetic research if it were widely adopted, its adoption in this case raises a wider question: as the lines between the discovery of new basic genetic knowledge and the development of personal genetic risk assessments blur, *(7) What sort of responsibilities to provide counseling and follow-up services should investigators expect to take on when they conduct studies to identify genes?*
   Investigators who believe that clinical follow-up services should be part of their planning often frame their proposals as including education for subjects. For example, one team reports that,

We believe that the major responsibility of this type of investigation (to their subjects' welfare) is formal education of the affected individuals, particularly those newly diagnosed, their families and their physicians. ... As part of the education component in our study, a detailed session is conducted during the study visit; all local subjects are afforded a clinical visit to review all data with the PKD physician; and all patients and all doctors receive a detailed letter describing the data obtained.[54]

Finally, a different kind of disclosure question comes up at the conclusion of a linkage study when investigators are preparing to publish their results. To present their data, investigators must publish the pedigrees on which they based their work. It is easy enough to present the pedigrees anonymously, but the family trees they provide are readily decipherable by family members and those who know them. It is thus possible for family members to learn not only about the carrier status of other relatives, but also other facts relevant to the genetic analysis, such as adoptions, stillbirths, and instances of misidentified paternity. This poses the question: *(8) What publishing conventions should be used to protect the privacy of families and individual family members involved in pedigree studies?*

One common practice within human genetics is to scramble pedigrees for publication by changing the gender and birth order of family members in order to disguise their identities, yet preserve the essential genetic story the pedigree tells.[55] The original data is then kept available for inspection only to other *bona fide* researchers. As linkage analysis spreads into other medical fields, this approach is meeting increased resistance: while the traditional publication practice of placing bars across the eyes of patients obscured information irrelevant to the topic, this approach also modifies the scientific data in question. One investigator complained:

When researchers say, "I am going to disguise the affection status and pedigree structure," they are really kidding themselves. They do not disguise it from the family. And if they have changed the raw data, then I think other researchers will feel uncomfortable. . . . You need to show pedigrees. You need to show segregation and affection status. You need to show sex ratios. . . . How else can anyone replicate the study? How else can anyone judge the paper? The way it is done now is a casual way of disguising pedigrees, which I do not think actually fools anybody.[56]

An NIH research team learned this lesson to its chagrin when it published a "disguised" pedigree of an Egyptian family that disclosed the existence of two children in which "paternal geno-type inconsistencies" were identified.[57] The results of this disclosure within the immediate family were disastrous, and led to new guidance to the NIH IRBs that, when misidentified paternity is uncovered in a genetic family study,

If the disease is rare with few subjects available, and it is scientifically impractical to discard the pedigree, then the results of the data analysis could be published without publishing the pedigree itself, with the pedigree made available to bona fide investigators who request it. If the pedigree must be included in the publication, the nuclear family in which the incompatibility occurs could be left out of the pedigree. If it is necessary to publish the complete pedigree, an approach could be made to the family to elicit admission of nonpaternity and to request permission to publish.[58]

This approach, in fact, is the one that would be most compatible with other existing guidelines for protecting the privacy of clinical research subjects in the medical literature.[59] But it challenges the time-honored convention of using pedigree diagrams as a convenient graphic summary of family study data, and it leaves open important ethical questions. From whom should the investigators solicit permission from within the family? Everyone represented in a pedigree? Only those who carry the mutation in question? Only family members with special interests at stake, like the Egyptian woman? While each of these approaches has its advocates, none is entirely satisfactory. Moreover, they all give rise to an additional question: What should investigators do in the face of intra-familial disagreements over permission to publish data about their family?

DISPOSITION AND REUSE OF DATA AND SAMPLES

The problem of how to handle an individual's or a family's decision to deny permission to publish data raises another set of policy questions that can emerge after the conclusion of a genetic family study. These questions revolve around the disposition of the information and DNA samples that investigators have gathered about their research subjects. Research subjects are routinely told that they are free to withdraw from studies at any time. Yet in genetic family studies, their participation consists of their presence on a pedigree and their DNA in a freezer. *(9) Does the subjects' right to end their association with a study oblige the investigator to expunge their information from the pedigree and to discard their DNA?*

Most teams treat DNA samples like other donated human biological material, as material over which the subjects no longer hold a claim. For example, one group draws on the *John Moore* case[60] to argue that "According to a 1990 California Supreme

Court case, a cell line is 'factually and legally distinct' from the cells taken from a subject, and therefore cannot be considered the 'property' of that subject."[61] However, unlike most donated tissue, DNA samples in a family collection gain their research value precisely to the extent that they continue to represent their donors. Thus, when another group of geneticists considered the issue, they determined the following:

Participants at the conference agreed that subjects in pedigree studies have the right to refuse to participate any further in the research, and should be able to have their names removed from a pedigree. There was also a consensus that the subjects could withdraw their personal DNA sample or require that it not be used in any further research, assuming that they had not formally transferred ownership to the researchers. However, subjects were not considered to have any control over the information obtained by investigators from their DNA samples, and researchers are free to use such information for further analysis consistent with approved research protocols.[62]

For investigators contemplating publication, this consensus yields mixed advice. The "names" of family members who deny permission to publish data should not be included: but does this extend to the anonymous symbols that signify them in the chart as well? Or are those symbols, conveying gender, genotype, and family relationships, simply "information obtained by the investigators," over which family members have no further control?[63]

Part of the reason the "ownership" of research data and materials becomes a question in genomic studies is that the pedigree information and DNA samples collected in the course of particular gene-hunting project often can be used to support subsequent projects. Traditionally, tissues and blood samples donated for research have been considered to be available for further study by researchers. Many consent forms for linkage studies make this assumption explicit to their subjects by having them provide blanket permission "for further research" with their samples. However, to the extent to which the familial relations between the samples' sources are retained for research purposes, these DNA collections will retain the signature of a particular family. Strictly speaking, any new molecular genetic study on a stored family collection is a new study with identifiable human subjects, even if the biologists involved never meet the persons who gave samples. Moreover, any studies that promise to uncover new genetic facts about the individuals can have significant implications for the subjects' interests and welfare, particularly when they produce clinically relevant information. This poses the question: *(10) What agreements are necessary to use stored materials for new studies or for clinical diagnoses?*

An increasingly common view is that "the day for informal donations of DNA samples is past,"[64] and that new molecular studies of collected samples should be subject to the same requirements as the original family study that generated the resource. The strongest view is that the subjects should know and agree to any molecular studies conducted on their DNA samples that were not specifically discussed under the initial consent without a "blanket consent" option. One statement of this position appears in the institutional guidelines developed by the IRB of Johns Hopkins University:

A subject cannot give consent to participate in a future experiment of unknown risk. Prior to recontacting donors who have either agreed to future testing or whose samples are stored and consent for future testing was not discussed, investigators must seek an opinion from the . . . IRB regarding the appropriateness of the risk:benefit ratio and possible impact of test results on the subjects. . . . If consent is given for genomic screening using a particular set of probes--identified as probes for a particular disease under study--probes identified with other diseases may not be used unless further consent is obtained for the study of the individual's DNA with those new probes.[65]

Of course, one category of research that has traditionally been exempt from the regulations that apply to research involving human subjects has been research with anonymous human tissue, and most of the human cell lines that are used for biomedical research are distributed through the genetic research community without any traditional personal identifiers attached.[66] As genetic mapping, DNA sequencing, and genotyping technologies progress, however, the adequacy of that practice will continue to be pressed by our increasing ability retrospectively to link samples to subjects. Because DNA samples are related in family studies and can serve to identify a particular family, it is almost impossible to "anonymize" the full family collection *and* have it serve a gene-hunting function. But even for studies that need not retain familial relationships (like efforts to sequence genes from samples known to carry specific mutations), we may reach the day when re-identification becomes possible. For those individuals who want to know the results of a study that used their DNA, it may simply become a matter of comparing their genetic fingerprint or profile with the research collection until a match is found, in the same way that the U.S. Army's DNA repository already identifies the anonymous fragments of war dead against its collection of stored and identified DNA samples from military personnel.[67] At the molecular level, a DNA sample is itself the ultimate identifier.[68]

CONCLUSION: AN AGENDA FOR MAKING POLICY

As the endnotes of this chapter indicate, over the last four years, the discussion of the ethical challenges posed by genetic family studies has begun in earnest. Gene hunters of different varieties (and their IRBs) have begun to gather to compare notes regarding their home-grown responses to shared questions.[69] Major institutional centers of human genetic research, such as the Johns Hopkins University, the University of Utah, and the National Institutes of Health, have developed internal guidance for their IRBs and investigators. In 1993, the national Office of Protection from Research Risk added a chapter to its IRB guidebook devoted to these issues.[70] And, perhaps most importantly, the feedback loop between investigators, IRBs, and research subjects is quickly being closed with respect to these issues. To complement the IRB guidebook, the major patient and family organization for people with genetic diseases, the Alliance for Genetic Support Groups, has produced a brochure for its constituency that recasts the OPRR's guidelines for IRBs into questions for families to ask investigators when approached about participating in genetic studies.[71] That brochure, distributed in bulk to the 200 different organizations that make up the Alliance for Genetic Support Groups, will help insure that if IRBs neglect to ask these questions of investigators, their subjects will.

On the other hand, while the research ethics discussion has begun in earnest in this area, it has not yet arrived at many policy conclusions. All of the 10 questions described above remain open for resolution. Collectively, they create an agenda for policy making on research involving human subjects that will be increasingly important for investigators and IRBs as the Human Genome Project propels the field into the next century.

Some of the questions posed here have not yet led to the formation of policy guidelines because they call into question some of *The Belmont Report's* ethical assumptions regarding ways to protect human subjects of research: Should the family as a whole, instead of as individuals, command our allegiance and respect? Other questions, like the choice of recruiting strategies or criteria to establish the eligibility of a subject, may have no univocal answers as matters of policy, but may have to be answered repeatedly, depending on the circumstances of particular studies and families. Given the operational flexibility required of genetic researchers in light of the range of traits and families, policy guidelines may need to be cast as questions that must be addressed in the design of a genetic family study, rather than as directives with particular solutions.

Still, some of the questions posed here might be resolved by the creation of more uniform policies by different organizations. No one policy-making body has the scope, authority, or expertise to address the full range of open policy questions in this area.[72] Yet policy making on these issues could still successfully develop if it flows in a coordinated way from all the different groups that are best equipped to provide guidance for different spheres.

For example, it should be possible for professional genetics societies, in concert with relevant lay organizations, to define criteria governing the clinical release of genotype data to research subjects. What prerequisites (in terms of the reliability of tests and their predictive power, information on their psychosocial impact, and their protection of their subjects' confidentiality), should a professionally responsible team meet before it discloses its findings to research subjects? Having prescribed the elements that should be in place before new genetic tests of different sorts are used clinically, some groups have already begun the process of identifying when research findings should be made available to research subjects.[73]

Similarly, the major funding sources for genetic research could be held accountable for supporting the education, counseling, and follow-up services that are needed to conduct genetic family studies in an ethically responsible fashion. In fact, NIH has already established the precedent of complementing molecular genetic studies with psychosocial research on the delivery of genetic testing services. While the focus is still on defining, rather than providing, clinical services, this comprehensive approach to gene identification research provides a way to integrate the molecular and clinical aspects of genetic studies within the research setting.[74]

Furthermore, well-publicized and well-reasoned publication policies within the biomedical literature could help investigators to avoid many of the pitfalls that they now encounter in their attempts to publish family data. It seems well within the province of editorial organizations like the International Council of Biology Editors to clarify whether the modification of pedigree data is an ethically acceptable practice, and what levels of familial permission might be required before studies can be published in good conscience.

Finally, questions concerning who controls the disposition and further research on DNA samples are not contingent on the details of particular studies. Much confusion could be avoided by a uniform policy regarding the rights of subjects to withdraw from ongoing studies and to give their consent to new studies involving their DNA and its bearing on their family. The OPRR, the federal office charged with interpreting current research regulations in the United States, might be appropriately charged with proposing guidelines on this topic.

Finally, an organization that can again take the lead in setting an example on all the issues in this area is the National Center for Human Genome Research. The policies and practices of its intramural genetic research laboratories should be codified and disseminated for discussion, in order to allow them to serve, eventually, as a model of good practice. After all, the renewed attention that genetic family studies are receiving are the result, in part, of the energy attracted to genetics by the Human Genome Project. To the extent that the Human Genome Project can help give shape to this discussion, its function as a lightning rod can be counted a success.

NOTES

1. J. Beckwith, "The Human Genome Initiative: Genetics' Lightning Rod," *American Journal of Law and Medicine* 17 (1991): 1-15.

2. DHHS, *Understanding Our Genetic Inheritance. The U.S. Human Genome Project: The First Five Years* (Bethesda, Md.: NIH, 1990, NIH publication no. 90-1590).

3. E.D. Green and R.H. Waterston, "The Human Genome Project: Prospects and Implications for Clinical Medicine," *Journal of the American Medical Association* 266 (1991): 1966-75.

4. D.N. Cooper and J. Schmidtke, "Molecular Genetic Approaches to the Analysis and Diagnosis of Human Inherited Disease: An Overview," *Annals of Medicine* 24 (1992): 29-42.

5. L. Andrews *et al.*, eds., *Assessing Genetic Risks: Implications for Health and Social Policy* (Washington, D.C.: National Academy Press, 1993), 59-99.

6. P.A. Futreal *et al.*, "BRCA1 Mutations in Primary Breast and Ovarian Carcinomas," *Science* 266 (1994): 120-22.

7. For a useful compilation of case studies of different approaches to genetic family studies and the issues they raise, see M. Frankel, ed., *Ethical and Legal Issues In Pedigree Research* (Washington, D.C.: American Association for the Advancement of Science, 1993).

8. CIOMS, *International Guidelines for Ethical Review of Epidemiological Studies* (Geneva: CIOMS, 1991). The prospect of a global DNA sampling effort to preserve representative genotypes from the world's vanishing indigenous populations pushes the discussion to still another level of difficulty. L. Cavalli-Sforza *et al.*, "Call for a Worldwide Survey of Human Genetic Diversity: A Vanishing Opportunity for the Human Genome Project," *Genomics* 11 (1991): 490-91; and M. Lock, "Interrogating the Human Diversity Genome Project," *Social Science & Medicine* 39 (1994): 603-06.

9. OPRR, "Human Genetic Research," in *Protecting Human Research Subjects: Institutional Review Board Guidebook* (Bethesda, Md.: OPRR, 1993), 5-46.

10. OPRR, "Recruitment of Subjects," in *Protecting Human Research Subjects: Institutional Review Board Guidebook*, 4-20.

11. S. Simpson, "Case Study on Bipolar Mood Disorder," in *Ethical and Legal Issues in Pedigree Research*, ed. M. Frankel (Washington D.C.: American Association for the Advancement of Science, 1993), 44-46.

12. D. Shore *et al.*, "Legal and Ethical Issues in Psychiatric Genetic Research," *American Journal of Medical Genetics* 48 (1993): 17-22.

13. *Ibid.*, 18.

14. For example, one investigator wrote:

In Utah, a family-facilitator approach has been very helpful to researchers. The facilitators, working closely with us, make phone calls to their relatives. They can then give us information, such as "I know this branch lives in Oklahoma." Facilitators are selected because they are "nosy" and they are good communicators. Once you begin to research a family, the facilitator will say, "I know who has colon cancer, I know which ones are going in for an operation." Therefore, I think we cannot be naive about issues of confidentiality within extended families.

M. Leppert, "Case Study on Colon Cancer," in *Ethical and Legal Issues in Pedigree Research*, 199.

15. N. Wexler, personal communication.

16. J. Gray, "Case study on Huntington's Disease," in *Ethical and Legal Issues in Pedigree Research*, 90.

17. R. Wachbroit, "Rethinking Medical Confidentiality: The Impact of Genetics," *Suffolk Law Review* (in press).

18. "Thus, unless IRBs take upon themselves the regulation of natural family affection and feelings of obligation, IRBs need not be especially concerned about familial pressures to participate in genetic studies." L.S. Parker and C.W. Lidz, "Familial Coercion to Participate in Genetic Family Studies: Is There Cause for IRB Intervention?" *IRB: A Review of Human Subjects Research* 16 (January-April, 1994): 6-12.

19. R. Wachbroit, "Who is the Patient? A Moral Problem," *Maryland Medical Journal* 38(1989):161-71; R. Shinn, "Family Relationships and Social Policy: An Ethical Inquiry," in *The Genetic Frontier: Ethics, Law and Policy*, in M. Frankel and A. Teich, eds. (Washington, D.C.: American Association for the Advancement of Science, 1993), 9-25; and R.J. Christie and C.B. Hoffmaster, *Ethical Issues in Family Medicine* (Oxford: Oxford University Press, 1986).

20. OPRR, "Recruitment of Subjects," 5-44.

21. S. Wiggins *et al.*, "The Psychological Consequences of Predictive Testing for Huntington's Disease," *New England Journal of Medicine* 327 (1992): 1401-5.

22. H. Markel, "The Stigma of Disease: Implications of Genetic Screening," *American Journal of Medicine* 939 (1992): 209-15; D. Nelkin and L. Tancredi, "Classify and Control: Genetic Information in the Schools," *American Journal of Law and Medicine* 17 (1991): 51-73.

23. P. Billings *et al.*, "Discrimination as a Consequence of Genetic Screening," *American Journal of Human Genetics* 50 (1992): 476-82; M. Rothstein, "Genetic Discrimination in Employment and the Americans

with Disabilities Act," *Houston Law Review* 29 (1992): 23-85; E. Draper, *Risky Business: Genetic Testing and Exclusionary Practices in the Hazardous Workplace* (New York: Cambridge University Press, 1991).

24. NIH/DOE Task Force on Genetic Information and Insurance, *Genetic Information and Health Insurance* (Washington, D.C.: U.S. Government Printing Office, 1992).

25. B. Gray, "Changing Federal Regulations of IRBs," *IRB: A Review of Human Subjects Research* 2 (January 1980): 1-5,12.

26. NIH, "Workshop on Population Screening for the Cystic Fibrosis Gene: Statement," *New England Journal of Medicine* 323 (1990): 70-71; F.P. Li *et al.*, "Recommendations on Predictive Testing for Germ Line P53 Mutations Among Cancer-Prone Individuals," *Journal of the National Cancer Institute* 84 (1992): 1156-60. (This is the statement by the American Society for Human Genetics on breast cancer testing.)

27. OPRR, "Recruitment of Subjects," 5-45.

28. H. Oster *et al.*, "Insurance and Genetic Testing: Where are We Now?" *American Journal of Human Genetics* 52 (1993): 565-77; J. McEwan *et al.*, "A Survey of Medical Directors of Life Insurance Companies Concerning Use of Genetic Information," *American Journal of Human Genetics* 52 (1993).

29. Li, "Recommendations on Predictive Testing," 1159.

30. NIH CF Studies Consortium, *June 1992 Workshop Report*, (unpublished report: National Center for Human Genome Research, NIH, Bethesda, Md., 3 June 1992).

31. D. Wertz *et al.*, "Genetic Testing for Children and Adolescents: Who Decides?" *Journal of the American Medical Association* 272 (1994): 875-881; C. Craufurd *et al.*, "Testing of Children for 'Adult' Genetic Diseases," *Lancet* 335 (1990): 1406.

32. Huntington's Disease Society of America, *Guidelines for Predictive Testing for Huntington's Disease* (New York: Huntington's Disease Society of America, 1989); P. Harper, "Research Samples from Families with Genetic Diseases: A Proposed Code of Conduct," *British Medical Journal* 306 (1993): 1391-99.

33. M. Bloch and M.R. Hayden, "Predictive Testing for Huntington Disease in Childhood: Challenges and Implications," *American Journal of Human Genetics* 46 (1990): 1-4.

34. Li, "Recommendations on Predictive Testing."

35. M. Green and A.J. Solnit, "Reactions to the Threatened Loss of a Child: A Vulnerable Child Syndrome," *Pediatrics* 34 (1964): 56-77.

36. E. Kodish, T. Murray, and S. Shurin, "Cancer Risk Research: What Should We Tell Subjects," *Clinical Research* (1994): 396-402, B. Biesecker *et al.*, "Genetic Counseling for Families with Inherited Susceptibility to Breast and Ovarian Cancer," *Journal of the American Medical Association* 269 (1993): 1970-74.

37. For his influential statement of the "descending order rule" for "conscripting" research subjects, see H. Jonas, "Philosophical Reflections on Experimentation with Human Subjects," in *Experimenting with Human Subjects*, ed. P. Freund (New York: George Braziller, 1970), 19.

38. E.G. Kodish, "Cancer Risk Research"; and Li, "Recommendations on Predictive Testing."

39. S.C. Harth *et al.*, "The Psychological Profile of Parents Who Volunteer Their Children for Clinical Research: A Controlled Study," *Journal of Medical Ethics* 18 (1992): 86-93.

40. Shore, "Legal and Ethical Issues in Psychiatric Genetic Research," 18. This group is even willing to ignore the dissent of incompetent patients in some cases. They argue, "When subjects are so demented or psychotic that they are not able to understand the purpose of the study (and they object to having blood drawn), an IRB may allow [with "appropriate substitute permission"] 'piggybacking' of research blood samples during venipuncture for clinically necessary studies."

41. The lod score is defined as the log of the likelihood of observing the co-inheritance of the disease and marker given chromosomal linkage, versus no linkage. Thus, a lod score of 3 indicates a likelihood ratio of 1,000 to 1 that the marker is linked to the causal disease gene in question. N. Risch, "Linkage Strategies for Genetically Complex Traits," *American Journal of Human Genetics* 46 (1990): 222-28.

42. C. MacKay, "Ethical Considerations in Research on Huntington's Disease," *Clinical Research* 25 (1977): 241-47 and C. MacKay, "Ethical Issues in Research Design and Conduct: Developing a Test to Detect Carriers of Huntington's Disease," *IRB: A Review of Human Subjects Research* 6 (July-August 1984): 1-5.

43. Biesecker, "Genetic Counseling."

44. D. Wertz and J. Fletcher, "Communicating Genetic Risks." *Science, Technology and Human Values* 4 (1987): 60-66.

45. M. Z. Pelias, "Duty to Disclose in Medical Genetics: A Legal Perspective," *American Journal of Medical Genetics* 39 (1991): 347-54.

46. P. Reilly, "When Should an Investigator Share Raw Data with the Subjects?" *IRB: A Review of Human Subjects Research* 2 (November 1980): 4-5,12.

47. C. MacKay, "Discussion Points to Consider in Research Related to the Human Genome," *Human Gene Therapy* 4 (1993): 489.

48. Kodish, "Cancer Risk Research"; and Li, "Recommendations on Predictive Testing."

49. B. LeRoy, "Where Theory Meets Practice: Challenges to the Field of Genetic Counseling," in *Prescribing Our Future: Ethical Challenges in Genetic Counseling*, eds. D. Bartels *et al.* (New York: Aldine de Gruyter, 1993), 39-54.

50. N. Holtzman, *Proceed With Caution: Predicting Genetic Risks in the Recombinant DNA Era* (Baltimore, Md.: Johns Hopkins University Press, 1989).

51. Shore, "Legal and Ethical Issues in Psychiatric Genetic Research," 18.

52. This includes the possibility of acquiring a federal "Certificate of Confidentiality" to protect research records from involuntary disclosure resulting from subpeonas and legal claims. Mackay, "Discussion Points to Consider in Research Related to the Human Genome," 492.

53. Biesecker, "Genetic Counseling."

54. M. Folstein *et al.*, *Report of the Clinical Genetic Research Guidelines Committee*, (Baltimore, Md.: Johns Hopkins University Hospital Joint Committee on Clinical Investigation, January, 1993).

55. Simpson, "Case Study on Bipolar Mood Disorder," 49.

56. Leppert, "Case Study on Colon Cancer." One wag has suggested that the only modification that might be successful in throwing families off the track and retaining the original data would be to change the names and institutions of the *investigators* for purposes of publication!

57. J.G. Compton *et al.*, "Linkage of Epidermolytic Hyperkeratosis to the Type II Keratin Gene Cluster on Chromosome 12Q," *Nature Genetics* 1 (1992): 301-05, 302.

58. H.A. Austin and M. Kaiser, *Summary Report to the Human Subjects Research Advisory Committee on the Meetings of the Intramural Working Group on Human Genetics Research* (unpublished report, Bethesda, Md., NIH, 23 August 1993.), 2-3.

59. M. Powers, "Publication-Related Risks to Privacy: Ethical Implications of Pedigree Studies," *IRB: A Review of Human Subjects Research* 15 (July-August 1993): 7-11.

60. *John Moore v. the Regents of the University of California.*, cited in W.J. Curran, "Scientific and Commercial Development of Human Cell Lines--Issues of Property, Ethics and Conflict of Interest," *New England Journal of Medicine* 324 (1991): 998-1000.

61. Shore, "Legal and Ethical Issues in Psychiatric Genetic Research," 19.

62. Shinn, "Family Relationships and Social Policy," 10-11.

63. One group recounts the following experience:

An example is the case in which a young woman, "Sharon," decided to join the HD roster. . . . This woman provided detailed family history information and good documentation of the medical histories of persons within her family who were affected. When asked to identify family members who would be best suited to complete

Affected Questionnaires on persons in the family who had HD, she . . . requested that her brother, "John," complete the Affected Questionnaire on their mother. . . . Several days after the questionnaire was mailed, a certified letter from John's attorney was received stating that John wanted "his family" removed from the Roster. A dilemma arose in the attempt to define "his family." The pedigree undoubtedly included "his mother," "his father," "his sister," and so forth, but this information belonged equally to his sister, who had originally provided the information.

Gray, "Case Study on Huntington's Disease," 96.

64. V. Hannig et al., "Whose DNA Is It, Anyway? Relationships Between Families and Researchers," American Journal of Medical Genetics 47 (1993): 257-60.

65. Folstein et al., Report of the Clinical Genetics Research Guidelines Committee, 3.

66. This excepts, of course, the first and most famous human tumour cell line, the "HeLa" cell line, which still goes by the name (Helen Lane) of the patient from whom it was taken. See G. Gey et al., "Tissue Culture Studies of the Proliferative Capacity of Cervical Carcinoma and Normal Epithelium," Cancer Research 12 (1952): 264-65.

67. N. Wilker et al., "DNA Data Banking and the Public Interest," in DNA on Trial: Genetic Identification and Criminal Justice, ed. P. Billings (Cold Spring Harbor, N.Y.: Cold Spring Harbor Press, 1992), 141-51.

68. See E. Lander, "DNA Fingerprinting: Science, Law and the Ultimate Identifier," in The Code of Codes: Scientific and Social Issues in the Human Genome Project, eds. D. Keules and L. Hood (Cambridge: Harvard University Press, 1992), 191-211.

69. See Frankel and Teich, Ethical and Legal Issues in Pedigree Research, for the proceedings of a conference in which strategies and practices regarding research with human subjects from five areas of genetic research were compared.

70. OPRR, "Recruitment of Subjects."

71. Alliance of Genetic Support Groups, Informed Consent: Participation in Genetic Research Studies (Chevy Chase, Md.: Alliance of Genetic Support Groups, 1993).

72. This is despite the recurrent call for a new federal body dedicated to addressing policy issues raised by advances in genetic research. See Andrews et al., eds., Assessing Genetics Risks, 290-309.

73. American Society for Human Genetics (ASHG), "Statement of the American Society of Human Genetics on Cystic Fibrosis Carrier

Screening," *American Journal of Human Genetics* 51 (1992): 1443-44; ASHG, "Statement of the American Society of Human Genetics on Genetic Testing for Cancer Risk," *American Journal of Human Genetics* 53 (1994).

74. National Heart, Lung, and Blood Institute, *Report of the Expert Panel on Genetic Strategies for Heart, Lung and Blood Diseases* (Bethesda, Md.: NIH, 1993).

The Nuremburg Code

1. The voluntary consent of the human subject is absolutely essential.

This means that the person involved should have legal capacity to give consent; should be so situated as to be able to exercise free power of choice, without the intervention of any element of force, fraud, deceit, duress, over-reaching, or other ulterior form of constraint or coercion; and should have sufficient knowledge and comprehension of the elements of the subject matter involved as to enable him to make an understanding and enlightened decision. This latter element requires that before the acceptance of an affirmative decision by the experimental subject there should be made known to him the nature, duration, and purpose of the experiment; the method and means by which it is to be conducted; all inconveniences and hazards reasonably to be expected; and the effects upon his health or person which may possibly come from his participation in the experiment.

The duty and responsibility for ascertaining the quality of the consent rests upon each individual who initiates, directs or engages in the experiment. It is a personal duty and responsibility which may not be delegated to another with impunity.

2. The experiment should be such as to yield fruitful results for the good of society, unprocurable by other methods or means of study, and not random and unnecessary in nature.

3. The experiment should be so designed and based on the results of animal experimentation and a knowledge of the natural history of the disease or other problem under study that the anticipated results will justify the performance of the experiment.

4. The experiment should be so conducted as to avoid all unnecessary physical and mental suffering and injury.

5. No experiment should be conducted where there is an *a priori* reason to believe that death or disabling injury will occur; except, perhaps, in those experiments where the experimental physicians also serve as subjects.

6. The degree of risk to be taken should never exceed that determined by the humanitarian importance of the problem to be solved by the experiment.

7. Proper preparations should be made and adequate facilities provided to protect the experimental subject against even remote possibilities of injury, disability, or death.

8. The experiment should be conducted only by scientifically qualified persons. The highest degree of skill and care should be required through all stages of the experiment of those who conduct or engage in the experiment.

9.   During the course of the experiment the human subject should be at liberty to bring the experiment to an end if he has reached the physical or mental state where continuation of the experiment seems to him to be impossible.

10. During the course of the experiment the scientist in charge must be prepared to terminate the experiment at any stage, if he has probable cause to believe, in the exercise of the good faith, superior skill and careful judgment required of him that a continuation of the experiment is likely to result in injury, disability, or death to the experimental subject.

Source: "Permissible Medical Experiments," *Trials of War Criminals before the Nuernberg Military Tribunals under Control Council Law No. 10: Nuernberg, October 1946-April 1949* (Washington: U.S. Government Printing Office, n.d., vol. 2), 181-82.

Declaration of Helsinki
WORLD MEDICAL ASSOCIATION
1964, revised 1975, 1983, 1989

The Declaration of Helsinki, which offers recommendations for conducting experiments using human subjects, was adopted in 1962 and revised by the 18th World Medical Assembly at Helsinki, Finland, in 1964. Subsequent revisions were approved in Tokyo (1975), Venice (1983), and Hong Kong (1989). The 1989 version is reprinted here.

The only significant changes between the 1975 revision, which was the most extensive, and the 1989 version are the addition of the requirement that, whenever possible, the consent of a minor child "must be obtained in addition to the consent of the minor's legal guardian" (I. 11) and the 1989 specification that the "specially appointed [independent] committee" (I. 2) be "independent of the investigator and the sponsor" and "in conformity with the laws and regulations of the country in which the research experiment is performed."

Introduction

It is the mission of the physician to safeguard the health of the people. His or her knowledge and conscience are dedicated to the fulfillment of this mission.

The Declaration of Geneva of The World Medical Association binds the physician with the words "The health of my patient will be my first consideration," and the International Code of Medical Ethics declares that, "A physician shall act only in the patient's interest when providing medical care which might have the effect of weakening the physical and mental condition of the patient."

The purpose of biomedical research involving human subjects must be to improve diagnostic, therapeutic and prophylactic procedures and the understanding of the aetiology and pathogenesis of disease.

In current medical practice most diagnostic, therapeutic or prophylactic procedures involve hazards. This applies especially to biomedical research.

Medical progress is based on research which ultimately must rest in part on experimentation involving human subjects.

In the field of biomedical research a fundamental distinction must be recognized between medical research in which the aim is essentially diagnostic or therapeutic for a patient, and medical research, the essential object of which is purely scientific and without implying direct diagnostic or therapeutic value to the person subjected to the research.

Special caution must be exercised in the conduct of research which may affect the environment, and the welfare of animals used for research must be respected.

Because it is essential that the results of laboratory experiments be applied to human beings to further scientific knowledge and to help suffering humanity, the World Medical Association has prepared the following recommendations as a guide to every physician in biomedical research involving human subjects. They should be kept under review in the future. It must be stressed that the standards as drafted are only a guide to physicians all over the world. Physicians are not relieved from criminal, civil and ethical responsibilities under the laws of their own countries.

I. Basic Principles

1. Biomedical research involving human subjects must conform to generally accepted scientific principles and should be based on adequately performed laboratory and animal experimentation and   a thorough knowledge of the scientific literature.

2. The design and performance of each experimental procedure involving human subjects should be clearly formulated in an experimental protocol which should be transmitted for consideration, comment and guidance to a specially appointed committee independent of the investigator and the sponsor, provided that this independent committee is in conformity with the laws and regulations of the country in which the research experiment is performed.

3. Biomedical research involving human subjects should be conducted only by scientifically qualified persons and under the supervision of a clinically competent medical person. The responsibility for the human subject must always rest with a medically qualified person and never rest on the subject of the research, even though the subject has given his or her consent.

4. Biomedical research involving human subjects cannot legitimately be carried out unless the importance of the objective is in proportion to the inherent risk to the subject.

5. Every biomedical research project involving human subjects should be preceded by careful assessment of predictable risks in comparison with foreseeable benefits to the subject or to others. Concern for the interests of the subject must always prevail over the interests of science and society.

6. The right of the research subject to safeguard his or her integrity must always be respected. Every precaution should be taken to respect the privacy of the subject and to minimize the impact of the study on the subject's physical and mental integrity and on the personality of the subject.

7. Physicians should abstain from engaging in research projects involving human subjects unless they are satisfied that the hazards involved are believed to be predictable. Physicians should cease any investigation if the hazards are found to outweigh the potential benefits.

8. In publication of the results of his or her research, the physician is obliged to preserve the accuracy of the results. Reports of experimentation not in accordance with the principles laid down in this Declaration should not be accepted for publication.

9. In any research on human beings, each potential subject must be adequately informed of the aims, methods, anticipated benefits and potential hazards of the study and the discomfort it may entail. He or she should be informed that he or she is at liberty to abstain from participation in the study and that he or she is free to withdraw his or her consent to participation at any time. The physician should then obtain the subject's freely-given informed consent, preferably in writing.

10. When obtaining informed consent for the research project the physician should be particularly cautious if the subject is in a dependent relationship to him or her or may consent under duress. In that case the informed consent should be obtained by a physician who is not engaged in the investigation and who is completely independent of this official relationship.

11. In the case of legal incompetence, informed consent should be obtained from the legal guardian in accordance with national legislation. Where physical or mental incapacity makes it impossible to obtain informed consent, or when the subject is a minor, permission from the responsible relative replaces that of the subject in accordance with national legislation. Whenever the minor child is in fact able to give consent, the minor's consent must be obtained in addition to the consent of the minor's legal guardian.

12. The research protocol should always contain a statement of the ethical considerations involved and should indicate that the principles enunciated in the present Declaration are complied with.

II. Medical Research Combined with Professional Care (Clinical research)

1. In the treatment of the sick person, the physician must be free to use a new diagnostic and therapeutic measure, if in his or her judgement

it offers hope of saving life, reestablishing health or alleviating suffering.

2. The potential benefits, hazards and discomfort of a new method should be weighed against the advantages of the best current diagnostic and therapeutic methods.

3. In any medical study, every patient--including those of a control group, if any--should be assured of the best proven diagnostic and therapeutic method.

4. The refusal of the patient to participate in a study must never interfere with the physician-patient relationship.

5. If the physician considers it essential not to obtain informed consent, the specific reasons for this proposal should be stated in the experimental protocol for transmission to the independent committee. (I,2).

6. The physician can combine medical research with professional care, the objective being the acquisition of new medical knowledge, only to the extent that medical research is justified by its potential diagnostic or therapeutic value for the patient.

III. Non-Therapeutic Biomedical Research Involving Human Subjects (Non-clinical biomedical research)

1. In the purely scientific application of medical research carried out on a human being, it is the duty of the physician to remain the protector of the life and health of that person on whom biomedical research is being carried out.

2. The subjects should be volunteers--either healthy persons or patients for whom the experimental design is not related to the patient's illness.

3. The investigator or the investigating team should discontinue the research if in his/her or their judgement it may, if continued, be harmful to the individual.

4. In research on man, the interest of science and society should never take precedence over considerations related to the well-being of the subject.

Source: The format of this text is that of the *Encyclopedia of Bioethics*, rev. ed. (New York: MacMillian, 1995), 2765-67.

The Belmont Report

OPRR Reports
NIH PHS HHS

Ethical Principles and Guidelines for the Protection of Human Subjects of Research

The National Commission for the Protection of Human Subjects of Biomedical and Behavioral Research

April 18, 1979

Belmont Report

Ethical Prinicples and Guidelines for Research Involving Human Subjects

Scientific research has produced substantial social benefits. It has also posed some troubling ethical questions. Public attention was drawn to these questions by reported abuses of human subjects in biomedical experiments, especially during the Second World War. During the Nuremberg War Crimes Trials, the Nuremberg code was drafted as a set of standards for judging physicians and scientists who had conducted biomedical experiments on concentration camp prisoners. This code became the prototype of many later codes[1] intended to assure that research involving human subjects would be carried out in an ethical manner.

The codes consist of rules, some general, others specific, that guide the investigators or the reviewers of research in their work. Such rules often are inadequate to cover complex situations; at times they come into conflict, and they are frequently difficult to interpret or apply. Broader ethical principles will provide a basis on which specific rules may be formulated, criticized and interpreted.

Three principles, or general prescriptive judgments, that are relevant to research involving human subjects are identified in this statement. Other principles may also be relevant. These three are comprehensive, however, and are stated at a level of generalization that should assist scientists, subjects, reviewers and interested citizens to understand the ethical issues inherent in research involving human subjects. These principles cannot always be applied so as to resolve beyond dispute particular ethical problems. The objective is to provide an analytical framework that will guide the resolution of ethical problems arising from research involving human subjects.

This statement consists of a distinction between research and practice, a discussion of the three basic ethical principles, and remarks about the application of these principles.

A. Boundaries Between Practice and Research

It is important to distinguish between biomedical and behavioral research, on the one hand, and the practice of accepted therapy on the other, in order to know what activities ought to undergo review for the protection of human subjects of research. The distinction between research and practice is blurred partly because both often occur together (as in research designed to evaluate a therapy) and partly because notable departures from standard practice are often called "experimental" when the terms "experimental" and "research" are not carefully defined.

For the most part, the term "practice" refers to interventions that are designed solely to enhance the well-being of an individual patient or client and that have a reasonable expectation of success. The purpose of medical or behavioral practice is to provide diagnosis, preventive treatment or therapy to particular individuals.[2] By contrast, the term "research" designates an activity designed to test an hypothesis, permit conclusions to be drawn, and thereby to develop or contribute to generalizable knowledge (expressed, for example, in theories, principles, and statements of relationships). Research is usually described in a formal protocol that sets forth an objective and a set of procedures designed to reach that objective.

When a clinician departs in a significant way from standard or accepted practice, the innovation does not, in and of itself, constitute research. The fact that a procedure is "experimental," in the sense of new, untested or different, does not automatically place it in the category of research. Radically new procedures of this description should, however, be made the object of formal research at an early stage in order to determine whether they are safe and effective. Thus, it is the responsibility of medical practice committees, for example, to insist that a major innovation be incorporated into a formal research project.[3]

Research and practice may be carried on together when research is designed to evaluate the safety and efficacy of a therapy. This need not cause any confusion regarding whether or not the activity requires review; the general rule is that if there is any element of research in an activity, that activity should undergo review for the protection of human subjects.

B. Basic Ethical Principles

The expression "basic ethical principles" refers to those general judgments that serve as a basic justification for the many particular ethical prescriptions and evaluations of human actions. Three basic principles, among those generally accepted in our cultural tradition, are particularly relevant to the ethics of research involving human subjects: the principles of respect for persons, beneficence and justice.

1. *Respect for Persons.*--Respect for persons incorporates at least two basic ethical convictions: first, that individuals should be treated as autonomous agents, and second, that persons with diminished autonomy are entitled to protection. The principle of respect for persons thus divides into two separate moral requirements: the requirement to acknowledge autonomy and the requirement to protect those with diminished autonomy.

An autonomous person is an individual capable of deliberation about personal goals and of acting under the direction of such deliberation. To respect autonomy is to give weight to autonomous persons' considered opinions and choices while refraining from obstructing their actions unless they are clearly detrimental to others. To show a lack of respect for an autonomous agent is to repudiate that person's considered judgements, to deny an individiual the freedom to act on those considered judgments, or to withhold information necessary to make a considered judgment, when there are no compelling reasons to do so.

However, not every human being is capable of self-determination. The capacity for self-determination matures during an individual's life, and some individuals lose this capacity wholly or in part because of illness, mental disability, or circumstances that severely restrict liberty. Respect for the immature and the incapacitated may require protecting them as they mature or while they are incapacitated.

Some persons are in need of extensive protection, even to the point of excluding them from activities which may harm them; other persons require little protection beyond making sure they undertake activities freely and with awareness of possible adverse consequences. The extent of protection afforded should depend upon the risk of harm and the likelihood of benefit. The judgment that any individual lacks autonomy should be periodically reevaluated and will vary in different situations.

In most cases of research involving human subjects, respect for persons demands that subjects enter into the research voluntarily and with adequate information. In some situations, however, application of the principle is not obvious. The involvement of prisoners as subjects of research provides an instructive example. On the one hand, it would seem that the principle of respect for persons requires that prisoners not be deprived of the opportunity to volunteer for research. On the other hand, under prison conditions they may be subtly coerced or unduly influenced to engage in research activities for which they would not otherwise volunteer. Respect for persons would then dictate that prisoners be protected. Whether to allow prisoners to "volunteer" or to "protect" them presents a dilemma. Respecting persons, in most hard cases, is often a matter of balancing competing claims urged by the principle of respect itself.

2. *Beneficence.*--Persons are treated in an ethical manner not only by respecting their decisions and protecting them from harm, but also by making efforts to secure their well-being. Such treatment falls under the principle of beneficence. The term "beneficence" is often understood to cover acts of kindness or charity that go beyond strict obligation. In this document, beneficence is understood in a stronger sense, as an obligation. Two general rules have been formulated as complementary expressions of beneficent actions in this sense: (1) do not harm and (2) maximize possible benefits and minimize possible harms.

The Hippocratic maxim "do no harm" has long been a fundamental principle of medical ethics. Claude Bernard extended it to the realm of research, saying that one should not injure one person regardless of the benefits that might come to others. However, even avoiding harm requires learning what is harmful; and, in the process of obtaining this information, persons may be exposed to risk of harm. Further, the Hippocratic Oath requires physicians to benefit their patients "according to their best judgment." Learning what will in fact benefit may require exposing persons to risk. The problem posed by these imperatives is to decide when it is justifiable to seek certain benefits despite the risks involved, and when the benefits should be foregone because of the risks.

The obligations of beneficence affect both individual investigators and society at large, because they extend both to particular research projects and to the entire enterprise of research. In the case of particular projects, investigators and members of their institutions are obliged to give forethought to the maximization of benefits and the reduction of risk that might occur from the research investigation. In the case of scientific research in general, members of the larger society are obliged to recognize the longer term benefits and risks that may result from the improvement of knowledge and from the development of novel medical, psychotherapeutic, and social procedures.

The principle of beneficence often occupies a well-defined justifying role in many areas of research involving human subjects. An example is found in research involving children. Effective ways of treating childhood diseases and fostering healthy development are benefits that serve to justify research involving children--even when individual research subjects are not direct beneficiaries. Research also makes it possible to avoid the harm that may result from the application of previously accepted routine practices that on closer investigation turn out to be dangerous. But the role of the principle of beneficence is not always so unambiguous. A difficult ethical problem remains, for example, about research that presents more than minimal risk without immediate prospect of direct benefit to the children involved. Some have argued that such research is inadmissible, while others have pointed out that this limit would rule out much research promising great benefit to children in the future. Here again, as with all hard cases, the different claims covered by the principle of beneficence may come into conflict and force difficult choices.

3. *Justice.*--Who ought to receive the benefits of research and bear its burdens? This is a question of justice, in the sense of "fairness in distribution" or "what is deserved." An injustice occurs when some benefit to which a person is entitled is denied without good reason or when some burden is imposed unduly. Another way of conceiving the principle of justice is that equals ought to be treated equally. However, this statement requires explication. Who is equal and who is unequal? What considerations justify departure from equal distribution? Almost all commentators allow that distinctions based on experience, age, deprivation, competence, merit and position do sometimes constitute criteria justifying differential treatment for certain purposes. It is necessary, then, to explain in what respects people should be treated equally. There are several widely accepted formulations of just ways to distribute burdens and benefits. Each formulation mentions some relevant property on the basis of which burdens and benefits should be distributed. These formulations are (1) to each person an equal share, (2) to each person according to individual need, (3) to each person according to individual effort, (4) to each person according to societal contribution, and (5) to each person according to merit.

Questions of justice have long been associated with social practices such as punishment, taxation and political representation. Until recently these questions have not generally been associated with scientific research. However, they are foreshadowed even in the earliest reflections on the ethics of research involving human subjects. For example, during the 19th and early 20th centuries the burdens of serving as research subjects fell largely upon poor ward patients, while the benefits of improved medical care flowed primarily to private patients. Subsequently, the exploitation of unwilling prisoners as research subjects in Nazi concentration camps was condemned as a particularly flagrant injustice. In this country, in the 1940s, the Tuskegee syphilis study used disadvantaged, rural black men to study the untreated course of a disease that is by no means confined to that population. These subjects were deprived of demonstrably effective treatment in order not to interrupt the project, long after such treatment became generally available.

Against this historical background, it can be seen how conceptions of justice are relevant to research involving human subjects. For example, the selection of research subjects needs to be scrutinized in order to determine whether some classes (e.g., welfare patients, particular racial and ethnic minorities, or persons confined to institutions) are being systematically selected simply because of their easy availability, their compromised position, or their manipulability, rather than for reasons directly related to the problem being studied. Finally, whenever research supported by public funds leads to the development of therapeutic devices and procedures, justice demands both that these not provide advantages only to those who can afford them and that such research should not unduly involve persons from groups unlikely to be among the beneficiaries of subsequent applications of the research.

C. Applications

Applications of the general principles to the conduct of research leads to consideration of the following requirements: informed consent, risk/benefit assessment, and the selection of subjects of research.

1. *Informed Consent.* Respect for persons requires that subjects, to the degree that they are capable, be given the opportunity to choose what shall or shall not happen to them. This opportunity is provided when adequate standards for informed consent are satisfied.

While the importance of informed consent is unquestioned, controversy prevails over the nature and possibility of an informed consent. Nonetheless, there is widespread agreement that the consent process can be analyzed as containing three elements: information, comprehension and voluntariness.

Information. Most codes of research establish specific items for disclosure intended to assure that subjects are given sufficient information. These items generally include: the research procedure, their purposes, risks and anticipated benefits, alternative procedures (where therapy is involved), and a statement offering the subject the opportunity to ask questions and to withdraw at any time from the research. Additional items have been proposed, including how subjects are selected, the person responsible for the research, etc.

However, a simple listing of items does not answer the question of what the standard should be for judging how much and what sort of information should be provided. One standard frequently invoked in medical practice, namely the information commonly provided by practitioners in the field or in the locale, is inadequate since research takes place precisely when a common understanding does not exist. Another standard, currently popular in malpractice law, requires the practitioner to reveal the information that reasonable persons would wish to know in order to make a decision regarding their care. This, too, seems insufficient since the research subject, being in essence a volunteer, may wish to know considerably more about risks gratuitously undertaken than do patients who deliver themselves into the hand of a clinician for needed care. It may be that a standard of "the reasonable volunteer" should be proposed: the extent and nature of information should be such that persons, knowing that the procedure is neither necessary for their care nor perhaps fully understood, can decide whether they wish to participate in the furthering of knowledge. Even when some direct benefit to them is anticipated, the subjects should understand clearly the range of risk and the voluntary nature of participation.

A special problem of consent arises where informing subjects of some pertinent aspect of the research is likely to impair the validity of the research. In many cases, it is sufficient to indicate to subjects that they are being invited to participate in research of which some features will not be revealed until the research is concluded. In all cases of research involving incomplete disclosure, such research is justified only if it is clear that (1) incomplete disclosure is truly necessary to accomplish the goals of the research, (2) there are no undisclosed risks to subjects that are more than minimal, and (3) there is an adequate plan for debriefing subjects, when appropriate, and for dissemination of research results to them. Information about risks should never be withheld for the purpose of eliciting the cooperation of subjects, and truthful answers should always be given to direct questions about the research. Care should be taken to distinguish cases in which disclosure would destroy or invalidate the research from cases in which disclosure would simply inconvenience the investigator.

Comprehension. The manner and context in which information is conveyed is as important as the information itself. For example, presenting information in a disorganized and rapid fashion, allowing too little time for consideration or curtailing opportunities for questioning, all may adversely affect a subject's ability to make an informed choice.

Because the subject's ability to understand is a function of intelligence, rationality, maturity and language, it is necessary to adapt the presentation of the information to the subject's capacities. Investigators are responsible for ascertaining that the subject has comprehended the information. While there is always an obligation to ascertain that the information about risk to subjects is complete and adequately comprehended, when the risks are more serious, that obligation increases. On occasion, it may be suitable to give some oral or written tests of comprehension.

Special provision may need to be made when comprehension is severely limited--for example, by conditions of immaturity or mental disability. Each class of subjects that one might consider as incompetent (e.g., infants and young children, mentally disabled patients, the terminally ill and the comatose) should be considered on its own terms. Even for these persons, however, respect requires giving them the opportunity to choose to the extent they are able, whether or not to participate in research. The objections of these subjects to involvement should be honored, unless the research entails providing them a therapy unavailable elsewhere. Respect for persons also requires seeking the permission of other parties in order to protect the subjects from harm. Such persons are thus respected both by acknowledging their own wishes and by the use of third parties to protect them from harm.

The third parties chosen should be those who are most likely to understand the incompetent subject's situation and to act in that person's best interest. The person authorized to act on behalf of the subject should be given an opportunity to observe the research as it proceeds in order to be able to withdraw the subject from the research, if such action appears in the subject's best interest.

Voluntariness. An agreement to participate in research constitutes a valid consent only if voluntarily given. This element of informed consent requires conditions free of coercion and undue influence. Coercion occurs when an overt threat of harm is intentionally presented by one person to another in order to obtain compliance. Undue influence, by contrast, occurs through an offer of an excessive, unwarranted, inappropriate or improper reward or other overture in order to obtain compliance. Also, inducements that would ordinarily be acceptable may become undue influences if the subject is especially vulnerable.

Unjustifiable pressures usually occur when persons in positions of authority or commanding influence--especially where possible sanctions are involved--urge a course of action for a subject. A continuum of such influencing factors exists, however, and it is impossible to state precisely where justifiable persuasion ends and undue influence begins. But undue influence would include actions such as manipulating a person's choice through the controlling influence of a close relative and threatening to withdraw health services to which an individual would otherwise be entitled.

2. *Assessment of Risks and Benefits.*--The assessment of risks and benefits requires a careful arrayal of relevant data, including, in some cases, alternative ways of obtaining the benefits sought in the research. Thus, the assessment presents both an opportunity and a responsibility to gather systematic and comprehensive information about proposed research. For the investigator, it is a means to examine whether the proposed research is properly designed. For a review committee, it is a method for determining whether the risks that will be presented to subjects are justified. For prospective subjects, the assessment will assist the determination whether or not to participate.

The Nature and Scope of Risks and Benefits. The requirement that research be justified on the basis of a favorable risk/benefit assessment bears a close relation to the principle of beneficence, just as the moral requirement that informed consent be obtained is derived primarily from the principle of respect for persons. The term "risk" refers to a possibility that harm may occur. However, when expressions such as "small risk" or "high risk" are used, they usually refer (often ambiguously) both to the chance (probability) of experiencing a harm and the severity (magnitude) of the envisioned harm.

The term "benefit" is used in the research context to refer to something of positive value related to health or welfare. Unlike "risk," "benefit" is not a term that expresses probabilities. Risk is properly contrasted to probability of benefits, and benefits are properly contrasted with harms rather than risks of harm. Accordingly, so-called risk/benefit assessments are concerned with the probabilities and magnitudes of possible harms and anticipated benefits. Many kinds of possible harms and benefits need to be taken into account. There are, for example, risks of psychological harm, physical harm, legal harm, social harm and economic harm and the corresponding benefits. While the most likely types of harm to research subjects are those of psychological or physical pain or injury, other possible kinds should not be overlooked.

Risks and benefits of research may affect the individual subjects, the families of the individual subjects, and society at large (or special groups of subjects in society). Previous codes and Federal regulations have required that risks to subjects be outweighed by the sum of both the anticipated benefit to the subject, if any, and the anticipated benefit to society in the form of the knowledge to be gained from the research. In balancing these different elements, the risks and benefits affecting the immediate research subject will normally carry special weight. On the other hand, interests other than those of the subject may on some occasions be sufficient by themselves to justify the risks involved in the research, so long as the subjects' rights have been protected. Beneficence thus requires that we protect against risk of harm to subjects and also that we be concerned about the loss of the substantial benefits that might be gained from research.

The Systematic Assessment of Risks and Benefits. It is commonly said that benefits and risks must be "balanced" and shown to be "in a favorable ratio." The metaphorical character of these terms draws attention to the difficulty of making precise judgments. Only on rare occasions will quantitative techniques be available for the scrutiny of research protocols. However, the idea of systematic, nonarbitrary analysis of risks and benefits should be emulated insofar as possible. This ideal requires those making decisions about the justifiability of research to be thorough in the accumulation and assessment of information about all aspects of the research, and to consider alternatives systematically. This procedure renders the assessment of research more rigorous and precise, while making communication between review board members and investigators less subject to misinterpretation, misinformation and conflicting judgments. Thus, there should first be a determination of the validity of the presuppositions of the research; then the nature, probability and magnitude of risk should be distinguished with as much clarity as possible. The method of ascertaining risks should be explicit, especially where there is no alternative to the use of such vague categories as small or slight risk. It should also be determined whether an investigator's estimates of the probability of harm or benefits are reasonable, as judged by known facts or other available studies.

Finally, assessment of the justifiability of research should reflect at least the following considerations: (i) Brutal or inhumane treatment of human subjects is never morally justified. (ii) Risks should be reduced to those necessary to achieve the research objective. It should be determined whether it is in fact necessary to use human subjects at all. Risk can perhaps never be entirely eliminated, but it can often be reduced by careful attention to alternative procedures. (iii) When research involves significant risk of serious impairment, review committees should be extraordinarily insistent on the justification of the risk (looking usually to the likelihood of benefit to the subject--or, in some rare cases, to the manifest voluntariness of the participation). (iv) When vulnerable populations are involved in research, the appropriateness of involving them should itself be demonstrated. A number of variables go into such judgments, including the nature and degree of risk, the condition of the particular population involved, and the nature and level of the anticipated benefits. (v) Relevant risks and benefits must be thoroughly arrayed in documents and procedures used in the informed consent process.

3. *Selection of Subjects.*--Just as the principle of respect for persons finds expression in the requirements for consent, and the principle of beneficence in risk/benefit assessment, the principle of justice gives rise to moral requirements that there be fair procedures and outcomes in the selection of research subjects.

Justice is relevant to the selection of subjects of research at two levels: the social and the individual. Individual justice in the selection of subjects would require that researchers exhibit fairness: thus, they should not offer potentially beneficial research only to some patients who are in their favor or select only "undesirable" persons for risky research. Social justice requires that distinction be drawn between classes of subjects that ought, and ought not, to participate in any particular kind of research, based on the ability of members of that class to bear burdens and on the appropriateness of placing further burdens on already burdened persons. Thus, it can be considered a matter of social justice that there is an order of preference in the selection of classes of subjects (e.g., adults before children) and that some classes of potential subjects (e.g., the institutionalized mentally infirm or prisoners) may be involved as research subjects, if at all, only on certain conditions.

Injustice may appear in the selection of subjects, even if individual subjects are selected fairly by investigators and treated fairly in the course of the research. This injustice arises from social, racial, sexual and cultural biases institutionalized in society. Thus, even if individual researchers are treating their research subjects fairly, and even if IRBs are taking care to assure that subjects are selected fairly within a particular institution, unjust social patterns may nevertheless appear in the overall distribution of the burdens and benefits of research. Although individual institutions or investigators may not be able to resolve a problem that is pervasive in their social setting, they can consider distributive justice in selecting research subjects.

Some populations, especially institutionalized ones, are already burdened in many ways by their infirmities and environments. When research is proposed that involves risks and does not include a therapeutic component, other less burdened classes of persons should be called upon first to accept these risks of research, except where the research is directly related to the specific conditions of the class involved. Also, even though public funds for research may often flow in the same directions as public funds for health care, it seems unfair that populations dependent on public health care constitute a pool of preferred research subjects if more advantaged populations are likely to be the recipients of the benefits.

One special instance of injustice results from the involvement of vulnerable subjects. Certain groups, such as racial minorities, the economically disadvantaged, the very sick, and the institutionalized may continually be sought as research subjects, owing to their ready availability in settings where research is conducted. Given their dependent status and their frequently compromised capacity for free consent, they should be protected against the danger of being involved in research solely for administrative convenience, or because they are easy to manipulate as a result of their illness or socioeconomic condition.

NOTES

1. Since 1945, various codes for the proper and responsible conduct of human experimentation in medical research have been adopted by different organizations. The best known of these codes are the Nuremberg Code of 1947, the Helsinki Declaration of 1964 (revised in 1975), and the 1971 Guidelines (codified into Federal Regulations in 1974) issued by the U.S. Department of Health, Education, and Welfare. Codes for the conduct of social and behavioral research have also been adopted, the best known being that of the American Psychological Association, published in 1973.

2. Although practice usually involves interventions designed solely to enhance the well-being of a particular individual, interventions are sometimes applied to one individual for the enhancement of the well-being of another (e.g., blood donation, skin grafts, organ transplants) or an intervention may have the dual purpose of enhancing the well-being of a particular individual, and, at the same time, providing some benefit to others (e.g., vaccination, which protects both the person who is vaccinated and society generally). The fact that some forms of practice have elements other than immediate benefit to the individual receiving an intervention, however, should not confuse the general distinction between research and practice. Even when a procedure applied in practice may benefit some other person, it remains an intervention designed to enhance the well-being of a particular individual or groups of individuals; thus, it is practice and need not be reviewed as research.

3. Because the problems related to social experimentation may differ substantially from those of biomedical and behavioral research, the Commission specifically declines to make any policy determination regarding such research at this time. Rather, the Commission believes that the problem ought to be addressed by one of its successor bodies.

Source: U.S. Government Printing Office: 1988--201/778-80319, GPO 887-809. Originally published in 44 *Federal Register* (18 April 1979), 23192-97.

APPENDIX D

Code of Federal Regulations

Title 45
Public Welfare

DEPARTMENT OF HEALTH AND HUMAN SERVICES
NATIONAL INSTITUTES OF HEALTH
OFFICE FOR PROTECTION FROM RESEARCH RISKS

Part 46 PROTECTION OF HUMAN SUBJECTS

Revised June 18, 1991

Subpart A--Federal Policy for the Protection of Human Subjects (Basic DHHS Policy for Protection of Human Research Subjects)

Sec.

46.101 To what does this policy apply?

46.102 Definitions.

46.103 Assuring compliance with this policy--research conducted or supported by any Federal Department or Agency.

46.104-46.106 [Reserved]

46.107 IRB membership.

46.108 IRB functions and operations.

46.109 IRB review of research.

46.110 Expedited review procedures for certain kinds of research involving no more than minimal risk, and for minor changes in approved research.

46.111 Criteria for IRB approval of research.

46.112 Review by institution.

46.113   Suspension or termination of IRB approval of research.
46.114   Cooperative Research.
46.115   IRB records.
46.116   General requirements for informed consent.
46.117   Documentation of informed consent.
46.118   Applications and proposals lacking definite plans for involvement of human subjects.
46.119   Research undertaken without the intention of involving human subjects.
46.120   Evaluation and disposition of applications and proposals for research to be conducted or supported by a Federal Department or Agency.
46.121   [Reserved]
46.122   Use of Federal funds.
46.123   Early termination of research support: Evaluation of applications and proposals.
46.124   Conditions.

Subpart B--Additional DHHS Protections Pertaining to Research, Development, and Related Activities Involving Fetuses, Pregnant Women, and Human In Vitro Fertilization

Sec.
46.201   Applicability.
46.202   Purpose.
46.203   Definitions.
46.204   Ethical Advisory Boards.
46.205   Additional duties of the Institutional Review Boards in connection with activities involving fetuses, pregnant women, or human in vitro fertilization.
46.206   General limitations.
46.207   Activities directed toward pregnant women as subjects.
46.208   Activities directed toward fetuses *in utero* as subjects.
46.209   Activities directed toward fetuses *ex utero*, including nonviable fetuses, as subjects.
46.210   Activities involving the dead fetus, fetal material, or the placenta.
46.211   Modification or waiver of specific requirements.

Subpart C--Additional DHHS Protections Pertaining to Biomedical and Behavioral Research Involving Prisoners as Subjects

Sec.
46.301   Applicability.
46.302   Purpose.
46.303   Definitions.
46.304   Composition of Institutional Review Boards where prisoners are involved.
46.305   Additional duties of the Institutional Review Boards where prisoners are involved.
46.306   Permitted research involving prisoners.

Subpart D--Additional DHHS Protections for Children Involved as Subjects in Research

Sec.
46.401   To what do these regulations apply?
46.402   Definitions.
46.403   IRB duties.
46.404   Research not involving greater than minimal risk.
46.405   Research involving greater than minimal risk but presenting the prospect of direct benefit to the individual subjects.
46.406   Research involving greater than minimal risk and no prospect of direct benefit to individual subjects, but likely to yield generalizable knowledge about the subject's disorder or condition.
46.407   Research not otherwise approvable which presents an opportunity to understand, prevent, or alleviate a serious problem affecting the health or welfare of children.
46.408   Requirements for permission by parents or guardians and for assent by children.
46.409   Wards.

Authority: 5 U.S.C. 301; Sec. 474(a), 88 Stat. 352 (42 U.S.C. 2891-3(a)).

Note: As revised, Subpart A of the DHHS regulations incorporates the Common Rule (Federal Policy) for the Protection of Human Subjects (56 FR 28003). Subpart D of the HHS regulations has been amended at Section 46.401(b) to reference the revised Subpart A.

The Common Rule (Federal Policy) is also codified at

7 CFR Part 1c Department of Agriculture
10 CFR Part 745 Department of Energy
14 CFR Part 1230 National Aeronautics and Space Administration
15 CFR Part 27 Department of Commerce
16 CFR Part 1028 Consumer Product Safety Commission
22 CFR Part 225 International Development Cooperation Agency,
    Agency for International Development
24 CFR Part 60 Department of Housing and Urban Development
28 CFR Part 46 Department of Justice
32 CFR Part 219 Department of Defense
34 CFR Part 97 Department of Education
38 CFR Part 16 Department of Veterans Affairs
40 CFR Part 26 Environmental Protection Agency
45 CFR Part 690 National Science Foundation
49 CFR Part 11 Department of Transportation

PART 46--PROTECTION OF HUMAN SUBJECTS

Subpart A--Federal Policy for the Protection of Human Subjects (Basic DHHS Policy for Protection of Human Research Subjects)

Source: 56 FR 28003, 18 June 1991.

§ 46.101 To what does this policy apply?

(a) Except as provided in paragraph (b) of this section, this policy applies to all research involving human subjects conducted, supported or otherwise subject to regulation by any Federal Department or Agency which takes appropriate administrative action to make the policy applicable to such research. This includes research conducted by Federal civilian employees or military personnel, except that each Department or Agency head may adopt such procedural modifications as may be appropriate from an administrative standpoint. It also includes research conducted, supported, or otherwise subject to regulation by the Federal Government outside the United States.

(1) Research that is conducted or supported by a Federal Department or Agency, whether or not it is regulated as defined in § 46.102(e), must comply with all sections of this policy.

(2) Research that is neither conducted nor supported by a Federal Department or Agency but is subject to regulation as defined in §. 46.102(e) must be reviewed and approved, in compliance with § 46.101, § 46.102, and § 46.107 through § 46.117 of this policy, by an Institutional Review Board (IRB) that operates in accordance with the pertinent requirements of this policy.

(b) Unless otherwise required by Department or Agency heads, research activities in which the only involvement of human subjects will be in one or more of the following categories are exempt from this policy:

(1) Research conducted in established or commonly accepted educational settings, involving normal educational practices, such as (i) research on regular and special education instructional strategies, or (ii) research on the effectiveness of or the comparison among instructional techniques, curricula, or classroom management methods.

(2) Research involving the use of educational tests (cognitive, diagnostic, aptitude, achievement), survey procedures, interview procedures or observation of public behavior, unless:

(i) information obtained is recorded in such a manner that human subjects can be identified, directly or through identifiers linked to the subjects; and (ii) any disclosure of the human subjects' responses outside the research could reasonably place the subjects at risk of criminal or civil liability or be damaging to the subjects' financial standing, employability, or reputation.

(3) Research involving the use of educational tests (cognitive, diagnostic, aptitude, achievement), survey procedures, interview procedures, or observation of public behavior that is not exempt under paragraph (b)(2)of this section, if:

(i) the human subjects are elected or appointed public officials or candidates for public office; or (ii) Federal statute(s) require(s) without exception that the confidentiality of the personally identifiable information will be maintained throughout the research and thereafter.

(4) Research involving the collection or study of existing data, documents, records, pathological specimens, or diagnostic specimens, if these sources are publicly available or if the information is recorded by the investigator in such a manner that subjects cannot be identified, directly or through identifiers linked to the subjects.

(5) Research and demonstration projects which are conducted by or subject to the approval of Department or Agency heads, and which are designed to study, evaluate, or otherwise examine:

(i) Public benefit or service programs; (ii) procedures for obtaining benefits or services under those programs; (iii) possible changes in or alternatives to those programs or procedures; or (iv) possible changes in methods or levels of payment for benefits or services under those programs.

(6) Taste and food quality evaluation and consumer acceptance studies, (i) if wholesome foods without additives are consumed or (ii) if a food is consumed that contains a food ingredient at or below the level and for a use found to be safe, or agricultural chemical or environmental contaminant at or below the level found to be safe, by the Food and Drug Administration or approved by the Environmental Protection Agency or the Food Safety and Inspection Services of the U.S. Department of Agriculture.

(c) Department or Agency heads retain final judgment as to whether a particular activity is covered by this policy.

(d) Department or Agency heads may require that specific research activities or classes of research activities conducted, supported, or otherwise subject to regulation by the Department or Agency but not otherwise covered by this policy, comply with some or all of the requirements of this policy.

(e) Compliance with this policy requires compliance with pertinent Federal laws or regulations which provide additional protections for human subjects.

(f) This policy does not affect any state or local laws or regulations which may otherwise be applicable and which provide additional protections for human subjects.

(g) This policy does not affect any foreign laws or regulations which may otherwise be applicable and which provide additional protections to human subjects of research.

(h) When research covered by this policy takes place in foreign countries, procedures normally followed in the foreign countries to protect human subjects may differ from those set forth in this policy. [An example is a foreign institution which complies with guidelines consistent with the World Medical Assembly Declaration (Declaration of Helsinki amended 1989) issued either by sovereign states or by an organization whose function for the protection of human research subjects is internationally recognized.] In these circumstances, if a Department or Agency head determines that the procedures prescribed by the institution afford protections that are at least equivalent to those provided in this policy, the Department or Agency head may approve the substitution of the foreign procedures in lieu of the procedural requirements provided in this policy. Except when otherwise required by statute, Executive Order, or the Department or Agency head, notices of these actions as they occur will be published in the **Federal Register** or will be otherwise published as provided in Department or Agency procedures.

(i) Unless otherwise required by law, Department or Agency heads may waive the applicability of some or all of the provisions of this policy to specific research activities or classes of research activities otherwise covered by this policy. Except when otherwise required by statute or Executive Order, the Department or Agency head shall forward advance notices of these actions to the Office for Protection from Research Risks, National Institutes of Health, Department of Health and Human Services (DHHS), and shall also publish them in the **Federal Register** or in such other manner as provided in Department or Agency procedures.[1]

§ 46.102 Definitions.

(a) *Department or Agency head* means the head of any Federal Department or Agency and any other officer or employee of any Department or Agency to whom authority has been delegated.

(b) *Institution* means any public or private entity or Agency (including Federal, State, and other agencies).

(c) *Legally authorized representative* means an individual or judicial or other body authorized under applicable law to consent on behalf of a prospective subject to the subject's participation in the procedure(s) involved in the research.

(d) *Research* means a systematic investigation, including research development, testing and evaluation, designed to develop or contribute to generalizable knowledge. Activities which meet this definition constitute research for purposes of this policy, whether or not they are conducted or supported under a program which is considered research for other purposes. For example, some demonstration and service programs may include research activities.

(e) *Research subject to regulation,* and similar terms are intended to encompass those research activities for which a Federal Department or Agency has specific responsibility for regulating as a research activity, (for example, Investigational New Drug requirements administered by

---

1. Institutions with DHHS-approved assurances on file will abide by provisions of Title 45 CFR Part 46 Subparts A-D. Some of the other departments and agencies have incorporated all provisions of Title 45 CFR Part 46 into their policies and procedures as well. However, the exemptions at 45 CFR 46.101(b) do not apply to research involving prisoners, fetuses, pregnant women, or human in vitro fertilization, Subparts B and C. The exemption at 45 CFR 46.101(b)(2), for research involving survey or interview procedures or observation of public behavior, does not apply to research with children, Subpart D, except for research involving observations of public behavior when the investigator(s) do not participate in the activities being observed.

the Food and Drug Administration). It does not include research activities which are incidentally regulated by a Federal Department or Agency solely as part of the Department's or Agency's broader responsibility to regulate certain types of activities whether research or non-research in nature (for example, Wage and Hour requirements administered by the Department of Labor).

(f) *Human subject* means a living individual about whom an investigator (whether professional or student)conducting research obtains

(1) data through intervention or interaction with the individual, or

(2) identifiable private information. *Intervention* includes both physical procedures by which data are gathered (for example, venipuncture) and manipulations of the subject or the subject's environment that are performed for research purposes. Interaction includes communication or interpersonal contact between investigator and subject. *Private information* includes information about behavior that occurs in a context in which an individual can reasonably expect that no observation or recording is taking place, and information which has been provided for specific purposes by an individual and which the individual can reasonably expect will not be made public (for example, a medical record). Private information must be individually identifiable (i.e., the identity of the subject is or may readily be ascertained by the investigator or associated with the information) in order for obtaining the information to constitute research involving human subjects.

(g) *IRB* means an Institutional Review Board established in accord with and for the purposes expressed in this policy.

(h) *IRB approval* means the determination of the IRB that the research has been reviewed and may be conducted at an institution within the constraints set forth by the IRB and by other institutional and Federal requirements.

(i) *Minimal risk* means that the probability and magnitude of harm or discomfort anticipated in the research are not greater in and of themselves than those ordinarily encountered in daily life or during the performance of routine physical or psychological examinations or tests.

(j) *Certification* means the official notification by the institution to the supporting Department or Agency, in accordance with the requirements of this policy, that a research project or activity involving human subjects has been reviewed and approved by an IRB in accordance with an approved assurance.

§ 46.103 Assuring compliance with this policy--research conducted or supported by any Federal Department or Agency.

(a) Each institution engaged in research which is covered by this policy and which is conducted or supported by a Federal Department or

Agency shall provide written assurance satisfactory to the Department or Agency head that it will comply with the requirements set forth in this policy. In lieu of requiring submission of an assurance, individual Department or Agency heads shall accept the existence of a current assurance, appropriate for the research in question, on file with the Office for Protection from Research Risks, National Institutes of Health, DHHS, and approved for Federalwide use by that office. When the existence of an DHHS-approved assurance is accepted in lieu of requiring submission of an assurance, reports (except certification) required by this policy to be made to Department and Agency heads shall also be made to the Office for Protection from Research Risks, National Institutes of Health, DHHS.

(b) Departments and agencies will conduct or support research covered by this policy only if the institution has an assurance approved as provided in this section, and only if the institution has certified to the Department or Agency head that the research has been reviewed and approved by an IRB provided for in the assurance, and will be subject to continuing review by the IRB. Assurances applicable to federally supported or conducted research shall at a minimum include:

(1) A statement of principles governing the institution in the discharge of its responsibilities for protecting the rights and welfare of human subjects of research conducted at or sponsored by the institution, regardless of whether the research is subject to Federal regulation. This may include an appropriate existing code, declaration, or statement of ethical principles, or a statement formulated by the institution itself. This requirement does not preempt provisions of this policy applicable to Department- or Agency-supported or regulated research and need not be applicable to any research exempted or waived under § 46.101 (b) or (i).

(2) Designation of one or more IRBs established in accordance with the requirements of this policy, and for which provisions are made for meeting space and sufficient staff to support the IRB's review and recordkeeping duties.

(3) A list of IRB members identified by name; earned degrees; representative capacity; indications of experience such as board certifications, licenses, etc., sufficient to describe each member's chief anticipated contributions to IRB deliberations; and any employment or other relationship between each member and the institution; for example: full-time employee, part-time employee, member of governing panel or board, stockholder, paid or unpaid consultant. Changes in IRB membership shall be reported to the Department or Agency head, unless in accord with § 46.103 (a) of this policy, the existence of a DHHS-approved assurance is accepted. In this case, change in IRB membership

shall be reported to the Office for Protection from Research Risks, National Institutes of Health, DHHS.

(4) Written procedures which the IRB will follow (i) for conducting its initial and continuing review of research and for reporting its findings and actions to the investigator and the institution; (ii) for determining which projects require review more often than annually and which projects need verification from sources other than the investigators that no material changes have occurred since previous IRB review; and (iii) for ensuring prompt reporting to the IRB of proposed changes in a research activity, and for ensuring that such changes in approved research, during the period for which IRB approval has already been given, may not be initiated without IRB review and approval except when necessary to eliminate apparent immediate hazards to the subject.

(5) Written procedures for ensuring prompt reporting to the IRB, appropriate institutional officials, and the Department or Agency head of (i) any unanticipated problems involving risks to subjects or others or any serious or continuing noncompliance with this policy or the requirements or determinations of the IRB; and (ii) any suspension or termination of IRB approval.

(c) The assurance shall be executed by an individual authorized to act for the institution and to assume on behalf of the institution the obligations imposed by this policy and shall be filed in such form and manner as the Department or Agency head prescribes.

(d) The Department or Agency head will evaluate all assurances submitted in accordance with this policy through such officers and employees of the Department or Agency and such experts or consultants engaged for this purpose as the Department or Agency head determines to be appropriate. The Department or Agency head's evaluation will take into consideration the adequacy of the proposed IRB in light of the anticipated scope of the institution's research activities and the types of subject populations likely to be involved, the appropriateness of the proposed initial and continuing review procedures in light of the probable risks, and the size and complexity of the institution.

(e) On the basis of this evaluation, the Department or Agency head may approve or disapprove the assurance, or enter into negotiations to develop an approvable one. The Department or Agency head may limit the period during which any particular approved assurance or class of approved assurances shall remain effective or otherwise condition or restrict approval.

(f) Certification is required when the research is supported by a Federal Department or Agency and not otherwise exempted or waived under § 46.101 (b) or (i). An institution with an approved assurance shall certify that each application or proposal for research covered by the assurance and by § 46.103 of this policy has been reviewed and approved by the IRB. Such certification must be submitted with the application or proposal or by such later date as may be prescribed by the Department or Agency to which the application or proposal is submitted. Under no condition shall research covered by § 46.103 of the policy be supported prior to receipt of the certification that the research has been reviewed and approved by the IRB. Institutions without an approved assurance covering the research shall certify within 30 days after receipt of a request for such a certification from the Department or Agency, that the application or proposal has been approved by the IRB. If the certification is not submitted within these time limits, the application or proposal may be returned to the institution.

(Approved by the Office of Management and Budget under Control Number 9999-0020.)

§§ 46.104-46.106 [Reserved]

§ 46.107 IRB membership.

(a) Each IRB shall have at least five members, with varying backgrounds to promote complete and adequate review of research activities commonly conducted by the institution. The IRB shall be sufficiently qualified through the experience and expertise of its members, and the diversity of the members, including consideration of race, gender, and cultural backgrounds and sensitivity to such issues as community attitudes, to promote respect for its advice and counsel in safeguarding the rights and welfare of human subjects. In addition to possessing the professional competence necessary to review specific research activities, the IRB shall be able to ascertain the acceptability of proposed research in terms of institutional commitments and regulations, applicable law, and standards of professional conduct and practice. The IRB shall therefore include persons knowledgeable in these areas. If an IRB regularly reviews research that involves a vulnerable category of subjects, such as children, prisoners, pregnant women, or handicapped or mentally disabled persons, consideration shall be given to the inclusion of one or more individuals who are knowledgeable about and experienced in working with these subjects.

(b) Every nondiscriminatory effort will be made to ensure that no IRB consists entirely of men or entirely of women, including the institution's consideration of qualified persons of both sexes, so long as no selection is made to the IRB on the basis of gender. No IRB may consist entirely of members of one profession.

(c) Each IRB shall include at least one member whose primary concerns are in scientific areas and at least one member whose primary concerns are in nonscientific areas.

(d) Each IRB shall include at least one member who is not otherwise affiliated with the institution and who is not part of the immediate family of a person who is affiliated with the institution.

(e) No IRB may have a member participate in the IRB's initial or continuing review of any project in which the member has a conflicting interest, except to provide information requested by the IRB.

(f) An IRB may, in its discretion, invite individuals with competence in special areas to assist in the review of issues which require expertise beyond or in addition to that available on the IRB. These individuals may not vote with the IRB.

§ 46.108 IRB functions and operations.

In order to fulfill the requirements of this policy each IRB shall:

(a) Follow written procedures in the same detail as described in § 46.103(b)(4) and to the extent required by § 46.103(b)(5).

(b) Except when an expedited review procedure is used (see § 46.110), review proposed research at convened meetings at which a majority of the members of the IRB are present, including at least one member whose primary concerns are in nonscientific areas. In order for the research to be approved, it shall receive the approval of a majority of those members present at the meeting.

§ 46.109 IRB review of research.

(a) An IRB shall review and have authority to approve, require modifications in (to secure approval), or disapprove all research activities covered by this policy.

(b) An IRB shall require that information given to subjects as part of informed consent is in accordance with § 46.116. The IRB may require that information, in addition to that specifically mentioned in § 46.116, be given to the subjects when in the IRB's judgment the information would meaningfully add to the protection of the rights and welfare of subjects.

(c) An IRB shall require documentation of informed consent or may waive documentation in accordance with § 46.117.

(d) An IRB shall notify investigators and the institution in writing of its decision to approve or disapprove the proposed research activity, or of modifications required to secure IRB approval of the research activity. If the IRB decides to disapprove a research activity, it shall include in its written notification a statement of the reasons for its decision and give the investigator an opportunity to respond in person or in writing.

(e) An IRB shall conduct continuing review of research covered by this policy at intervals appropriate to the degree of risk, but not less than once per year, and shall have authority to observe or have a third party observe the consent process and the research.

(Approved by the Office of Management and Budget under Control Number 9999-0020.)

§ 46.110 Expedited review procedures for certain kinds of research involving no more than minimal risk, and for minor changes in approved research.

(a) The Secretary, HHS, has established, and published as a Notice in the **Federal Register**, a list of categories of research that may be reviewed by the IRB through an expedited review procedure. The list will be amended, as appropriate, after consultation with other departments and agencies, through periodic republication by the Secretary, HHS, in the **Federal Register**. A copy of the list is available from the Office for Protection from Research Risks, National Institutes of Health, DHHS, Bethesda, Maryland 20892.

(b) An IRB may use the expedited review procedure to review either or both of the following:

(1) some or all of the research appearing on the list and found by the reviewer(s) to involve no more than minimal risk,

(2) minor changes in previously approved research during the period (of one year or less) for which approval is authorized.

Under an expedited review procedure, the review may be carried out by the IRB chairperson or by one or more experienced reviewers designated by the chairperson from among members of the IRB. In reviewing the research, the reviewers may exercise all of the authorities of the IRB except that the reviewers may not disapprove the research. A research activity may be disapproved only after review in accordance with the non-expedited procedure set forth in § 46.108(b).

(c) Each IRB which uses an expedited review procedure shall adopt a method for keeping all members advised of research proposals which have been approved under the procedure.

(d) The Department or Agency head may restrict, suspend, terminate, or choose not to authorize an institution's or IRB's use of the expedited review procedure.

§ 46.111 Criteria for IRB approval of research.

(a) In order to approve research covered by this policy the IRB shall determine that all of the following requirements are satisfied:

(1) Risks to subjects are minimized: (i) by using procedures which are consistent with sound research design and which do not unnecessarily expose subjects to risk, and (ii) whenever appropriate, by using procedures already being performed on the subjects for diagnostic or treatment purposes.

(2) Risks to subjects are reasonable in relation to anticipated benefits, if any, to subjects, and the importance of the knowledge that may reasonably be expected to result. In evaluating risks and benefits, the IRB should consider only those risks and benefits that may result from the research (as distinguished from risks and benefits of therapies subjects would receive even if not participating in the research). The IRB should not consider possible long-range effects of applying knowledge gained in the research (for example, the possible effects of the research on public policy) as among those research risks that fall within the purview of its responsibility.

(3) Selection of subjects is equitable. In making this assessment the IRB should take into account the purposes of the research and the setting in which the research will be conducted and should be particularly cognizant of the special problems of research involving vulnerable populations, such as children, prisoners, pregnant women, mentally disabled persons, or economically or educationally disadvantaged persons.

(4) Informed consent will be sought from each prospective subject or the subject's legally authorized representative, in accordance with, and to the extent required by § 46.116.

(5) Informed consent will be appropriately documented, in accordance with, and to the extent required by § 46.117.

(6) When appropriate, the research plan makes adequate provision for monitoring the data collected to ensure the safety of subjects.

(7) When appropriate, there are adequate provisions to protect the privacy of subjects and to maintain the confidentiality of data.

(b) When some or all of the subjects are likely to be vulnerable to coercion or undue influence, such as children, prisoners, pregnant women, mentally disabled persons, or economically or educationally disadvantaged persons, additional safeguards have been included in the study to protect the rights and welfare of these subjects.

§ 46.112 Review by institution.

Research covered by this policy that has been approved by an IRB may be subject to further appropriate review and approval or disapproval by officials of the institution. However, those officials may not approve the research if it has not been approved by an IRB.

§ 46.113 Suspension or termination of IRB approval of research.

An IRB shall have authority to suspend or terminate approval of research that is not being conducted in accordance with the IRB's requirements or that has been associated with unexpected serious harm to subjects. Any suspension or termination of approval shall include a statement of the reasons for the IRB's action and shall be reported promptly to the investigator, appropriate institutional officials, and the Department or Agency head.
(Approved by the Office of Management and Budget under Control Number 9999-0020.)

§ 46.114 Cooperative research.

Cooperative research projects are those projects covered by this policy which involve more than one institution. In the conduct of cooperative research projects, each institution is responsible for safeguarding the rights and welfare of human subjects and for complying with this policy. With the approval of the Department or Agency head, an institution participating in a cooperative project may enter into a joint review arrangement, rely upon the review of another qualified IRB, or make similar arrangements for avoiding duplication of effort.

§ 46.115 IRB records.

(a) An institution, or when appropriate an IRB, shall prepare and maintain adequate documentation of IRB activities, including the following:
(1) Copies of all research proposals reviewed, scientific evaluation, if any, that accompany the proposals, approved sample consent documents, progress reports submitted by investigators, and reports of injuries to subjects.
(2) Minutes of IRB meetings which shall be in sufficient detail to show attendance at the meetings; actions taken by the IRB; the vote on these actions including the number of members voting for, against, and abstaining; the basis for requiring changes in or disapproving research; and a written summary of the discussion of controverted issues and their resolution.
(3) Records of continuing review activities.
(4) Copies of all correspondence between the IRB and the investigators.

(5) A list of IRB members in the same detail as described in §
46.103(b)(3).

(6) Written procedures for the IRB in the same detail as described in
§ 46.103(b)(4) and § 46.103(b)(5).

(7) Statements of significant new findings provided to subjects, as
required by § 46.116(b)(5).

(b) The records required by this policy shall be retained for at least
3 years, and records relating to research which is conducted shall be
retained for at least 3 years after completion of the research. All records
shall be accessible for inspection and copying by authorized representatives of the Department or Agency at reasonable times and in a
reasonable manner.

((Approved by the Office of Management and Budget under Control
Number 9999-0020.)

§ 46.116 General requirements for informed consent.

Except as provided elsewhere in this policy, no investigator may
involve a human being as a subject in research covered by this policy
unless the investigator has obtained the legally effective informed
consent of the subject or the subject's legally authorized representative.
An investigator shall seek such consent only under circumstances that
provide the prospective subject or the representative sufficient opportunity to consider whether or not to participate and that minimize the
possibility of coercion or undue influence. The information that is given
to the subject or the representative shall be in language understandable
to the subject or the representative. No informed consent, whether oral
or written, may include any exculpatory language through which the
subject or the representative is made to waive or appear to waive any of
the subject's legal rights, or releases or appears to release the investigator,
the sponsor, the institution or its agents from liability for negligence.

(a) Basic elements of informed consent. Except as provided in
paragraph (c) or (d) of this section, in seeking informed consent the
following information shall be provided to each subject:

(1) a statement that the study involves research, an explanation of
the purposes of the research and the expected duration of the subject's
participation, a description of the procedures to be followed, and identification of any procedures which are experimental;

(2) a description of any reasonably foreseeable risks or discomforts
to the subject;

(3) a description of any benefits to the subject or to others which
may reasonably be expected from the research;

(4) a disclosure of appropriate alternative procedures or courses of
treatment, if any, that might be advantageous to the subject;

(5) a statement describing the extent, if any, to which confidentiality of records identifying the subject will be maintained;

(6) for research involving more than minimal risk, an explanation as to whether any compensation and an explanation as to whether any medical treatments are available if injury occurs and, if so, what they consist of, or where further information may be obtained;

(7) an explanation of whom to contact for answer to pertinent questions about the research and research subjects' rights, and whom to contact in the event of a research-related injury to the subject; and

(8) a statement that participation is voluntary, refusal to participate will involve no penalty or loss of benefits to which the subject is otherwise entitled, and the subject may discontinue participation at any time without penalty or loss of benefits to which the subject is otherwise entitled.

(b) additional elements of informed consent. When appropriate, one or more of the following elements of information shall also be provided to each subject:

(1) a statement that the particular treatment or procedure may involve risks to the subject (or to the embryo or fetus, if the subject is or may become pregnant) which are currently unforeseeable;

(2) anticipated circumstances under which the subject's participation may be terminated by the investigator without regard to the subject's consent;

(3) any additional costs to the subject that may result from participation in the research;

(4) the consequences of a subject's decision to withdraw from the research and procedures for orderly termination of participation by the subject;

(5) A statement that significant new findings developed during the course of the research which may relate to the subject's willingness to continue participation will be provided to the subject; and

(6) the approximate number of subjects involved in the study.

(c) An IRB may approve a consent procedure which does not include, or which alters, some or all of the elements of informed consent set forth above, or waive the requirement to obtain informed consent provided the IRB finds and documents that:

(1) the research or demonstration project is to be conducted by or subject to the approval of state or local government officials and is designed to study, evaluate, or otherwise examine: (i) public benefit or service programs; (ii) procedures for obtaining benefits or services under those programs; (iii) possible changes in or alternatives to those programs or procedures; or (iv) possible changes in methods or levels of payment for benefits or services under those programs; and

(2) the research could not practicably be carried out without the waiver or alteration.

(d) An IRB may approve a consent procedure which does not include, or which alters, some or all of the elements of informed consent set forth in this section, or waive the requirements to obtain informed consent provided the IRB finds and documents that:

(1) the research involves no more than minimal risk to the subjects;

(2) the waiver or alteration will not adversely affect the rights and welfare of the subjects;

(3) the research could not practicably be carried out without the waiver or alteration; and

(4) whenever appropriate, the subjects will be provided with additional pertinent information after participation.

(e) The informed consent requirements in this policy are not intended to preempt any applicable Federal, State, or local laws which require additional information to be disclosed in order for informed consent to be legally effective.

(f) Nothing in this policy is intended to limit the authority of a physician to provide emergency medical care, to the extent the physician is permitted to do so under applicable Federal, State, or local law. (Approved by the Office of Management and Budget under Control Number 9999-0020.)

§ 46.117 Documentation of informed consent.

(a) Except as provided in paragraph (c) of this section, informed consent shall be documented by the use of a written consent form approved by the IRB and signed by the subject or the subject's legally authorized representative. A copy shall be given to the person signing the form.

(b) Except as provided in paragraph (c) of this section, the consent form may be either of the following:

(1) A written consent document that embodies the elements of informed consent required by § 46.116. This form may be read to the subject or the subject's legally authorized representative, but in any event, the investigator shall give either the subject or the representative adequate opportunity to read it before it is signed; or

(2) A short form written consent document stating that the elements of informed consent required by § 46.116 have been presented orally to the subject or the subject's legally authorized representative. When this method is used, there shall be a witness to the oral presentation. Also, the IRB shall approve a written summary of what is to be said

to the subject or the representative. Only the short form itself is to be signed by the subject or the representative. However, the witness shall sign both the short form and a copy of the summary, and the person actually obtaining consent shall sign a copy of the summary. A copy of the summary shall be given to the subject or the representative, in addition to a copy of the short form.

(c) An IRB may waive the requirement for the investigator to obtain a signed consent form for some or all subjects if it finds either:

(1) That the only record linking the subject and the research would be the consent document and the principal risk would be potential harm resulting from a breach of confidentiality. Each subject will be asked whether the subject wants documentation linking the subject with the research, and the subject's wishes will govern; or

(2) That the research presents no more than minimal risk of harm to subjects and involves no procedures for which written consent is normally required outside of the research context.

In cases in which the documentation requirement is waived, the IRB may require the investigator to provide subjects with a written statement regarding the research.

(Approved by the Office of Management and Budget under Control Number 9999-0020.)

§ 46.118 Applications and proposals lacking definite plans for involvement of human subjects.

Certain types of applications for grants, cooperative agreements, or contracts are submitted to departments or agencies with the knowledge that subjects may be involved within the period of support, but definite plans would not normally be set forth in the application or proposal. These include activities such as institutional type grants when selection of specific projects is the institution's responsibility; research training grants in which the activities involving subjects remain to be selected; and projects in which human subjects' involvement will depend upon completion of instruments, prior animal studies, or purification of compounds. These applications need not be reviewed by an IRB before an award may be made. However, except for research exempted or waived under § 46.101 (b) or (i), no human subjects may be involved in any project supported by these awards until the project has been reviewed and approved by the IRB, as provided in this policy, and certification submitted, by the institution, to the Department or Agency.

§ 46.119 Research undertaken without the intention of involving human subjects.

In the event research is undertaken without the intention of involving human subjects, but it is later proposed to involve human subjects in the research, the research shall first be reviewed and approved by an IRB, as provided in this policy, a certification submitted, by the institution, to the Department or Agency, and final approval given to the proposed change by the Department or Agency.

§ 46.120 Evaluation and disposition of applications and proposals for research to be conducted or supported by a Federal Department or Agency.

(a) The Department or Agency head will evaluate all applications and proposals involving human subjects submitted to the Department or Agency through such officers and employees of the Department or Agency and such experts and consultants as the Department or Agency head determines to be appropriate. This evaluation will take into consideration the risks to the subjects, the adequacy of protection against these risks, the potential benefits of the research to the subjects and others, and the importance of the knowledge gained or to be gained.

(b) On the basis of this evaluation, the Department or Agency head may approve or disapprove the application or proposal, or enter into negotiations to develop an approvable one.

§ 46.121 [Reserved]

§ 46.122 Use of Federal Funds

Federal funds administered by a Department or Agency may not be expended for research involving human subjects unless the requirements of this policy have been satisfied.

§ 46.123 Early termination of research support: Evaluation of applications and proposals.

(a) The Department or Agency head may require that Department or Agency support for any project be terminated or suspended in the manner prescribed in applicable program requirements, when the Department or Agency head finds an institution has materially failed to comply with the terms of this policy.

(b) In making decisions about supporting or approving applications or proposals covered by this policy the Department or Agency head may take into account, in addition to all other eligibility requirements and program criteria, factors such as whether the applicant has been subject to a termination or suspension under paragraph (a) of this section and whether the applicant or the person or persons who would direct or has/have directed the scientific and technical aspects of an activity has/have, in the judgment of the Department or Agency head, materially failed to discharge responsibility for the protection of the rights and welfare of human subjects (whether or not the research was subject to Federal regulation).

§ 46.124 Conditions

With respect to any research project or any class of research projects the Department or Agency head may impose additional conditions prior to or at the time of approval when in the judgment of the Department or Agency head additional conditions are necessary for the protection of human subjects.

Subpart B--Additional DHHS Protections Pertaining to Research, Development, and Related Activities Involving Fetuses, Pregnant Women, and Human In Vitro Fertilization

Source: 40 FR 33528, 8 August 1975, 43 FR 1758, 11 January 1978; 43 FR 51559, 3 November 1978.

§ 46.201 Applicability.

(a) The regulations in this subpart are applicable to all Department of Health and Human Services grants and contracts supporting research, development, and related activities involving: (1) the fetus, (2) pregnant women, and (3) human *in vitro* fertilization.

(b) Nothing in this subpart shall be construed as indicating that compliance with the procedures set forth herein will in any way render inapplicable pertinent State or local laws bearing upon activities covered by this subpart.

(c) The requirements of this subpart are in addition to those imposed under the other subparts of this part.

§ 46.202 Purpose.

It is the purpose of this subpart to provide additional safeguards in reviewing activities to which this subpart is applicable to assure that they conform to appropriate ethical standards and relate to important societal needs.

§ 46.203 Definitions.

As used in this subpart:

(a) "Secretary" means the Secretary of Health and Human Services and any other officer or employee of the Department of Health and Human Services (DHHS) to whom authority has been delegated.

(b) "Pregnancy" encompasses the period of time from confirmation of implantation (through any of the presumptive signs of pregnancy, such as missed menses, or by a medically acceptable pregnancy test), until expulsion or extraction of the fetus.

(c) "Fetus" means the product of conception from the time of implantation (as evidenced by any of the presumptive signs of pregnancy, such as missed menses, or a medically acceptable pregnancy test), until a determination is made, following expulsion or extraction of the fetus, that it is viable.

(d) "Viable" as it pertains to the fetus means being able, after either spontaneous or induced delivery, to survive (given the benefit of available medical therapy) to the point of independently maintaining heart beat and respiration. The Secretary may from time to time, taking into account medical advances, publish in the **Federal Register** guidelines to assist in determining whether a fetus is viable for purposes of this subpart. If a fetus is viable after delivery, it is a premature infant.

(e) "Nonviable fetus" means a fetus *ex utero* which although living, is not viable.

(f) "Dead fetus" means a fetus *ex utero* which exhibits neither heartbeat, spontaneous respiratory activity, spontaneous movement of voluntary muscles, nor pulsation of the umbilical cord (if still attached).

(g) "*In vitro* fertilization" means any fertilization of human ova which occurs outside the body of a female, either through admixture of donor human sperm and ova or by any other means.

§ 46.204 Ethical Advisory Boards.

(a) One or more Ethical Advisory Boards shall be established by the Secretary. Members of these Board(s) shall be so selected that the

Board(s) will be competent to deal with medical, legal, social, ethical, and related issues and may include, for example, research scientists, physicians, psychologists, sociologists, educators, lawyers, and ethicists, as well as representatives of the general public. No Board member may be a regular, full-time employee of the Department of Health and Human Services.

(b) At the request of the Secretary, the Ethical Advisory Board shall render advice consistent with the policies and requirements of this part as to ethical issues, involving activities covered by this subpart, raised by individual applications or proposals. In addition, upon request by the Secretary, the Board shall render advice as to classes of applications or proposals and general policies, guidelines, and procedures.

(c) A Board may establish, with the approval of the Secretary, classes of applications or proposals which: (1) must be submitted to the Board, or (2) need not be submitted to the Board. Where the Board so establishes a class of applications or proposals which must be submitted, no application or proposal within the class may be funded by the Department or any component thereof until the application or proposal has been reviewed by the Board and the Board has rendered advice as to its acceptability from an ethical standpoint.

(d) No application or proposal involving human *in vitro* fertilization may be funded by the Department or any component thereof until the application or proposal has been reviewed by the Ethical Advisory Board and the Board has rendered advice as to its acceptability from an ethical standpoint.

§ 46.205 Additional duties of the Institutional Review Boards in connection with activities involving fetuses, pregnant women, or human in vitro fertilization.

(a) In addition to the responsibilities prescribed for Institutional Review Boards under Subpart A of this part, the applicant's or offeror's Board shall, with respect to activities covered by this subpart, carry out the following additional duties:

(1) determine that all aspects of the activity meet the requirements of this subpart;

(2) determine that adequate consideration has been given to the manner in which potential subjects will be selected, and adequate provision has been made by the applicant or offeror for monitoring the actual informed consent process (e.g, through such mechanisms, when appropriate, as participation by the Institutional Review Board or subject advocates in: (i) overseeing the actual process by which individ-

ual consents required by this subpart are secured either by approving induction of each individual into the activity or verifying, perhaps through sampling, that approved procedures for induction of individuals into the activity are being followed, and (ii) monitoring the progress of the activity and intervening as necessary through such steps as visits to the activity site and continuing evaluation to determine if any unanticipated risks have arisen);

(3) carry out such other responsibilities as may be assigned by the Secretary.

(b) No award may be issued until the applicant or offeror has certified to the Secretary that the Institutional Review Board has made the determinations required under paragraph (a) of this section and the Secretary has approved these determinations, as provided in § 46.120 of Subpart A of this part.

(c) Applicants or offerors seeking support for activities covered by this subpart must provide for the designation of an Institutional Review Board, subject to approval by the Secretary, where no such Board has been established under Subpart A of this part.

§ 46.206 General limitations.

(a) No activity to which this subpart is applicable may be undertaken unless:

(1) appropriate studies on animals and nonpregnant individuals have been completed;

(2) except where the purpose of the activity is to meet the health needs of the mother or the particular fetus, the risk to the fetus is minimal and, in all cases, is the least possible risk for achieving the objectives of the activity;

(3) individuals engaged in the activity will have no part in: (i) any decisions as to the timing, method, and procedures used to terminate the pregnancy, and (ii) determining the viability of the fetus at the termination of the pregnancy; and

(4) no procedural changes which may cause greater than minimal risk to the fetus or the pregnant woman will be introduced into the procedure for terminating the pregnancy solely in the interest of the activity.

(b) No inducements, monetary or otherwise, may be offered to terminate pregnancy for purposes of the activity.

Source: 40 FR 33528, 8 August 1975, as amended at 40 FR 51638, 6 November 1975.

§ 46.207 Activities directed toward pregnant women as subjects.

(a) No pregnant woman may be involved as a subject in an activity covered by this subpart unless: (1) the purpose of the activity is to meet the health needs of the mother and the fetus will be placed at risk only to the minimum extent necessary to meet such needs, or (2) the risk to the fetus is minimal.

(b) An activity permitted under paragraph (a) of this section may be conducted only if the mother and father are legally competent and have given their informed consent after having been fully informed regarding possible impact on the fetus, except that the father's informed consent need not be secured if: (1) the purpose of the activity is to meet the health needs of the mother; (2) his identity or whereabouts cannot reasonably be ascertained; (3) he is not reasonably available; or (4) the pregnancy resulted from rape.

§ 46.208 Activities directed toward fetuses *in utero* as subjects.

(a) No fetus *in utero* may be involved as a subject in any activity covered by this subpart unless: (1) the purpose of the activity is to meet the health needs of the particular fetus and the fetus will be placed at risk only to the minimum extent necessary to meet such needs, or (2) the risk to the fetus imposed by the research is minimal and the purpose of the activity is the development of important biomedical knowledge which cannot be obtained by other means.

(b) An activity permitted under paragraph (a) of this section may be conducted only if the mother and father are legally competent and have given their informed consent, except that the father's consent need not be secured if: (1) his identity or whereabouts cannot reasonably be ascertained, (2) he is not reasonably available, or (3) the pregnancy resulted from rape.

§ 46.209 Activities directed toward fetuses *ex utero* including non-viable fetuses, as subjects.

(a) Until is has been ascertained whether or not a fetus *ex utero* is viable, a fetus *ex utero* may not be involved as a subject in an activity covered by this subpart unless:

(1) there will be no added risk to the fetus resulting from the activity, and the purpose of the activity is the development of important biomedical knowledge which cannot be obtained by other means, or

(2) the purpose of the activity is to enhance the possibility of survival of the particular fetus to the point of viability.

(b) No nonviable fetus may be involved as a subject in an activity covered by this subpart unless:

(1) vital functions of the fetus will not be artificially maintained,

(2) experimental activities which of themselves would terminate the heartbeat or respiration of the fetus will not be employed, and

(3) the purpose of the activity is the development of important biomedical knowledge which cannot be obtained by other means.

(c) In the event the fetus *ex utero* is found to be viable, it may be included as a subject in the activity only to the extent permitted by and in accordance with the requirements of other subparts of this part.

(d) An activity permitted under paragraph (a) or (b) of this section may be conducted only if the mother and father are legally competent and have given their informed consent, except that the father's informed consent need not be secured if: (1) his identity or whereabouts cannot reasonably be ascertained, (2) he is not reasonably available, or (3) the pregnancy resulted from rape.

§ 46.210 Activities involving the dead fetus, fetal material, or the placenta.

Activities involving the dead fetus, mascerated fetal material, or cells, tissue, or organs excised from a dead fetus shall be conducted only in accordance with any applicable State or local laws regarding such activities.

§ 46.211 Modification or waiver of specific requirements.

Upon the request of an applicant or offeror (with the approval of its Institutional Review Board), the Secretary may modify or waive specific requirements of this subpart, with the approval of the Ethical Advisory Board after such opportunity for public comment as the Ethical Advisory Board considers appropriate in the particular instance. In making such decisions, the Secretary will consider whether the risks to the subject are so outweighed by the sum of the benefit to the subject and the importance of the knowledge to be gained as to warrant such modification or waiver and that such benefits cannot be gained except through a modification or waiver. Any such modifications or waivers will be published as notices in the **Federal Register**.

Subpart C--Additional DHHS Protections Pertaining to Biomedical and Behavioral Research Involving Prisoners as Subjects

Source: 43 FR 53655, 16 November 1978.

§ 46.301 Applicability.

(a) The regulations in this subpart are applicable to all biomedical and behavioral research conducted or supported by the Department of Health and Human Services involving prisoners as subjects.

(b) Nothing in this subpart shall be construed as indicating that compliance with the procedures set forth herein will authorize research involving prisoners as subjects, to the extent such research is limited or barred by applicable State or local law.

(c) The requirements of this subpart are in addition to those imposed under the other subparts of this part.

§ 46.302 Purpose.

Inasmuch as prisoners may be under constraints because of their incarceration which could affect their ability to make a truly voluntary and uncoerced decision whether or not to participate as subjects in research, it is the purpose of this subpart to provide additional safeguards for the protection of prisoners involved in activities to which this subpart is applicable.

§ 46.303 Definitions.

As used in this subpart:

(a) "Secretary" means the Secretary of Health and Human Services and any other officer or employee of the Department of Health and Human Services to whom authority has been delegated.

(b) "DHHS" means the Department of Health and Human Services.

(c) "Prisoner" means any individual involuntarily confined or detained in a penal institution. The term is intended to encompass individuals sentenced to such an institution under a criminal or civil statute, individuals detained in other facilities by virtue of statutes or commitment procedures which provide alternatives to criminal prosecution or incarceration in a penal institution, and individuals detained pending arraignment, trial, or sentencing.

(d) "Minimal risk" is the probability and magnitude of physical or psychological harm that is normally encountered in the daily lives, or in the routine medical, dental, or psychological examination of healthy persons.

§ 46.304 Composition of Institutional Review Boards where prisoners are involved.

In addition to satisfying the requirements in §46.107 of this part, an Institutional Review Board, carrying out responsibilities under this part with respect to research covered by this subpart, shall also meet the following specific requirements:

(a) A majority of the Board (exclusive of prisoner members)shall have no association with the prison(s) involved, apart from their membership on the Board.

(b) At least one member of the Board shall be a prisoner, or a prisoner representative with appropriate background and experience to serve in that capacity, except that where a particular research project is reviewed by more than one Board only one Board need satisfy this requirement.

§ 46.305 Additional duties of the Institutional Review Boards where prisoners are involved.

(a) In addition to all other responsibilities prescribed for Institutional Review Boards under this part, the Board shall review research covered by this subpart and approve such research only if it finds that:

(1) the research under review represents one of the categories of research permissible under § 46.306(a)(2);

(2) any possible advantages accruing to the prisoner through his or her participation in the research, when compared to the general living conditions, medical care, quality of food, amenities and opportunity for earnings in the prison, are not of such a magnitude that his or her ability to weigh the risks of the research against the value of such advantages in the limited choice environment of the prison is impaired;

(3) the risks involved in the research are commensurate with risks that would be accepted by nonprisoner volunteers;

(4) procedure for the selection of subjects within the prison are fair to all prisoners and immune from arbitrary intervention by prison authorities or prisoners. Unless the principal investigator provides to the Board justification in writing for following some other procedures, control subjects must be selected randomly from the group of available prisoners who meet the characteristics needed for that particular re-

search project;

(5) the information is presented in language which is understandable to the subject population;

(6) adequate assurance exists that parole boards will not take into account a prisoner's participation in the research in making decisions regarding parole, and each prisoner is clearly informed in advance that participation in the research will have no effect on his or her parole; and

(7) where the Board finds there may be a need for follow-up examination or care of participants after the end of their participation, adequate provision has been made for such examination or care, taking into account the varying lengths of individual prisoners' sentences, and for informing participants of this fact.

(b) The Board shall carry out such other duties as may be assigned by the Secretary.

(c) The institution shall certify to the Secretary, in such form and manner as the Secretary may require, that the duties of the Board under this section have been fulfilled.

§ 46.306 Permitted research involving prisoners.

(a) Biomedical or behavioral research conducted or supported by DHHS may involve prisoners as subjects only if:

(1) the institution responsible for the conduct of the research has certified to the Secretary that the Institutional Review Board has approved the research under §46.305 of this subpart; and

(2) in the judgment of the Secretary the proposed research involves solely the following:

(A) study of the possible causes, effects, and processes of incarceration and of criminal behavior, provided that the study presents no more than minimal risk and no more than inconvenience to the subjects;

(B) study of prisons as institutional structures or of prisoners as incarcerated persons, provided that the study presents no more than minimal risk and no more than inconvenience to the subjects;

(C) research on conditions particularly affecting prisoners as a class (for example, vaccine trials and other research on hepatitis which is much more prevalent in prisons than elsewhere; and research on social and psychological problems such as alcoholism, drug addiction, and sexual assaults) provided that the study may proceed only after the Secretary has consulted with appropriate experts including experts in penology, medicine, and ethics, and published notice, in the **Federal Register**, of his intent to approve such research; or

(D) research on practices, both innovative and accepted, which have the intent and reasonable probability of improving the health or well-being of the subject. In cases in which those studies require the assignment of prisoners in a manner consistent with protocols approved by the IRB to control groups which may not benefit from the research, the study may proceed only after the Secretary has consulted with appropriate experts, including experts in penology, medicine, and ethics, and published notice, in the **Federal Register**, of the intent to approve such research.

(b) Except as provided in paragraph (a) of this section, biomedical or behavioral research conducted or supported by DHHS shall not involve prisoners as subjects.

Subpart D--Additional DHHS Protections for Children Involved as Subjects in Research.

Source: 48 FR 9818, 8 March 1983; 56 FR 28032, 18 June 1991.

§ 46.401 To what do these regulations apply?

(a) This subpart applies to all research involving children as subjects, conducted or supported by the Department of Health and Human Services.

(1) This includes research conducted by Department employees, except that each head of an Operating Division of the Department may adopt such nonsubstantive, procedural modifications as may be appropriate from an administrative standpoint.

(2) It also includes research conducted or supported by the Department of Health and Human Services outside the United States, but in appropriate circumstances, the Secretary may, under paragraph (e) of § 46.101 of Subpart A, waive the applicability of some or all of the requirements of these regulations for research of this type.

(b) Exemptions at § 46.101(b)(1) and (b)(3) through (b)(6) are applicable to this subpart. The exemption at § 46.101(b)(2) regarding educational tests is also applicable to this subpart. However, the exemption at § 46.101(b)(2)for research involving survey or interview procedures or observations of public behavior does not apply to research covered by this subpart, except for research involving observation of public behavior when the investigator(s) do not participate in the activities being observed.

(c) The exceptions, additions, and provisions for waiver as they appear in paragraphs (c) through (i) of § 46.101 of Subpart A are applicable to this subpart.

§ 46.402 Definitions.

The definitions in § 46.102 of Subpart A shall be applicable to this subpart as well. In addition, as used in this subpart:

(a) "Children" are persons who have not attained the legal age for consent to treatments or procedures involved in the research, under the applicable law of the jurisdiction in which the research will be conducted.

(b) "Assent" means a child's affirmative agreement to participate in research. Mere failure to object should not, absent affirmative agreement, be construed as assent.

(c) "Permission" means the agreement of parent(s) or guardian to the participation of their child or ward in research.

(d) "Parent" means a child's biological or adoptive parent.

(e) "Guardian" means an individual who is authorized under applicable State or local law to consent on behalf of a child to general medical care.

§ 46.403 IRB duties.

In addition to other responsibilities assigned to IRBs under this part, each IRB shall review research covered by this subpart and approve only research which satisfies the conditions of all applicable sections of this subpart.

§ 46.404 Research not involving greater than minimal risk.

DHHS will conduct or fund research in which the IRB finds that no greater than minimal risk to children is presented, only if the IRB finds that adequate provisions are made for soliciting the assent of the children and the permission of their parents or guardians, as set forth in §46.408.

§ 46.405 Research involving greater than minimal risk but presenting the prospect of direct benefit to the individual subjects.

DHHS will conduct or fund research in which the IRB finds that more than minimal risk to children is presented by an intervention or procedure that holds out the prospect of direct benefit for the individual subject, or by a monitoring procedure that is likely to contribute to the subject's well-being, only if the IRB finds that:

(a) the risk is justified by the anticipated benefit to the subjects;

(b) the relation of the anticipated benefit to the risk is at least as favorable to the subjects as that presented by available alternative approaches; and

(c) adequate provisions are made for soliciting the assent of the children and permission of their parents or guardians, as set forth in § 46.408.

§ 46.406 Research involving greater than minimal risk and no prospect of direct benefit to individual subjects, but likely to yield generalizable knowledge about the subject's disorder or condition.

DHHS will conduct or fund research in which the IRB finds that more than minimal risk to children is presented by an intervention or procedure that does not hold out the prospect of direct benefit for the individual subject, or by a monitoring procedure which is not likely to contribute to the wellbeing of the subject, only if the IRB finds that:

(a) the risk represents a minor increase over minimal risk;

(b) the intervention or procedure presents experiences to subjects that are reasonably commensurate with those inherent in their actual or expected medical, dental, psychological, social, or educational situations;

(c) the intervention or procedure is likely to yield generalizable knowledge about the subjects' disorder or condition which is of vital importance for the understanding or amelioration of the subjects' disorder or condition; and

(d) adequate provisions are made for soliciting assent of the children and permission of their parents or guardians, as set forth in § 46.408.

§ 46.407 Research not otherwise approvable which presents an opportunity to understand, prevent, or alleviate a serious problem affecting the health or welfare of children.

DHHS will conduct or fund research that the IRB does not believe meets the requirements of § 46.404, § 46.405, or § 46.406 only if:

(a) the IRB finds that the research presents a reasonable opportunity to further the understanding, prevention, or alleviation of a serious problem affecting the health or welfare of children; and

(b) the Secretary, after consultation with a panel of experts in pertinent disciplines (for example: science, medicine, education, ethics, law) and following opportunity for public review and comment, has determined either:

(1) that the research in fact satisfies the conditions of § 46.404, § 46.405, or § 46.406, as applicable, or (2) the following:

(i) the research presents a reasonable opportunity to further the understanding, prevention, or alleviation of a serious problem affecting the health or welfare of children;

(ii) the research will be conducted in accordance with sound ethical principles;

(iii) adequate provisions are made for soliciting the assent of children and the permission of their parents or guardians, as set forth in § 46.408.

§ 46.408 Requirements for permission by parents or guardians and for assent by children.

(a) In addition to the determinations required under other applicable sections of this subpart, the IRB shall determine that adequate provisions are made for soliciting the assent of the children, when in the judgment of the IRB the children are capable of providing assent. In determining whether children are capable of assenting, the IRB shall take into account the ages, maturity, and psychological state of the children involved. This judgment may be made for all children to be involved in research under a particular protocol, or for each child, as the IRB deems appropriate. If the IRB determines that the capability of some or all of the children is so limited that they cannot reasonably be consulted or that the intervention or procedure involved in the research holds out a prospect of direct benefit that is important to the health or well-being of the children and is available only in the context of the research, the assent of the children is not a necessary condition for proceeding with the research. Even where the IRB determines that the subjects are capable of assenting, the IRB may still waive the assent requirement under circumstances in which consent may be waived in accord with § 46.116 of Subpart A.

(b) In addition to the determinations required under other applicable sections of this subpart, the IRB shall determine, in accordance with and to the extent that consent is required by § 46.116 of Subpart A, that adequate provisions are made for soliciting the permission of each child's parents or guardian. Where parental permission is to be obtained, the IRB may find that the permission of one parent is sufficient for research to be conducted under § 46.404 or § 46.405. Where research is covered by § 46.406 and § 46.407 and permission is to be obtained from parents, both parents must give their permission unless one parent is deceased, unknown, incompetent, or not reasonably available, or when only one parent has legal responsibility for the care and custody of the child.

(c) In addition to the provisions for waiver contained in § 46.116 of Subpart A, if the IRB determines that a research protocol is designed for conditions or for a subject population for which parental or guardian permission is not a reasonable requirement to protect the subjects (for example, neglected or abused children), it may waive the consent requirements in Subpart A of this part and paragraph (b) of this section, provided an appropriate mechanism for protecting the children who will participate as subjects in the research is substituted, and provided further that the waiver is not inconsistent with Federal, State, or local law. The choice of an appropriate mechanism would depend upon the nature and purpose of the activities described in the protocol, the risk and anticipated benefit to the research subjects, and their age, maturity, status, and condition.

(d) Permission by parents or guardians shall be documented in accordance with and to the extent required by § 46.117 of Subpart A.

(e) When the IRB determines that assent is required, it shall also determine whether and how assent must be documented.

§ 46.409 Wards.

(a) Children who are wards of the State or any other agency, institution, or entity can be included in research approved under § 46.406 or § 46.407 only if such research is:

(1) related to their status as wards; or

(2) conducted in schools, camps, hospitals, institutions, or similar settings in which the majority of children involved as subjects are not wards.

(b) If the research is approved under paragraph (a) of this section, the IRB shall require appointment of an advocate for each child who is a ward, in addition to any other individual acting on behalf of the child as guardian or in loco parentis. One individual may serve as advocate for more than one child. The advocate shall be an individual who has the background and experience to act in, and agrees to act in, the best interests of the child for the duration of the child's participation in the research and who is not associated in any way (except in the role as advocate or member of the IRB) with the research, the investigator(s), or the guardian organization.

RESEARCH ACTIVITIES WHICH MAY BE REVIEWED THROUGH EXPEDITED REVIEW PROCEDURES

Research activities involving no more than minimal risk *and* in which the only involvement of human subjects will be in one or more of the following categories (carried out through standard methods) may be reviewed by the Institutional Review Board through the expedited review procedure authorized in § 46.110 of 45 CFR Part 46.

(1) Collection of: hair and nail clippings, in a nondisfiguring manner; deciduous teeth; and permanent teeth if patient care indicates a need for extraction.

(2) Collection of excreta and external secretions including sweat, un-cannulated saliva, placenta removed at delivery, and amniotic fluid at the time of rupture of the membrane prior to or during labor.

(3) Recording of data from subjects 18 years of age or older using noninvasive procedures routinely employed in clinical practice. This includes the use of physical sensors that are applied either to the surface of the body or at a distance and do not involve input of matter or significant amounts of energy into the subject or an invasion of the subject's privacy. It also includes such procedures as weighing, testing sensory acuity, electrocardiography, electroencephalography, thermography, detection of naturally occurring radioactivity, diagnostic echography, and electroretinography. It does not include exposure to electromagnetic radiation outside the visible range (for example, x-rays, microwaves).

(4) Collection of blood samples by venipuncture, in amounts not exceeding 450 milliliters in an eight-week period and no more often than two times per week, from subjects 18 years of age or older and who are in good health and not pregnant.

(5) Collection of both supra-and subgingival dental plaque and calculus, provided the procedure is not more invasive than routine prophylactic scaling of the teeth and the process is accomplished in accordance with accepted prophylactic techniques.

(6) Voice recordings made for research purposes such as investigations of speech defects.

(7) Moderate exercise by healthy volunteers.

(8) The study of existing data, documents, records, pathological specimens, or diagnostic specimens.

(9) Research on individual or group behavior or characteristics of individuals, such as studies of perception, cognition, game theory, or test development, where the investigator does not manipulate subjects' behavior and the research will not involve stress to subjects.

(10) Research on drugs or devices for which an investigational new drug exemption or an investigational device exemption is not required.

Source: 46 FR 8392, 26 January 1981.

NIH Guidelines on the Inclusion of Women and Minorities as Subjects in Clinical Research

AGENCY: National Institute of Health. PHS, DHHS

SUPPLEMENTARY INFORMATION: NIH Guidelines on the Inclusion of Women and Minorities as Subjects in Clinical Research

I. Introduction

This document sets forth guidelines on the inclusion of women and members of minority groups and their subpopulations in clinical research, including clinical trials, supported by the National Institutes of Health (NIH). For the purposes of this document, clinical research is defined as NIH-supported biomedical and behavioral research involving human subjects. These guidelines, implemented in accordance with section 492B of the Public Health Service Act, added by the NIH Revitalization Act of 1993, Public Law (Pub.L.) 103-43, supersede and strengthen the previous policies, NIH/ADAMHA Policy Concerning the Inclusion of Women in Study Populations, and ADAMHA/NIH Policy Concerning the Inclusion of Minorities in Study Populations, published in the NIH GUIDE FOR GRANTS AND CONTRACTS, 1990.

The 1993 guidelines continue the 1990 guidelines with three major additions. The new policy requires that, in addition to the continuing inclusion of women and members of minority groups in all NIH-supported biomedical and behavioral research involving human subjects, the NIH must:

- Ensure that women and members of minorities and their subpopulations are included in all human subject research.
- For Phase III clinical trials, ensure that women and minorities and their subpopulations must be included such that valid analyses of differences in intervention effect can be accomplished:
- Not allow cost as an acceptable reason for excluding these groups; and,

● Initiate programs and support for outreach efforts to recruit these groups into clinical studies.

Since a primary aim of research is to provide scientific evidence leading to a change in health policy or a standard of care, it is imperative to determine whether the intervention or therapy being studied affects women or men or members of minority groups and their subpopulations differently. To this end, the guidelines published here are intended to ensure that all future NIH-supported biomedical and behavioral research involving human subjects will be carried out in a manner sufficient to elicit information about individuals of both genders and the diverse racial and ethnic groups and, in the case of clinical trials, to examine differential effects on such groups. Increased attention, therefore, must be given to gender, race, and ethnicity in earlier stages of research to allow for informed decisions at the Phase III clinical trial stage.

These guidelines reaffirm NIH's commitment to the fundamental principles of inclusion of women and racial and ethnic minority groups and their subpopulations in research. This policy should result in a variety of new research opportunities to address significant gaps in knowledge about health problems that affect women and racial/ethnic minorities and their subpopulations.

The NIH recognizes that issues will arise with the implementation of these guidelines and thus welcomes comments. During the first year of implementation, NIH will review the comments, and consider modifications, within the scope of the statute, to the guidelines.

II. Background

The NIH Revitalization Act of 1993, PL 103-43, signed by President Clinton on June 10, 1993, directs the NIH to establish guidelines for inclusion of women and minorities in clinical research. This guidance shall include guidelines regarding--

(A) the circumstances under which the inclusion of women and minorities as subjects in projects of clinical research is inappropriate * * *;

(B) the manner in which clinical trials are required to be designed and carried out * * *; and

(C) the operation of outreach programs * * * 492B(d)(1)

The statute states that

In conducting or supporting clinical research for the purposes of this title, the Director of NIH shall * * * ensure that--

A. women are included as subjects in each project of such research; and

B. members of minority groups are included in such research. 492B(a)(1)

The statute further defines "clinical research" to include "clinical trials" and states that

In the case of any clinical trial in which women or members of minority groups will be included as subjects, the Director of NIH shall ensure that the trial is designed and carried out in a manner sufficient to provide for valid analysis of whether the variables being studied in the trial affect women or members of minority groups, as the case may be, differently than other subjects in the trial. 492B(C)

Specifically addressing the issue of minority groups, the statute states that

The term "minority group" includes subpopulations of minority groups. The Director of NIH shall, through the guidelines established * * * define the terms "minority group" and "subpopulation" for the purposes of the preceding sentence. 492B(g)(2)

The statute speaks specifically to outreach and states that

The Director of NIH, in consultation with the Director of the Office of Research of Women's Health and the Director of the Office of Research on Minority Health, shall conduct or support outreach programs for the recruitment of women and members of minority groups as subjects in the projects of clinical research. 492B(a)(2)

The statute includes a specific provision pertaining to the cost of clinical research and, in particular clinical trials.

(A)(i) In the case of a clinical trial, the guidelines shall provide that the costs of such inclusion in the trial is (sic) not a permissible consideration in determining whether such inclusion is inappropriate. 492B(d)(2)

(ii) In the case of other projects of clinical research, the guidelines shall provide that the costs of such inclusion in the project is (sic) not a permissible consideration in determining whether such inclusion is inappropriate unless the data regarding women or members of minority groups, respectively, that would be obtained in such project (in the event that such inclusion were required) have been or are being obtained through other means that provide data of comparable quality. 492B(d)(2)

Exclusions to the requirement for inclusion of women and minorities are stated in the statute, as follows:

The requirements established regarding women and members of minority groups shall not apply to the project of clinical research if the inclusion, as subjects in the project, of women and members of minority groups, respectively--

(1) Is inappropriate with respect to the health of the subjects;

(2) Is inappropriate with respect to the purpose of the research; or

(3) Is inappropriate under such other circumstances as the Director of NIH may designate. 492B(b)

(B) In the case of a clinical trial, the guidelines may provide that such inclusion in the trial is not required if there is substantial scientific data demonstrating that there is no significant difference between--

(i) The effects that the variables to be studied in the trial have on women or members of minority groups, respectively; and

(ii) The effects that variables have on the individuals who would serve as subjects in the trial in the event that such inclusion were not required 492B(d)(2)

III. Policy

A. Research Involving Human Subjects

It is the policy of NIH that women and members of minority groups and their subpopulations must be included in all NIH-supported biomedical and behavioral research projects involving human subjects, unless a clear and compelling rationale and justification establishes to the satisfaction of the relevant Institute/Center Director that inclusion is inappropriate with respect to the health of the subjects or the purpose of the research. Exclusion under other circumstances may be made by the Director, NIH, upon the recommendation of an Institute/Center Director based on a compelling rationale and justification. Cost is not an acceptable reason for exclusion except when the study would duplicate data from other sources. Women of childbearing potential should not be routinely excluded from participation in clinical research. All NIH-supported biomedical and behavioral research involving human subjects is defined as clinical research. This policy applies to research subjects of all ages.

The inclusion of women and members of minority groups and their subpopulations must be addressed in developing a research design appropriate to the scientific objectives of the study. The research plan should describe the composition of the proposed study population in terms of gender and racial/ethnic group, and provide a rationale for selection of such subjects. Such a plan should contain a description of the proposed outreach programs for recruiting women and minorities as participants.

B. Clinical Trials

Under the statute, when a Phase III clinical trial (see Definitions, Section V-A) is proposed, evidence must be reviewed to show whether or not clinically important gender or race/ethnicity differences in the intervention effect are to be expected. This evidence may include, but is not limited to, data derived from prior animal studies, clinical observations, metabolic studies, genetic studies, pharmacology studies, and observational, natural history, epidemiology and other relevant studies.

As such, investigators must consider the following when planning a Phase III clinical trial for NIH support.

• If the data from prior studies strongly indicate the existence of significant differences of clinical or public health importance in intervention effect among subgroups (gender and/or racial/ethnic subgroups), the primary question(s) to be addressed by the proposed Phase III trial and the design of that trial must specifically accommodate this. For example, if men and women are thought to respond differently to an intervention, then the Phase III trial must be designed to answer two separate primary questions, one for men and the other for women, with adequate sample size for each.

• If the data from prior studies strongly support no significant differences of clinical or public health importance in intervention effect between subgroups, then gender or race/ethnicity will not be required as subject selection criteria. However, the inclusion of gender or racial/ ethnic subgroups is still strongly encouraged.

• If the data from prior studies neither support strongly nor negate strongly the existence of significant differences of clinical or public health importance in intervention effect between subgroups, then the Phase III trial will be required to include sufficient and appropriate entry of gender and racial/ethnic subgroups, so that valid analysis of the intervention effect in subgroups can be performed. However, the trial will not be required to provide high statistical power for each subgroup.

Cost is not an acceptable reason for exclusion of women and minorities from clinical trials.

C. Funding

NIH funding components will not award any grant, cooperative agreement or contract or support any intramural project to be conducted or funded in Fiscal Year 1995 and thereafter which does not comply with this policy. For research awards that are covered by this policy, awardees will report annually on enrollment of women and men, and on the race and ethnicity of research participants.

IV. Implementation

A. Date of Implementation

This policy applies to all applications/proposals and intramural projects to be submitted on and after June 1, 1994 (the date of full implementation) seeking Fiscal Year 1995 support. Projects funded prior to June 10, 1993, must still comply with the 1990 policy and report annually on enrollment of subjects using gender and racial/ethnic categories as required in the Application for Continuation of a Public Health Service Grant (PHS Form 2590), in contracts and in intramural projects.

B. Transition Policy

NIH-supported biomedical and behavioral research projects involving human subjects, with the exception of Phase III clinical trial projects as discussed below, that are awarded between June 10, 1993, the date of enactment, and September 30, 1994, the end of Fiscal Year 1994, shall be subject to the requirements of the 1990 policy and the annual reporting requirements on enrollment using gender and racial/ethnic categories.

For all Phase III clinical trial projects proposed between June 10, 1993 and June 1, 1994, and those awarded between June 10, 1993 and September 30, 1994, Institute/Center staff will examine the applications/proposals, pending awards, awards and intramural projects to determine if the study was developed in a manner consistent with the new guidelines. If it is deemed inconsistent, NIH staff will contact investigators to discuss approaches to accommodate the new policy. Administrative actions may be needed to accommodate or revise the pending trials. Institutes/Centers may need to consider initiating a complementary activity to address any gender or minority representation concerns.

The NIH Director will determine whether the Phase III clinical trial being considered during this transition is in compliance with this policy, whether acceptable modifications have been made, or whether the Institute/Center will initiate a complementary activity that addresses the gender or minority representation concerns. Pending awards will not be funded without this determination.

Solicitations issued by the NIH planned for release after the date of publication of the guidelines in the **Federal Register** will include the new requirements.

C. Roles and Responsibilities

While this policy applies to all applicants for NIH-supported biomedical and behavioral research involving human subjects, certain individuals and groups have special roles and responsibilities with regard to the adoption and implementation of these guidelines.

The NIH staff will provide educational opportunities for the extramural and intramural community concerning this policy; monitor its implementation during the development, review, award and conduct of research; and manage the NIH research portfolio to address the policy.

1. Principal Investigators

Principal investigators should assess the theoretical and/or scientific linkages between gender, race/ethnicity, and their topic of study. Following this assessment, the principal investigator and the applicant institution will address the policy in each application and proposal, providing the required information on inclusion of women and minorities and their subpopulations in research projects, and any required justifications for exceptions to the policy. Depending on the purpose of the study, NIH recognizes that a single study may not include all minority groups.

2. Institutional Review Boards (IRBs)

As the IRBs implement the guidelines, described herein, for the inclusion of women and minorities and their subpopulations, they must also implement the regulations for the protection of human subjects as described in title **45 CFR** part 46, "Protection of Human Subjects."

They should take into account the Food and Drug Administration's "Guidelines for the Study and Evaluation of Gender Differences in the Clinical Evaluation of Drugs." Vol. 58, **Federal Register** 39406.

3. Peer Review Groups

In conducting peer review for scientific and technical merit, appropriately constituted initial review groups (including study sections), technical evaluation groups, and intramural review panels will be instructed, as follows:

● To evaluate the proposed plan for the inclusion of minorities and both genders for appropriate representation or to evaluate the proposed justification when representation is limited or absent,

● To evaluate the proposed exclusion of minorities and women on the basis that a requirement for inclusion is inappropriate with respect to the health of the subjects,

● To evaluate the proposed exclusion of minorities and women on the basis that a requirement for inclusion is inappropriate with respect to the purpose of the research,

● To determine whether the design of clinical trials is adequate to measure differences when warranted,

● To evaluate the plans for recruitment/outreach for study, participants, and

● To include these criteria as part of the scientific assessment and assigned score.

4. NIH Advisory Councils

In addition to its current responsibilities for review of projects where the peer review groups have raised questions about the appropriate inclusion of women and minorities, the Advisory Council/Board of each Institute/Center shall prepare biennial reports, for inclusion in the overall NIH Director's biennial report, describing the manner in which the Institute/Center has complied with the provisions of the statute.

5. Institute/Center Directors

Institute/Center Directors and their staff shall determine whether: (a) The research involving human subjects, (b) the Phase III clinical trials, and (c) the exclusions meet the requirements of the statute and these guidelines.

6. NIH Director

The NIH Director may approve, on a case-by-case basis, the exclusion of projects, as recommended by the Institute/Center Director, that may be inappropriate to include within the requirements of these guidelines on the basis of circumstances other than the health of the subjects, the purpose of the research, or costs.

7. Recruitment Outreach by Extramural and Intramural Investigators

Investigators and their staff(s) are urged to develop appropriate and culturally sensitive outreach programs and activities commensurate with the goals of the study. The objective should be to actively recruit the most diverse study population consistent with the purposes of the research project. Indeed, the purpose should be to establish a relationship between the investigator(s) and staff(s) and populations and community(ies) of interest such that mutual benefit is derived for participants in the study. Investigator(s) and staff(s) should take precautionary measures to ensure that ethical concerns are clearly noted, such that there is minimal possibility of coercion or undue influence in the incentives or rewards offered in recruiting into or retaining participants in studies. It is also the responsibility of the IRBs to address these ethical concerns.

Furthermore, while the statute focuses on recruitment outreach, NIH staff underscore the need to appropriately retain participants in clinical studies, and thus, the outreach programs and activities should address both recruitment and retention.

To assist investigators and potential study participants, NIH staff have prepared a notebook, "NIH Outreach Notebook On the Inclusion of Women and Minorities in Biomedical and Behavioral Research." The notebook addresses both recruitment and retention of women and minorities in clinical studies, provides relevant references and case studies, and discusses ethical issues. It is not intended as a definitive text on this subject, but should assist investigators in their consideration of an appropriate plan for recruiting and retaining participants in clinical studies. The notebook is expected to be available early in 1994.

8. Educational Outreach by NIH to Inform the Professional Community

NIH staff will present the new guidelines to investigators, IRB members, peer review groups, and Advisory Councils in a variety of public educational forums.

9. Applicability to Foreign Research Involving Human Subjects

For foreign awards, the NIH policy on inclusion of women in research conducted outside the U.S. is the same as that for research conducted in the U.S.

However, with regard to the population of the foreign country, the definition of the minority groups may be different than in the U.S. If there is scientific rationale for examining subpopulation group differences within the foreign population, investigators should consider designing their studies to accommodate these differences.

V. Definitions

Throughout the section of the statute pertaining to the inclusion of women and minorities, terms are used which require definition for the purpose of implementing these guidelines. These terms, drawn directly from the statute, are defined below.

A. Clinical Trial

For the purpose of these guidelines, a "clinical trial" is a broadly based prospective Phase III clinical investigation, usually involving several hundred or more human subjects, for the purpose of evaluating an experimental intervention in comparison with a standard or control intervention or comparing two or more existing treatments. Often the aim of such investigation is to provide evidence leading to a scientific basis for consideration of a change in health policy or standard of care. The definition includes pharmacologic, non-pharmacologic, and behavioral interventions given for disease prevention, prophylaxis, diagnosis, or therapy. Community trials and other population-based intervention trials are also included.

B. Research Involving Human Subjects

All NIH-supported biomedical and behavioral research involving human subjects is defined as clinical research under this policy. Under this policy, the definition of human subjects in title 45 **CFR** part 46, the Department of Health and Human Services regulations for the protection of human subjects applies: "Human subject means a living individual about whom an investigator (whether professional or student) conducting research obtains: (1) Data through intervention or interaction with the individual, or (2) identifiable private information." These regulations specifically address the protection of human subjects from research risks. It should be noted that there are research areas (Exemptions 1-6) that are exempt from these regulations. However, under these guidelines, NIH-supported biomedical and behavioral research projects involving human subjects which are exempt from the human subjects regulations should still address the inclusion of women and minorities in their study design. Therefore, all biomedical and behavioral research projects involving human subjects will be evaluated for compliance with this policy.

C. Valid Analysis

The term "valid analysis" means an unbiased assessment. Such an assessment will, on average, yield the correct estimate of the difference in outcomes between two groups of subjects. Valid analysis can and should be conducted for both small and large studies. A valid analysis does not need to have a high statistical power for detecting a stated effect. The principal requirements for ensuring a valid analysis of the question of interest are:

- Allocation of study participants of both genders and from different racial/ethnic groups to the intervention and control groups by an unbiased process such as randomization,

- Unbiased evaluation of the outcome(s) of study participants, and

- Use of unbiased statistical analyses and proper methods of inference to estimate and compare the intervention effects among the gender and racial/ethnic groups.

D. Significant Difference

For purposes of this policy, a "significant difference" is a difference that is of clinical or public health importance, based on substantial scientific data. This definition differs from the commonly used "statistically significant difference," which refers to the event that, for a given set of data, the statistical test for a difference between the effects in two groups achieves statistical significance. Statistical significance depends upon the amount of information in the data set. With a very large amount of information, one could find a statistically significant, but clinically small difference that is of very little clinical importance. Conversely, with less information one could find a large difference of potential importance that is not statistically significant.

E. Racial and Ethic Categories

1. Minority Groups

A minority group is a readily identifiable subset of the U.S. population which is distinguished by either racial, ethnic, and/or cultural heritage.

The Office of Management and Budget (OMB) Directive No. 15 defines the minimum standard of basic racial and ethnic categories, which are used below. NIH has chosen to continue the use of these definitions because they allow comparisons to many national data bases, especially national health data bases. Therefore, the racial and ethnic categories described below should be used as basic guidance, cognizant of the distinction based on cultural heritage.

American Indian or Alaskan Native: A person having origins in any of the original peoples of North America, and who maintains cultural identification through tribal affiliation or community recognition.

Asian or Pacific Islander: A person having origins in any of the original peoples of the Far East, Southeast Asia, the Indian subcontinent, or the Pacific Islands. This area includes, for example, China, India, Japan, Korea, the Philippine Islands and Samoa.

Black, not of Hispanic Origin: A person having origins in any of the black racial groups of Africa.

Hispanic: A person of Mexican, Puerto Rican, Cuban, Central or South American or other Spanish culture or origin, regardless of race.

2. Majority Group

White, not of Hispanic Origin: A person having origins in any of the original peoples of Europe, North Africa, or the Middle East.

NIH recognizes the diversity of the U.S. population and that changing demographics are reflected in the changing racial and ethnic composition of the population. The terms "minority groups" and "minority subpopulations" are meant to be inclusive, rather than exclusive, of differing racial and ethnic categories.

3. Subpopulations

Each minority group contains subpopulations which are delimited by geographic origins, national origins and/or cultural differences. It is recognized that there are different ways of defining and reporting racial and ethnic subpopulation data. The subpopulation to which an individual is assigned depends on self-reporting of specific racial and ethnic origin. Attention to subpopulations also applies to individuals of mixed racial and/or ethnic parentage. Researchers should be cognizant of the possibility that these racial/ethnic combinations may have biomedical and/or cultural implications related to the scientific question under study.

F.   Outreach Strategies

These are outreach efforts by investigators and their staff(s) to appropriately recruit and retain populations of interest into research studies. Such efforts should represent a thoughtful and culturally sensitive plan of outreach and generally include involvement of other individuals and organizations relevant to the populations and communities of interest, e.g., family, religious organizations, community leaders and informal gatekeepers, and public and private institutions and organizations. The objective is to establish appropriate lines of communication and cooperation to build mutual trust and cooperation such that both the study and the participants benefit from such collaboration.

G.   Research Portfolio

Each Institute and Center at the NIH has its own research portfolio, i.e., its "holdings" in research grants, cooperative agreements, contracts and intramural studies. The Institute or Center evaluates the research awards in its portfolio to identify those areas where there are knowledge gaps or which need special attention to advance the science involved. NIH may consider funding projects to achieve a research portfolio reflecting diverse study populations. With the implementation of this new policy, there will be a need to ensure that sufficient resources are provided within a program to allow for data to be developed for a smooth transition from basic research to Phase III clinical trials that meet the policy requirements.

VI. Discussion--Issues in Scientific Plans and Study Designs

A.   Issues in Research Involving Human Subjects

The biomedical and behavioral research process can be viewed as a stepwise process progressing from discovery of new knowledge through research in the laboratory, research involving animals, research involving human subjects, validation of interventions through clinical trials, and broad application to improve the health of the public.

All NIH-supported biomedical and behavioral research involving human subjects is defined broadly in this guidance as clinical research. This is broader than the definition provided in the 1990 NIH Guidance and in many program announcements, requests for applications, and requests for proposals since 1990.

The definition was broadened because of the need to obtain data about minorities and both genders early in the research process when hypotheses are being formulated, baseline data are being collected, and various measurement instruments and intervention strategies are being developed. Broad inclusion at these early stages of research provides valuable information for designing broadly based clinical trials, which are a subset of studies under the broad category of research studies.

The policy on inclusion of minorities and both genders applies to all NIH-supported biomedical and behavioral research involving human subjects so that the maximum information may be obtained to understand the implications of the research findings on the gender or minority group.

Investigators would consider the types of information concerning gender and minority groups which will be required when designing future Phase III clinical trials, and try to obtain it in their earlier stages of research involving human subjects. NIH recognizes that the understanding of health problems and conditions of different U.S. populations may require attention to socioeconomic differences involving occupation, education, and income gradients.

B. Issues in Clinical Trials

The statute requires appropriate representation of subjects of different gender and race/ethnicity in clinical trials so as to provide the opportunity for detecting major qualitative differences (if they exist) among gender and racial/ethnic subgroups and to identify more subtle differences that might, if warranted, be explored in further specifically targeted studies. Other interpretations may not serve as well the health needs of women, minorities, and all other constituencies.

Preparatory to any Phase III clinical trial, certain data are typically obtained. Such data are necessary for the design of an appropriate Phase III trial and include observational clinical study data, basic laboratory (i.e. *in vitro* and animal) data, and clinical, physiologic, pharmacokinetic, or biochemical data from Phase I and Phase II studies. Genetic studies, behavioral studies, and observational, natural history, and epidemiological studies may also contribute data.

It is essential that data be reviewed from prior studies on a diverse population, that is, in subjects of both genders and from different racial/ethnic groups. These data must be examined to determine if there are significant differences of clinical or public health importance observed between the subgroups.

While data from prior studies relating to possible differences among intervention effects in different subgroups must be reviewed, evidence of this nature is likely to be less convincing than that deriving from the subgroup analyses that can be performed in usual-sized Phase III trials. This is because the evidence from preliminary studies is likely to be of a more indirect nature (e.g., based on surrogate endpoints), deriving from uncontrolled studies (e.g., nonrandomized Phase II trials), and based on smaller numbers of subjects than in Phase III secondary analyses. For this reason, it is likely that data from preliminary studies will, in the majority of cases, neither clearly reveal significant differences of clinical or public health importance between subgroups of patients, nor strongly negate them.

In these cases, Phase III trials should still have appropriate gender and racial/ethnic representation, but they would not need to have the large sample sizes necessary to provide a high statistical power for detecting differences in intervention effects among subgroups. Nevertheless, analyses of subgroup effects must be conducted and comparisons between the subgroups must be made. Depending on the results of these analyses, the results of other relevant research, and the results of meta-analyses of clinical trials, one might initiate subsequent trials to examine more fully these subgroup differences.

C. Issues Concerning Appropriate Gender Representation

The "population at risk" may refer to only one gender where the disease, disorders, or conditions are gender specific. In all other cases, there should be approximately equal numbers of both sexes in studies of populations or subpopulations at risk, unless different proportions are appropriate because of the known prevalence, incidence, morbidity, mortality rates, or expected intervention effect.

D. Issues Concerning Appropriate Representation of Minority Groups and Subpopulations in All Research Involving Human Subjects Including Phase III Clinical Trials

While the inclusion of minority subpopulations in research is a complex and challenging issue, it nonetheless provides the opportunity for researchers to collect data on subpopulations where knowledge gaps exist. Researchers must consider the inclusion of subpopulations in all stages of research design. In meeting this objective, they should be aware of concurrent research that addresses specific subpopulations, and consider potential collaborations which may result in complementary subpopulation data.

At the present time, there are gaps in baseline and other types of data necessary for research involving certain minority groups and/or subpopulations of minority groups. In these areas, it would be appropriate for researchers to obtain such data, including baseline data, by studying a single minority group.

It would also be appropriate for researchers to test survey instruments, recruitment procedures, and other methodologies used in the majority or other population(s) with the objective of assessing their feasibility, applicability, and cultural competence/relevance to a particular minority group or subpopulation. This testing may provide data on the validity of the methodologies across groups. Likewise, if an intervention has been tried in the majority population and not in certain minority groups, it would be appropriate to assess the intervention effect on a single minority group and compare the effect to that obtained in the majority population. These types of studies will advance scientific research and assist in closing knowledge gaps.

A complex issue arises over how broad or narrow the division into different subgroups should be, given the purpose of the research. Division into many racial/ethnic subgroups is tempting in view of the cultural and biological differences that exist among these groups and the possibility that some of these differences may in fact impact in some way upon the scientific question. Alternatively, from a practical perspective, a limit has to be placed on the number of such subgroups that can realistically be studied in detail for each intervention that is researched. The investigator should clearly address the rationale for inclusion or exclusion of subgroups in terms of the purpose of the research. Emphasis should be placed upon inclusion of subpopulations in which the disease manifests itself or the intervention operates in an appreciable different way. Investigators should report the subpopulations included in the study.

An important issue is the appropriate representation of minority groups in research, especially in geographical locations which may have limited numbers of racial/ethnic population groups available for study. The investigator must address this issue in terms of the purpose of the research, and other factors, such as the size of the study, relevant characteristics of the disease, disorder or condition, and the feasibility of making a collaboration or consortium or other arrangements to include

minority groups. A justification is required if there is limited representation. Peer reviewers and NIH staff will consider the justification in
their evaluations of the project.

NIH interprets the statute in a manner that leads to feasible and real
improvements in the representativeness of different racial/ethnic groups
in research and places emphasis on research in those subpopulations that
are disproportionately affected by certain diseases or disorders.

Source: National Institutes of Health, "NIH Guidelines on the Inclusion of Women and Minorities as Subjects in Clinical Research," *Federal
Register* 59 (28 March 1994), 14508-13.

International Ethical Guidelines for Biomedical Research Involving Human Subjects

The Council for International Organizations
of Medical Sciences (CIOMS) in
Collaboration with the
World Health Organization (WHO)

Geneva
1993

PREAMBLE

The term "research" refers to a class of activities designed to develop or contribute to generalizable knowledge. Generalizable knowledge consists of theories, principles or relationships, or the accumulation of information on which they are based, that can be corroborated by accepted scientific methods of observation and inference. In the present context "research" includes both medical and behavioural studies pertaining to human health. Usually "research" is modified by the adjective "biomedical" to indicate that the reference is to health-related research.

Progress in medical care and disease prevention depends upon an understanding of physiological and pathological processes or epidemiological findings, and requires at some time research involving human subjects. The collection, analysis and interpretation of information obtained from research involving human beings contribute significantly to the improvement of human health.

Research involving human subjects includes that undertaken together with patient care (clinical research) and that undertaken on patients or other subjects, or with data pertaining to them, solely to contribute to generalizable knowledge (non-clinical biomedical research). Research is defined as "clinical" if one or more of its components is designed to be diagnostic, prophylactic or therapeutic for the individual subject of the research. Invariably, in clinical research, there are also components designed not to be diagnostic, prophylactic or therapeutic for the subject; examples include the administration of placebos and the performance of laboratory tests in addition to those required to serve the purposes of medical care. Hence the term "clinical research" is used here rather than "therapeutic research".

Research involving human subjects includes:

- studies of a physiological, biochemical or pathological process, or of the response to a specific intervention--whether physical, chemical or psychological--in healthy subjects or patients;
- controlled trials of diagnostic, preventive or therapeutic measures in larger groups of persons, designed to demonstrate a specific generalizable response to these measures against a background of individual biological variation;
- studies designed to determine the consequences for individuals and communities of specific preventive or therapeutic measures; and
- studies concerning human health-related behaviour in a variety of circumstances and environments.

Research involving human subjects may employ either observation or physical, chemical or psychological intervention; it may also either generate records or make use of existing records containing biomedical or other information about individuals who may or may not be identifiable from the records or information. The use of such records and the protection of the confidentiality of data obtained from those records are discussed in *International Guidelines for Ethical Review of Epidemiological Studies* (CIOMS, 1991).

Research involving human subjects includes also research in which environmental factors are manipulated in a way that could affect incidentally-exposed individuals. Research is defined in broad terms in order to embrace field studies of pathogenic organisms and toxic chemicals under investigation for health-related purposes.

Research involving human subjects is to be distinguished from the practice of medicine, public health and other forms of health care, which is designed to contribute directly to the health of individuals or communities. Prospective subjects may find it confusing when research and practice are to be conducted simultaneously, as when research is designed to obtain new information about the efficacy of a drug or other therapeutic, diagnostic or preventive modality.

Research involving human subjects should be carried out only by, or strictly supervised by, suitably qualified and experienced investigators and in accordance with a protocol that clearly states: the aim of the research; the reasons for proposing that it involve human subjects; the nature and degree of any known risks to the subjects; the sources from which it is proposed to recruit subjects; and the means proposed for ensuring that subjects' consent will be adequately informed and voluntary. The protocol should be scientifically and ethically appraised by one or more suitably constituted review bodies, independent of the investigators.

New vaccines and medicinal drugs, before being approved for general use, must be tested on human subjects in clinical trials; such trials, which constitute a substantial part of all research involving human subjects, are described in Annex 2.

THE GUIDELINES

Informed Consent of Subjects

Guideline 1: Individual informed consent

For all biomedical research involving human subjects, the investigator must obtain the informed consent of the prospective subject or, in the case of an individual who is not capable of giving informed consent, the proxy consent of a properly authorized representative.

Guideline 2: Essential information for prospective research subjects

Before requesting an individual's consent to participate in research, the investigator must provide the individual with the following information, in language that he or she is capable of understanding:

- that each individual is invited to participate as a subject in research, and the aims and methods of the research;
- the expected duration of the subject's participation;
- the benefits that might reasonably be expected to result to the subject or to others as an outcome of the research;
- any foreseeable risks or discomfort to the subject, associated with participation in the research;
- any alternative procedures or courses of treatment that might be as advantageous to the subject as the procedure or treatment being tested;
- the extent to which confidentiality of records in which the subject is identified will be maintained;
- the extent of the investigator's responsibility, if any, to provide medical services to the subject;

- that therapy will be provided free of charge for specified types of research-related injury;
- whether the subject or the subject's family or dependants will be compensated for disability or death resulting from such injury; and
- that the individual is free to refuse to participate and will be free to withdraw from the research at any time without penalty or loss of benefits to which he or she would otherwise be entitled.

Guideline 3: Obligations of investigators regarding informed consent

The investigator has a duty to:
- communicate to the prospective subject all the information necessary for adequately informed consent;
- give the prospective subject full opportunity and encouragement to ask questions;
- exclude the possibility of unjustified deception, undue influence and intimidation;
- seek consent only after the prospective subject has adequate knowledge of the relevant facts and the consequences of participation, and has had sufficient opportunity to consider whether to participate;
- as a general rule, obtain from each prospective subject a signed form as evidence of informed consent; and
- renew the informed consent of each subject if there are material changes in the conditions or procedures of the research.

Guideline 4: Inducement to participate

Subjects may be paid for inconvenience and time spent, and should be reimbursed for expenses incurred, in connection with their participation in research; they may also receive free medical services. However, the payments should not be so large or the medical services so extensive as to induce prospective subjects to consent to participate in the research against their better judgment ("undue inducement"). All payments, reimbursements and medical services to be provided to research subjects should be approved by an ethical review committee.

Guideline 5: Research involving children

Before undertaking research involving children, the investigator must ensure that:

- children will not be involved in research that might equally well be carried out with adults;
- the purpose of the research is to obtain knowledge relevant to the health needs of children;
- a parent or legal guardian of each child has given proxy consent;
- the consent of each child has been obtained to the extent of the child's capabilities;
- the child's refusal to participate in research must always be respected unless according to the research protocol the child would receive therapy for which there is no medically-acceptable alternative;
- the risk presented by interventions not intended to benefit the individual child-subject is low and commensurate with the importance of the knowledge to be gained; and
- interventions that are intended to provide therapeutic benefit are likely to be at least as advantageous to the individual child-subject as any available alternative.

Guideline 6: Research involving persons with mental or behavioural disorders

Before undertaking research involving individuals who by reason of mental or behavioural disorders are not capable of giving adequately informed consent, the investigator must ensure that:

- such persons will not be subjects of research that might equally well be carried out on persons in full possession of their mental faculties;
- the purpose of the research is to obtain knowledge relevant to the particular health needs of persons with mental or behavioural disorders;
- the consent of each subject has been obtained to the extent of that subject's capabilities, and a prospective subject's refusal to participate in non-clinical research is always respected;
- in the case of incompetent subjects, informed consent is obtained from the legal guardian or other duly authorized person;
- the degree of risk attached to interventions that are not intended to benefit the individual subject is low and commensurate with the importance of the knowledge to be gained; and
- interventions that are intended to provide therapeutic benefit are likely to be at least as advantageous to the individual subject as any alternative.

Guideline 7: Research involving prisoners

Prisoners with serious illness or at risk of serious illness should not arbitrarily be denied access to investigational drugs, vaccines or other agents that show promise of therapeutic or preventive benefit.

Guideline 8: Research involving subjects in underdeveloped communities

Before undertaking research involving subjects in underdeveloped communities, whether in developed or developing countries, the investigator must ensure that:

- persons in underdeveloped communities will not ordinarily be involved in research that could be carried out reasonably well in developed communities;
- the research is responsive to the health needs and the priorities of the community in which it is to be carried out;
- every effort will be made to secure the ethical imperative that the consent of individual subjects be informed; and
- the proposals for the research have been reviewed and approved by an ethical review committee that has among its members or consultants persons who are thoroughly familiar with the customs and traditions of the community.

Guideline 9: Informed consent in epidemiological studies

For several types of epidemiological research individual informed consent is either impracticable or inadvisable. In such cases the ethical review committee should determine whether it is ethically acceptable to proceed without individual informed consent and whether the investigator's plans to protect the safety and respect the privacy of research subjects and to maintain the confidentiality of the data are adequate.

Selection of Research Subjects

Guideline 10: Equitable distribution of burdens and benefits

Individuals or communities to be invited to be subjects of research should be selected in such a way that the burdens and benefits of the research will be equitably distributed. Special justification is required for inviting vulnerable individuals and, if they are selected, the means of protecting their rights and welfare must be particularly strictly applied.

Guideline 11: Selection of pregnant or nursing (breastfeeding) women as research subjects

Pregnant or nursing women should in no circumstances be the subjects of non-clinical research unless the research carries no more than minimal risk to the fetus or nursing infant and the object of the research is to obtain new knowledge about pregnancy or lactation. As a general rule, pregnant or nursing women should not be subjects of any clinical trails except such trials as are designed to protect or advance the health of pregnant or nursing women or fetuses or nursing infants, and for which women who are not pregnant or nursing would not be suitable subjects.

Confidentiality of Data

Guideline 12: Safeguarding confidentiality

The investigator must establish secure safeguards of the confidentiality of research data. Subjects should be told of the limits to the investigators' ability to safeguard confidentiality and of the anticipated consequences of breaches of confidentiality.

Compensation of Research Subjects for Accidental Injury

Guideline 13: Right of subjects to compensation

Research subjects who suffer physical injury as a result of their participation are entitled to such financial or other assistance as would compensate them equitably for any temporary or permanent impairment or disability. In the case of death, their dependants are entitled to material compensation. The right to compensation may not be waived.

Review Procedures

Guideline 14: Constitution and responsibilities of ethical review committees

All proposals to conduct research involving human subjects must be submitted for review and approval to one or more independent ethical and scientific review committees. The investigator must obtain such approval of the proposal to conduct research before the research is begun.

Externally Sponsored Research

Guideline 15: Obligations of sponsoring and host countries

Externally sponsored research entails two ethical obligations:
- An external sponsoring agency should submit the research protocol to ethical and scientific review according to the standards of the country of the sponsoring agency, and the ethical standards applied should be no less exacting than they would be in the case of research carried out in that country.
- After scientific and ethical approval in the country of the sponsoring agency, the appropriate authorities of the host country, including a national or local ethical review committee or its equivalent, should satisfy themselves that the proposed research meets their own ethical requirements.

ANNEX II

THE PHASES OF CLINICAL TRIALS OF VACCINES AND DRUGS

Vaccine development

Phase I refers to the first introduction of a candidate vaccine into a human population for initial determination of its safety and biological effects, including immunogenicity. This phase may include studies of dose and route of administration, and usually involves fewer than 100 volunteers.

Phase II refers to the initial trials examining effectiveness in a limited number of volunteers (usually between 200 and 500); the focus of this phase is immunogenicity.

Phase III trials are intended for a more complete assessment of safety and effectiveness in the prevention of disease, involving a larger number of volunteers in a multicentre adequately controlled study.

Drug development

Phase I refers to the first introduction of a drug into humans. Normal volunteer subjects are usually studied to determine levels of drugs at which toxicity is observed. Such studies are followed by dose-ranging studies in patients for safety and, in some cases, early evidence of effectiveness.

Phase II investigation consists of controlled clinical trials designed to demonstrate effectiveness and relative safety. Normally, these are performed on a limited number of closely monitored patients.

Phase III trials are performed after a reasonable probability of effectiveness of a drug has been established and are intended to gather additional evidence of effectiveness for specific indications and more precise definition of drug-related adverse effects. This phase includes both controlled and uncontrolled studies.

Phase IV trials are conducted after the national drug registration authority has approved a drug for distribution or marketing. These trials may include research designed to explore a specific pharmacological effect, to establish the incidence of adverse reactions, or to determine the effects of long-term administration of a drug. Phase IV trials may also be designed to evaluate a drug in a population not studied adequately in the premarketing phases (such as children or the elderly) or to establish a new clinical indication for a drug. Such research is to be distinguished from marketing research, sales promotion studies, and routine post-marketing surveillance for adverse drug reactions in that these categories ordinarily need not be reviewed by ethical review committees (see Guideline 14).

   In general, Phase I drug trials and Phase I and Phase II vaccine trials should be conducted according to the articles of the Declaration of Helsinki that refer to non-clinical research. However, some exceptions can be justified. For example, it is customary and ethically justifiable to conduct Phase I studies of highly toxic chemotherapies of cancer in patients with cancer, rather than in normal volunteers as prescribed in the Declarations of Helsinki, Article III.2. Similarly, it may be ethically justifiable to involve HIV-seropositive individuals as subjects in Phase II trials of candidate vaccines.

   Phase II and Phase III drug trials should be conducted according to the articles of the Declaration of Helsinki that refer to "medical research combined with professional care (clinical research)". However, the Declaration does not provide for controlled clinical trials. Rather, it assures the freedom of the physician "to use a new diagnostic and therapeutic measure, if in his or her judgment it offers hope of saving life, reestablishing health or alleviating suffering" (Article II.1). Also in regard to Phase II and Phase III drug trials there are customary and ethically justified exceptions to the requirements of the Declaration of Helsinki. A placebo given to a control group, for example, cannot be justified by its "potential diagnostic or therapeutic value for the patient", as Article II.6 prescribes. Many other interventions and procedures characteristic of late-phase drug development have no possible diagnostic or therapeutic value for the patients and thus must be justified on other grounds; usually such justification consists of a reasonable expectation that they carry little or no risk and that they will contribute materially to the achievement of the goals of the research.

Phase III trials of vaccines do not use "a new diagnostic and therapeutic measure" that offers "hope of saving life, reestablishing health or alleviating suffering" (clinical research). Yet administration of the vaccine is intended to be a benefit to the subject rather than "the purely scientific application of medical research carried out on a human being" (non-clinical biomedical research). Thus, Phase III vaccine-trials do not conform to either of the categories defined in the Declaration of Helsinki.

Source: The Council for International Organizations of Medical Sciences (Geneva: CIOMS, 1993).

INDEX

Abortion
embryo research, 168, 309-10
fetal research
fetal tissue, 165, 309, 374, 382-85.
See also Fetal tissue/tissue
transplants
fetuses, 372, 390. *See also* Fetus
and national/public policies regarding research, 158, 162-66, 169,
371-74. *See also* Politics, influ-
ence of
Abortifacients, research on, 138, 164,
166
Abuses of research subjects, 4-10, 159-
60. *See also* Harm(s), of research;
Wrongs
Academic freedom. *See* Freedom, aca-
demic
Ackerman, Terrence F., 51, 54, 360
Adolescent(s), research, 49
AIDS, research. *See* HIV/AIDS
Alexander, Leo, 20n. 22, 240
Alliance for Genetic Support Groups,
420-21
Alzheimer's disease, 182n. 55, 192, 384
American College of Obstetricians and
Gynecologists, 375
American Fertility Society, 375
American Medical Association, 111,
149, 207, 211
Animal rights advocates, 130-31
Animals, research on, 130-31
Anthropology. *See* Cross-cultural re-
search, ethics of
Aquinas, Thomas, 72-73
Aristotle, 72-73, 81
Assent to involvement in research. *See*
Children, research; Mentally in-
firm, assent
Assurance of compliance agreements/

contracts, 10, 130, 456-59
Autonomy. *See also* Ethics, rights;
Freedom; Informed consent, ethical and legal bases; Respect for
persons, and autonomy; Selec-
tion/recruitment of subjects
as basis of rights of researchers, 56-
57
as basis of rights of subjects, 56
and beneficence/social benefit, 47-
51, 54
of children, 359-61
complexity of in genetics research,
404-11, 421
cultural/historical roots, 67-68, 70,
239-42, 245, 248-51, 255, 264.
See also Values/goods, types of,
cultural
and deontology, 51-57
ethical priority of, defenses and
debates, 35-36, 46-57, 79, 101
ethical weight of, 66
free power/voluntarism, 56, 431,
440, 444
and informed/voluntary consent,
46, 282
of non-Western subjects. *See*
Cross -cultural research, ethics
overriding of, 51-55

"*Baby Doe* Rules," 164
Balancing ethical principles. *See* Eth-
ics, judgments concerning
Balancing risks and probable benefits.
See Risk(s), and benefits
Battery, legal views of, and informed
consent, 42n. 12
Beauchamp, Tom L., 43n. 15, 61-62
Beecher, Henry K., 8-9, 12-13, 210,

243, 340

Behavioral research. *See* Research, behavioral

Bellah, Robert, 67

Belmont Report, The [Reprinted as Appendix C], 33-36, 52-53, 64, 84-85, 106-7, 305-7, 310, 323-25
historical background, 324-25
limitations/flaws of, 36, 106-7, 136-39, 161, 179n. 23, 125-26, 307, 421

Beneficence. *See also* Research, justifications; Selection/recruitment of subjects
duty to conduct research, 93-99
duty to maximize probable benefits and minimize possible harms, 440-41, 445-47, 462. *See also* Risk(s), and benefits
duty to participate in research, 43n. 16, 96-98, 101, 343
duty to protect from harm. *See* "Do no harm"/nonmaleficence
duty to rescue/help resolve serious health problems, 96-98, 346-47
ethical principle of, 34, 440-41
ethical priority in research, 84
justifying compromises to subjects' interests, 91, 96-99
justifying research risks. *See* Risk(s), justification
as overruling autonomy, 228
protection from harm, 83-89, 283, 325, 442-43. *See also* "Do no harm"/nonmaleficence

Benefits (probable or anticipated)
of biomedical research on prevention and control of disease, 7-11, 86, 91. *See also* Research, justifications for; Values/goods, types of, of technological/scientific
direct benefits as justifications of research, 436
ethics, relation to, 34. *See* Beneficence
inequitable distribution of. *See* Jus-

tice
participation in clinical trials perceived as, 10-11, 91-96, 110-17, 123, 199
and risks, balance of. *See* Risk(s), and benefits

Bernard, Claude, 45

Bias(es)
institutional review boards, 50
physicians, 94
researchers, 50-55. *See also* Researchers
social. *See* Stigmatization, social

Bioethics, modern. *See also* Ethics and ethical theory
as distinct from non-Western medical ethics, 268-69
national agenda for, 166-68, 172-73
national policy making, need of. *See* Public bioethics
nature and values of, 61-62, 70, 172-73, 269-71

Biomedical Ethics Advisory Committee (BEAC), 163, 373

Bone marrow research, 379

Brock, Dan W., 351

Canada, research and regulations. *See* Regulations, research

Canadian Medical Association, 216

Cancer
breast, 321, 333-34
history, 306
patients' access to new therapies, 56-57, 323. *See also* Multicenter clinical trials; Parallel track research; Randomized clinical trials; Terminal illness research
comprehensive ethical analysis of, 328-36. *See also* Research, design of
as forerunner of changes in clinical trials, 320-23
as medical treatment/"best therapy," 199, 320-21
and multicenter trials, 322

National Surgical Adjuvant Breast and Bowel Cancer Project (NSABP), 321, 333-34
Phase I trials, 306-7, 326-30
phases of, 321. *See also* Phases of clinical trials; Research, design
routinization of research, 199
and serious risks, 321
Case studies in the ethics of research. *See* Ethics, case studies/examples
Children
best interest of, 339-45, 353-59
with HIV/AIDS, 116-17
privacy of, 346
regulations of research involving. *See also* Regulations
U.S. federal regulations, 345-49, 478-82
criticisms/limitations, 345-47
research. *See also* Institutional review boards, children
assent of subjects, 53, 308, 345, 347, 356-66, 435, 479, 481-82. *See also* Informed consent, as a process of communication; Nonconsenting/assenting subjects; Parental permission
assent forms, 360-61
elements of, 360-61
child's right to refuse, 347, 358-59
coercion, 352-53, 358-60
consent, presumptive, 342
debates over ethics and regulations, 64-66, 339-66
genetics research, 410-11
growth hormone trials, questions about, 361-65
justifications of, 63-66, 76, 308, 340-66
international guidelines, 513
minimal risk to, 65, 74, 308
minimal risk, debates over definitions, 64-66, 342-43, 348-56. *See also under* Minimal risk
nonassenting/consenting, 339
nontherapeutic, 341-46. *See also*

Nontherapeutic research, with children
more than minimal risk, 346, 348, 362, 441, 479-80
"no discernible risk," 341-43
for serious health problems, 79-80, 346, 441, 480-81
permission to be subject. *See* Parental permission/consent
respect for childrens'
choice/moral agency, 358-59
experiences/perspectives, 308, 353-56, 359
moral development, 344, 353, 358-59
therapeutic, 342-46, 359
minimal risk, 65, 74, 308, 342-43
more than minimal risk, 65-66, 346, 410, 479-80
potential overall benefit, 342, 363
underrepresented in, 117
venipunctures, 355-56, 483
Childress, James F., 43n. 15, 61-62, 382
Choice. *See* Autonomy; Informed consent
Christakis, Nicholas A., 291
CIOMS. *See* Codes/codifications of research ethics, Council for International Organizations of Medical Sciences
Clinical trials. *See* Phases of clinical trials; Randomized clinical trials; Research
Clinton, William F., 165, 374
Cloning. *See under* Embryo
Codes/codifications of research ethics
Council for International Organizations of Medical Sciences (CIOMS) and World Health Organization (WHO) *International Ethical Guidelines for Biomedical Research Involving Human Subjects* [Reprinted as Appendix F], 16, 225-26, 235-39, 243-49, 253-55, 291-93
limitations/flaws, 227, 245-55,

262-63, 291-93
Federal (U.S.) regulations. *See* Regulations, *Code of U.S. Federal Regulations*
in Germany (1931), 6, 22n. 34, 177n. 10
Helsinki Declaration, [Reprinted as Appendix B], 16, 63, 85-86, 89, 224, 235-46, 252-54
  influence of, 242-43
  limitations/flaws, 227, 236, 242-44, 252-54, 262-63
Nuremberg Code, [Reprinted as Appendix A], 7-8, 16, 45-46, 63, 85-86, 89, 177n. 10, 237-42, 250-53. *See also* Subject(s), coercion
  influence, 241-42
  limitations/flaws, 227, 235-36, 240-43, 250-52, 262-63, 365
Coercion. *See* Subject(s), coercion
Committee, research review. *See* Institutional review boards
Common Federal Rule, 132-34. *See* Regulations, *Code of U.S. Federal Regulations*
Commissions, bioethics. *See* Public bioethics
Community
  based research, 114-16
  involvement in research design and conducting, 114-16
  representation on review committees, 459-60
Compensation for injuries caused by research, 140-41
  disclosure of availability of compensation, 465
  effects on federal policy, 141
  required in international guidelines, 507
Competence. *See also* Incompetence
  of children. *See* Children, research involving, respect for childrens'
  and comprehension, 286-87, 446-47
  of investigators. *See* Researchers, competency
  of non-Western subjects, 286-88

Comprehension. *See* Competence
Confidentiality, 435, 462, 507
  breaches of in fetal tissue research, 383
  for child subjects, 346
  ethical/moral grounding. *See* Respect for persons
  of families in genetics research, 404-6
  of individuals in genetics research, 406-9
Conflict of interest, possible. *See also* Financial issues; Industrial/manufacturers' sponsorship; Institutional review boards; Post-marketing research
  in comparison to other interests, 198
  defined, 147-49
  financial. *See* Financial issues
  governmental, 13
  guidelines concerning, 149, 207
  institutional, 13, 197-98
  institutional review boards, 148
  personal, 13
  physicians', 186, 207-8
  researchers', 148-49, 193, 198
Conscription of persons into research, 54. *See also* Selection/recruitment of subjects
Consent forms, 466-67. *See also* Informed consent, information needed; Informed consent, lay language
  institutional review boards' focus on, 319
  for Phase I cancer protocols, 327
  signing/not signing, 291, 466-67, 504
Consent, informed. *See* Informed Consent
Consequentialism, ethical. *See* Ethics, consequentialism
Contracts of assurance of compliance. *See* Assurance of compliance
Council for International Organizations of Medical Sciences (CIOMS). *See under* Codes/codifications

Costs of research. *See* Research, costs
Covenants, moral, 339-45
Cross-cultural research. *See also under*
    Institutional review boards; Ge-
    netics research
abuses, 274-76
and AIDS vaccine research, 140, 261,
    275, 286
and anthropology/ethnology, 246-
    47, 255, 268-71, 276, 288-94
described, 261-62
and epidemiology. *See* Epidemiol-
    ogical research
ethics. *See* Ethics, pluralism; Ethics,
    principles; Ethics, universal-
    ism/absolutism; Values/goods,
    types of, cultural
autonomy and informed consent,
    controversies, 137, 225-28,
    243-49, 254-55, 263-66, 281-
    95
beneficence, 289
self-esteem/worth, 292
exploitation/injustice, 244-46, 291
goals/ultimate goals of, 247-49,
    281, 284-86, 292-95
harms/risks, 266
protection from, 288
imperialism of Western ethics,
    223, 237, 284, 290, 294-95
international guidelines for under-
    developed communities, 507
proxy consent, 285, 288-89
respect for persons, 248, 255, 281-
    84, 291-95
sexist bias, 289
genetics. *See* Genetics, research
guidelines. *See* Codes/codifications,
    CIOMS
industry/drug manufacturers' spon-
    sorship, 245-46
negotiations over approval, 227, 249-
    50, 272-74, 508

Data and Safety Monitoring Com-
    mittees. *See under* National
Data-faking. *See* Researchers, scientific
    integrity

Deception. *See* Wrongs, of deception
Decision making
ethical. *See* Ethics, as discerning/
    reasoned judgments; Ethics, judg-
    ments concerning within institu-
    tional review boards. *See* Institu-
    tional review boards
Deontology. *See* Ethics, deontology
Department of Health and Human
    Services (DHHS). *See under*
    U.S.A.
Design of research. *See* Randomized
    clinical trials; Research, design
Diabetes, 378-79, 384-86
Diagnosis/diagnostic testing. *See un-*
    der Embryo; Fetus; Genetics
Dingell, John, 131-32
Disadvantaged persons. *See* Vulner-
    able persons
Disclosure of
availability of compensation for in-
    juries. *See* Compensation
information to subjects. *See* In-
    formed Consent, information
research findings. *See under* Genet-
    ics research, ethics of
research funding. *See* Financial is-
    sues
risks and benefits. *See* Informed con-
    sent, information needed;
    Risk(s)
sponsorship of research. *See also*
    Sponsorship of research
to colleagues, 206-7
to subjects, 194-95, 328
Discrimination, cultural, racial, reli-
    gious, social, 6-10, 37-38, 120-21,
    244-46, 291
Distribution of harms and benefits.
    See Justice
Distrust. *See also* Trust
of physicians, 209-10
of researchers and institutional re-
    view boards, 12, 130-32
DNA research, recombinant. *See* Hu-
    man Genome Project
"Do no harm"/nonmaleficence, 77-
    78, 330, 343-44, 440. *See also* Be-

neficence, protection from harm; Risk(s); Subject(s), protection
duty to minimize risks. *See* Minimal risk; Risk(s)
duty to overcome/prevent social harms, 94-96, 120, 440-41. *See also* Harm(s)
duty to protect subjects from harms, 83-89, 283, 325, 440-41
as overruling autonomy, 228
as overruling beneficence, 344
Doctor-patient relationships. *See* Physician-patient
Documentation. *See* Consent forms
Double-blind studies. *See* Randomized clinical trials
Drug research. *See* Phases of clinical trials
Duty
to conduct research. *See* Beneficence and deontology. *See* Ethics, deontology/deontological
ethical. *See* Ethics, duties/obligations; principles of
to participate in human research, 35-36, 91, 96-99
prima facie moral duties. *See* Ethics, *prima facie*
Dying persons/patients. *See* Terminal illness

Embryo
cloning of, 374, 376, 393-94
embryoscopy, 390
moral status, 309
nongovernmental guidelines, 375, 393-94
regulations, governmental, 392-93. *See also* Regulations
research
and abortion controversy, 168, 309
described, 390-92
diagnosis/testing, 392
limitations, 309-10
payments to donors prohibited, 394
permitted/prohibited research, 393-94
relation to gamete research, 390-92. *See also under* Gametes, research; Genetics, research
Employment, risk of losing in genetics research, 408-9
Epidemiological research
ethics and regulations, 93, 251-52, 502, 506
genetics, 403-4
in non-Western settings, 289
Equipoise. *See* Randomized clinical trials
Equity. *See* Justice
Ethics. *See also* Bioethics, modern; Moral/morality; Values/goods, types of
and anthropology/ethnology. *See* Cross-cultural research, ethics
authoritative tradition(s), relation to, 18n. 5
and autonomy. *See* Autonomy
case studies/examples of ethics of research, 5-11, 47-48, 79-80, 118-20, 361-65, 416-17. *See also* Institutional review boards, examples of ethical problems
casuistry, 4, 35, 59-81, 226, 290-91. *See also under* Ethics, judgments concerning
consequentialism, 4
and culture. *See* Ethics, pluralism; Ethics, universalism/absolutism; Values/goods, types of
deontology/deontological duties, 4, 35, 51, 61-62. *See also* Ethics, duties/obligations
definitions of. *See* Ethics, nature and areas of
as delimiting research, 45-57; 83-84, 347, 358-59
descriptive versus normative, 5-6
as discerning/reasoned judgments, 2-3, 80-81
and practical reasoning, 81
by virtuous and prudent persons, 80-81
duties/obligations, 3-4, 51-57, 83-

87, 93-99, 123-25, 339-45. *See also* Ethics, deontology/deontological duties; Ethics, principles of; Ethics, *prima facie* ethics

as limiting/constraining research, 83-84, 347, 358-59

and facts/accurate information, 2, 306

harms to persons, 35

in contrast to wrongs, 35

ideal observer theory, 76

judgments concerning. *See also* Ethics, rationality

balancing values and moral principles, 50, 68-72. *See also* Ethics, casuistry; Values/goods, types of

the relations and/or fit between moral principles, cultural values, specific situations, 59-60, 68-76

the weighing/prioritizing of moral principles, 34-36, 45-57, 67-71, 83-99, 323-25, 339-45

and law, 42n. 12, 74

metaphorical nature of, 59, 60, 67-70, 75-76, 95

and moral character. *See* Ethics, virtue ethics

nature and areas of, 1-4, 61-66, 83-87, 98-99, 323-25, 339-45

nonconsequentialism. *See* Ethics, deontology/deontological

paternalism, 228, 426

pluralism, 227-29, 237-39, 245, 248-50, 262, 268-76, 283. *See also* Cross-cultural research, ethics; Ethics, relativism; Ethics, universalism/absolutism

criticisms of, 228, 288-91

prima facie ethics/duties, 19n. 15, 56-57, 62, 64-65. *See also* Ethics, duties/obligations

principles, 4, 51, 61-62, 64-79, 247-50, 255, 281-82, 287-89, 323-25, 339-45. *See also* Ethics, duties/

obligations; Ethics, universalism/absolutism

autonomy. *See* Autonomy; Respect for persons

beneficence. *See* Beneficence

"do no harm"/nonmaleficence. *See* "Do no harm"/nonmaleficence

gratitude, 88, 91-92

fidelity, 339-45

humanness and humanity, 247-48

justice. *See* Justice

respect for persons. *See* Respect for persons

truth-telling/veracity. *See* Disclosure of; Wrongs, of deception

professional and codified. *See* Codes/codifications

rationality, 2-4, 69-71. *See also* Ethics, judgments concerning

and regulation(s), relation between, 3, 38-39, 442-48

relativism, 228-29, 266-67, 283. *See also* Ethics, pluralism

criticisms of, 227, 267-68, 276

ethical versus contextual, 228

rights, human, 56-57. *See also* Autonomy; Freedom; Respect for persons

as subjective or not, 78

and trust. *See* Distrust; Trust

and ultimate goals/goods, 3, 20n. 22, 148

and ultimate/transcending moral principles, 248-49, 255

universalism/absolutism of principles, 36, 64-66, 79-80, 227-29, 235-38, 244-49, 283-84, 292-95. *See also* Cross-cultural research, ethics; Ethics, pluralism; Ethics, principles

criticisms of, 227, 245-49, 254-55, 262-66, 270-71, 276

utilitarianism, 4, 20n. 22, 46-48, 74-75, 98

and value(s), types of, 3, 5-10. *See*

also Values/goods, types of
virtue ethics/human virtues, 3, 68,
    80-81
wrongs versus harms, 35
Ethics advisory boards/committees/
    panels, 163, 168-70, 374, 377, 389
    See also National, Ethics Advi-
    sory Board; Public bioethics
Expedited review, 20n. 57, 461
    activities subject to, 482-83
Experimentation. *See* History of ex-
    perimentation; Research, defini-
    tions and terminology
Exploitation, 4-10, 244-46, 291

Faden, Ruth, 50-51, 246-47
Fairness, justice as. *See* Justice
Family/families
    parental permission. *See* Parental
        permission
    as unit of consideration in genetics
        research, 137, 311, 403, 407-8,
        421
Fertilization, *in vitro*. *See In vitro* fer-
    tilization
Fetal tissue/tissue transplant research.
    See also Abortion; Institutional
    review boards, fetal tissue; Tis-
    sue, human; Transplantation
    brain cell, 373, 377-80, 384
    described, 377-78
    ethics of
        and abortion, 163-65, 309, 381-
            84, 472
        confidentiality, 383
        informed consent, 381
        patents, 385-86
        right of woman to designate re-
            cipient of donation, 382-84
        risks, 473
        sale of prohibited, 374, 381
    federal tissue banks, 384-85
    gonadal, 386-87
    moratorium on, 163-65, 373-74
    pancreas, thymus, liver, 378-79
    and political turmoil. *See* Politics,
        influence
    regulations, federal and state, 380-

81, 469-74. *See also* Regulations
Fetoscopy. *See* Fetus, research
Fetus. *See also* Abortion; Politics, in-
    fluence of on research; Vulner-
    able persons/subjects
    moral status, 138, 309
        in comparison to women's au-
            tonomy, 123
    protection of, 113, 122
    research
        and abortion controversy, 163,
            309
        about-to-be-aborted, 77-78, 373-
            74, 389
        described, 387-90
        diagnosis/fetal diagnosis, 162, 164,
            387-90
        drug studies, 387
        ethics of
            benefits, 388
            informed permission/consent,
                388, 474
            respect for, 122-23
            risks, nature of, 77-78, 122, 164,
                388, 473
                more than minimal, 122-23,
                    388-89, 474
        ex utero, 388, 473-74
        fetoscopy, 162, 373, 387
        following abortion. *See* Fetal tis-
            sue/tissue transplant
        in utero, 388-89, 473
        moratorium on non-minimal risk
            research, 373
        nongovernmental guidelines, 374-
            76
        regulations, national, 372-74. *See
            also* Regulations
        surgery, 387-88, 390
        therapy, 164, 388, 390
        umbilical cord sampling/transfus-
            ing, 387-90
Financial issues, 142, 148, 185-200. *See
    also* Conflicts of interest, possible;
    Institutional review boards, finan-
    cial issues; Post-marketing re-
    search; Research, costs; Selection/
    recruitment of subjects

between investigators and physician
recruiters
"finders" fees for recruiting, 142,
196-97
between researchers and subjects
inducements/payments for subjects' involvement, 187-89,
504
disclosures of sponsors, 194-95, 210-
11
as incentive for medical institutions'
research, 13, 197-98
increasing significance, 150, 198-99.
See also Values/goods, financial
patient-funded/paid research, 191-
93
reimbursements by insurance and
managed care, 189-90, 196
Fletcher, John C., 310
Food and Drug Administration (FDA),
U.S.A. See under U.S.A.
Forms, assent and consent. See Children, research; Consent forms
Freedman, Benjamin, 353
Fraud. See Researchers', scientific integrity
Freedom. See also Autonomy; Ethics,
rights, human; Respect for persons
academic freedom of researchers,
149, 166, 169, 179n. 23
procreative, 383-84
to refuse to participate in research,
347, 358-59
to withdraw from research, 432, 465,
504
Funding of research. See Conflicts of
interest; Financial issues; Research, costs, extent of

Gametes, research on, 168, 390-92. See
also under Embryo; In vitro fertilization; Ova and oocyte research; Sperm research
sex selection/control of gender, 392
Geertz, Clifford, 264-65, 269
Gender bias. See Women

Gene therapy, 162, 311
Genetic testing, 311, 414, 422
Genetics research. See also Human Genome Project; Institutional review boards, genetics
research
counseling during, 414-15
cross-cultural, 403-4. See also Cross-
cultural research
described, 310-11, 404, 412
diagnosis/testing, 311, 399, 402
disease etiology, 402
embryological/gamete research,
392-94. See also under Embryo
ethics of
children, involvement of, 410-11
coercion/undue pressure, 406-8
confidentiality/privacy
of families, 404-8, 415-20
of individuals, 404-9, 417, 420
disclosure of results to subjects,
412-15
ethical guidelines, diversity of, 403
family-centered, import of. See
Family/families, as unit
history of, 162, 164
incompetent subjects, 411
informed consent, 317n. 35, 408-
9, 413-20
to publish results, 417
publishing findings, 416-18
recruitment strategies, 404-9
undue pressure/coercion, 406-
7
risks
for children, 410-11
discrimination, 409
economic: lost employment
and insurability, 408-09
psychological and social, 311,
406, 408, 413-15. See also
Stigmatization, social
public perceptions, 414
subjects' "ownership"/control
over subsequent research,
417-20
support groups' involvement,
407, 420-21

Genome. *See* Human Genome Project/research
Germ line cells. *See* Gametes, research
Germany. *See* Codes/codifications, in Germany
Governmental regulations of research. *See* Regulations
Guardian. *See* Proxy consent

Harm(s). *See also* "Do no harm"/non-maleficence; Risk(s)
in cancer research, risks of. *See under* Cancer
of deception. *See under* Wrongs
ethical, 35. *See also* Harm(s), of research; Wrongs, ethical
of lost trust in physicians, 209-10
minimization. *See under* "Do no harm"/nonmaleficence
of research. *See also* Abuses; Wrongs
in non-Western cultures. *See* Cross-cultural research, abuses
in past/in history, 5-10, 118-21, 159-60
recent/present-day research, 11, 26 nn. 52 and 54, 110, 128
timely detection of, 136
Hastings Center, The, and *Hastings Center Report*, 173, 343, 353
Heart transplants, 175n. 2
Helsinki, Declaration of. See Codes/codifications
Hepatitis, infectious, study of at Willowbrook, 9
Hippocratic Oath/ethics, 45, 151n. 9, 240, 270, 440
History of. *See also* Public bioethics
ethical violations, 6-10, 118-20, 159-60, 324-25
experimentation/medical research, 4-5, 151n. 3, 306
value conflicts in, 3
federal regulations in U.S., 10-11, 159
research ethics involving children, 339-49
HIV/AIDS. *See also* Justice

patients/subjects
access to clinical trials, 108-16
access to experimental therapies, 56-57, 323. *See also* Parallel-track drugs
as catalysts for reframing research ethics, 107-9, 137-38, 325, 330
influence on design of research, 109, 330-31
research
AIDS vaccine, 140, 168, 286, 288
as changing clinical trials, 108-10, 116-17
combined with treatment/therapy, 55, 109
delay due to bias and politics, 164-65
and new awareness of disease threats, 108
Human Genome Project/research, 162, 164, 199, 311, 401-2, 414, 422-23. *See also* Genetics research
Ethical, Legal and Social Implications (ELSI) division, 168, 311
Human Investigation Committees. *See* Institutional review boards
Huntington's disease, 413, 428n. 63

IJsselmuiden, Carel B., 246-47
Immunodeficiencies, 379
Incapacitated persons. *See* Mentally infirm
Incompetence. *See also* Competence
assent for mentally incompetent, 167, 287
protection of subjects, 324-25
proxy permission in genetics research, 411
Individualism, Western. *See under* Values/goods, types of
Inducements for physicians to recruit. *See* Financial issues
Inducements to subjects. *See* Financial issues; Subject(s)
Industrial/manufacturers' sponsorship of research, 13, 148, 194. *See also* Conflicts of interest, possible
Informed consent, 7

adolescents, 49
and autonomy. *See* Autonomy
battery, legal, relationship to, 42n. 12
"blank check" or "blanket" consent,
    48-49, 418-19
and misinformation, 48-49
communication/explanations to
    subjects, 287-88
    and comprehension. *See* Compe-
        tence
    cultural roots to. *See* Values, cul-
        tural/social, Western
    delegation of authority for. *See*
        Proxy
    differing assessments of by pro-
        fessionals and lay persons, 50-51
documentation of, 466-67
elements of, 464-65
ethical and legal bases, 34, 37, 46, 324,
    442. *See also* Autonomy; Respect
    for persons
exceptions to. *See* Informed consent,
    waivers; Research, nonconsenting
forms. *See* consent forms
in genetics research. *See* Genetics re-
    search, informed consent
information needed for, 47-51, 287,
    325-28, 435, 442-43, 464-66, 503-
    4. *See also* consent forms
lack of. *See* Post-marketing research/
    clinical trials; Subject(s), aware-
    ness
lay language, 464. *See also* consent
    forms
and maximum tolerated dose (MTD)
    agents, 329-30
and minority groups, 287
in non-Western cultures. *See* Cross-
    cultural
and placebo-controlled trials. *See*
    Placebos
in post-marketing research, lack of,
    150
as a process of communication and
    negotiation, 308, 443-44, 471-
    72, 504. *See also* Children, re-
    search
proxy or surrogate. *See* Proxy con-

sent
and "reasonable person" standard,
    48-49
"reasonable volunteer" standard,
    442-43
requirements of, 86
scepticism over, 210-11
timing of, 443-44
validity/determinations of, 50
voluntary nature of, 431, 440, 444-
    45
waivers or alterations of, 43n. 14,
    89-90, 292, 443, 464-65. *See also*
    Nonconsenting/assenting sub-
    jects
Injury. *See* Harm(s); Compensation for
    research-caused injuries
Institute of Medicine (IOM). *See under*
    National, Academy of Sciences
Institutional review boards (IRBs), 10.
    See also Regulations
authority of, 306, 460, 463
biases of, 50
cancer research protocols. *See under*
    Cancer
children, protocols concerning, 345-
    47, 349, 353-56, 359-60. *See also*
    Children, research
composition/membership, 37, 459-
    60
    ethical basis for, 37
and conflict of interest, possible. *See*
    also Conflict of interest
    IRB roles, 148
    payments to subjects, 187-88
    researchers' interests. *See* Conflict
        of interest, researchers'
and cross-cultural/ multi-national
    research, 139-40, 272-75, 292.
    See also Cross-cultural research
disclosure of sponsor(s) of research.
    See under Disclosure of
embryo research. *See* Embryo, re-
    search
ethical responsibilities of, 33-38, 64,
    88-89, 119-20, 323-36
    design of clinical trials. *See* Re-
        search, design of

search, design of
expanded responsibilities, present need of, 328-35
examples of ethical problems encountered by, 47-48, 326-27, 329-30, 354-56, 361-65. *See also* Ethics, case studies
fetal tissue, 310. *See also* Fetal tissue/tissue transplant research
fetus. *See* Fetus, research
financial issues over payments/sponsorship, 193, 211. *See also* Financial issues
focus on consent forms, 325-28
for-profit, 13
genetics research, 403, 405, 407, 420-21. *See also* Genetics, research
history of, 10, 127, 159-61
in vitro fertilization. *See In vitro* fertilization
litigation against, 335
maximum tolerated dose (MTD) drug decisions. *See under* Informed consent
multicenter trials, 134-36
names for, 24n. 47, 319
normal analysis/roles, 36, 134, 323-28
responsibilities and functions, 10, 43n. 23, 131-35, 306
self-regulation, 132-33
surveillance of. *See* Surveillance of institutional review boards
Institutionalized subjects. *See* Mentally infirm and/or institutionalized
Insurance companies' payments for research, 189-90
International research. *See* Cross-cultural research
Investigator(s). *See* Researchers
In vitro fertilization, 161, 164, 310, 373, 375, 391-92, 469-71. *See also* Gametes, research
IRB: A Review of Human Subjects Research, 324
Ivy, Andrew, 240-41

Japan, research by during World War

II, 21n. 25
Jewish Chronic Disease Hospital Study, 9, 159
John Moore v. Regents of the University of California, 418
Jonas, Hans, 87
Jonsen, Albert R., 34, 51, 54, 99
Judgments, ethical. *See* Ethics, judgments concerning; Ethics, nature and areas of; Ethics, principles of; Ethics, rationality of
Justice. *See also* HIV/AIDS; Minority groups; Selection/recruitment of subjects; Vulnerable persons/subjects; Women
changing views of burdens and benefits of research, 37-38, 107-24. *See also* Research, benefits and burdens
equal access to benefits, 109-17, 123, 486
ethical principle of, 34, 53-55, 106-23
and federal (U.S.) regulations, 35
and selection/access of subjects, 38-39, 123
racial minorities. *See* Minority groups
women. *See* Women
sharing of burdens and benefits, 440-41, 462, 506
theories of, 52, 441-42

Kant, Immanuel, 4, 48, 248
Katz, Jay, 9, 59-60, 66, 79, 314n. 18, 337n. 6, 363
Kelsey, Frances, 119
Kleinman, Arthur, 261-62
Kopelman, Loretta M., 349-50

Labelling/stigmatizing of persons. *See* Stigmatization
Law(s). *See* Ethics, and law; Negligence; Regulations
Leiken, Sanford L., 357
Levine, Carol, 100
Levine, Robert J., 226-27, 310, 389
Liberty. *See* Freedom

Loyalty. *See* Conflict of interest, researchers'; Researchers, scientific integrity
Lying. *See* Wrongs, of deception

Macklin, Ruth, 247-48
Maximum tolerated dose (MTD) drugs. *See under* Informed consent
May, William, 342
McCormick, Richard A., 339-45
Media hype, 314n. 20
Medical
  care
    as basic social good, 95-97
    of persons with terminal illness, 162, 168
  ethics. *See* Bioethics
  injuries/injurious nature of, 93-94
    correction of as justification for research, 93-94
  practice
    for the benefit of the sick, 45-46, 208
    conflicts of interests in, 207-8
    post-marketing (Phase IV) research. *See* Post-marketing research/clinical trials
    relation to research. *See* Research, definitions
  professional ethics, 210, 238, 243, 330, 344, 433, 436
  specializations. *See under* names of specialties
Mentally infirm and/or institutionalized persons, 167, 356. *See also* Proxy consent
  abuses, 8-9
  assent, 314n. 18
  comprehension of, 443-44
  international guidelines, 505
  problems in genetics research, 411
  proxy consent, 444
  respect for, 439-40, 444
Meslin, Eric M., 350-51
Minimal risk
  definitions of, 28n. 57, 65, 308, 456. *See also* Children, research; Risk(s), classification of

ethical roots. *See* "Do no harm"/ nonmaleficence
  meaning of/debates over, 64-66, 85, 342-43, 348-56
  children. *See* Children, research, minimal
  fetuses, 77-78
  minor increases over, 66-74, 99
  more than minimal. *See* Children, research
  regulations regarding, 314n. 17
Minimization of research risks. *See* Risk(s)
Minority groups. *See also* Justice
  active recruitment of, 492-93, 496-500
  defined and described, 486, 495
  and discrimination, 37-38, 447. *See also* Public Health Service Syphilis Study; Stigmatization
  greater/equal access to clinical trials, 114-16, 138, 484-88
    compared to access to medical care, 121, 123
  guidelines regarding. *See* National, Institutes of Health, *Guidelines on the Inclusion of Women and Minorities as Subjects in Clinical Research*
  and informed consent, 287
  and justice in burdens and benefits of research, 37-38, 107-24
  underrepresented in research, 115-16, 449-500
Misconduct, academic. *See* Researchers, scientific integrity
Moral/morality. *See also* Ethics; Values/goods, types of
  common morality and local customs, 232n. 31
  metaphors. *See* Ethics, metaphorical nature of
  obligations. *See* Ethics
  status of embryos, fetus, and persons. *See under* Embryo; Fetus; Persons/personhood; Respect for persons
Multicenter clinical trials. *See also*

Cancer; Randomized clinical trials; Research, design
descriptions of, 135
increase of, 322
and local institutional review board review, 134-36, 322, 463
Mustard Gas experiments, 7

National. See also U.S.A.
Academy of Sciences
Institute of Medicine (IOM), 375-76, 389, 391, 393
Advisory Board on Ethics in Reproduction (NABER), 168, 171, 375-76, 385, 393-94
bioethics policy commissions. See Public bioethics
Commission for Protection of Human Subjects of Behavioral and Biomedical Research, 10, 62-66, 87-88, 160-62
ethics of, 35, 52-53, 63-66, 88-92, 100-101
in contrast to Nuremberg Code and Helsinki Declaration, 92, 101
history of, 62-64
work regarding
children, 52-53, 63-66, 72, 74, 77, 339-49, 356-58
criticisms of, 356, 366
fetuses, 77-78, 310, 372-73
mentally infirm, 356
Data and Safety Monitoring Committees, 40, 135-36
Ethics Advisory Board, 53, 66, 79, 161-63, 347, 373, 470-71, 474
See also Ethics advisory boards
Institute for Bioethics and Public Policy, proposals for, 173-75, 376-77
Institute of Neurological and Communicative Disorders and Stroke, 373
Institutes of Health (NIH), 10, 37, 111-12, 163-66, 181n. 38, 373-74, 422, 485-90
Growth hormone clinical trials,

361-65
Guidelines on the Inclusion of Women and Minorities as Subjects in Clinical Research [Reprinted as Appendix E], 37, 39, 111-12
Human Tissue Transplantation Research Panel, 374, 383, 394
Office for Protection from Research Risks. See Office for Protection from Research Risks (OPRR)
Science Foundation, 149
Surgical Adjuvant Breast and Bowel Project (NSABP). See under Cancer
Nazi/National Socialist German research, 6, 63-64
Negligence, laws of, 42n. 12
Nonconsenting/assenting subjects, 66, 250-55, 340. See also Children, research; Informed consent, waivers; Parental permission; Proxy consent
Nondisclosure of purpose of research. See Subjects
Nonmaleficence. See "Do no harm"/nonmaleficence
Nontherapeutic research, 85, 89
with children, 90. See also Children, research, nontherapeutic
definitions, 436, 480
and minimal risks, 89
and more than minimal risks, 89-90
placebos. See Placebo
Norms, moral. See Ethics; Moral/morality
Nuremberg Code [Reprinted in Appendix A]. See Codes/codifications
Nuremberg Military Tribunal, 7, 177n. 10

Obligations, moral. See Duty
Obstetrics and gynecology, 375
Office for Protection from Research Risks (OPRR), 10, 12-13, 40n. 1, 124-25, 132, 136, 405, 422. See also

Surveillance of institutional review boards
Guidebook(s) of, 10, 26n. 51, 224, 310, 420
Office of Technology Assessment. See under U.S.A.
Ohnuki-Tierney, Emiko, 247
Oncology. See Cancer
Ova and oocyte research, 386-87, 391, 394. See also Gametes, research

Pappworth, M.H., 87, 325
Parallel-track drugs, 56, 113-14, 137. See also under Cancer; HIV/AIDS
questions regarding, 137-38
Parental permission/consent, 53, 347, 481-82. See also Children, research; Nonconsenting/assenting subjects; Proxy consent
forms for, 360
by foster parents, 117
in genetics research, problematic nature of, 410-11
parents as vulnerable to permission requests, 360, 411
subjects without parental permission, 117
waiver for research with children, 117, 348
Parenthood, 344, 364
Parkinson's disease. See Fetal tissue/ tissue transplant, brain cell
Patient-physician relationships. See Physician-patient relationships
Patients. See also Subject(s)
unknowing involvement in clinical trials, 47-49, 207-8
Payers, third party. See Industry/ manufacturers; Insurance companies' payments
Payment, cash. See Financial issues
Pediatrics. See Children
Penicillin, 7, 9
Personal self-esteem/sense of worth. See Worth
Persons/personhood. See also Respect for persons; Values/goods, types of

personhood of embryo or fetus, 388
respect for. See Respect for persons
Western and non-Western views of, 264-65
Pharmaceutical industry. See Industrial/manufacturers' sponsorship
Phases of clinical trials. See also under Cancer
drug trials defined and described, 204, 321, 508-10
Phase I trials, 326-30
Phase II trials, 321
Phase III trials, 488-90, 497-98
Phase IV trials. See Post-marketing research
for vaccine development, 508
Physician-investigators. See Researchers
Physician-patient relationships, 186, 359
Placebos
and controlled trials, 321
with children, 364
Placental tissue. See Tissue, human
Politics, influence of on research, 158-66, 309. See also Abortion; Fetus; Public Bioethics
fetal, fetal tissue, and embryo research, 162-68
history of, 159-66
Post-marketing research/clinical trials. See also Conflicts of interest, possible; Financial issues
conflicts of interest, 150, 207-8, 211-12
ways of resolving, 213-14
costs to patients, 207
described, 203-5
informed consent, 210-11
lack of consent, 207-8
lack of regulatory oversight, 150, 214
as marketing, 204, 209
prevalence of, 205-6
risks of, 209
scientific validity of, 153n. 14, 215-16
Poverty/research on poor persons, 7-

10. *See also* Vulnerable persons/
subjects
Practice, medical. *See* Medical, prac-
tice
Pregnant women. *See* Women, preg-
nant
Prenatal diagnosis. *See* Fetus, research
involving
President's Commission for the Study
of Ethical Problems in Medicine
and Biomedical and Behavioral
Research, 110, 160, 162
Prima facie moral duties. *See* Ethics,
prima facie ethics/duties
Primam non nocere. *See* "Do no harm"
PRIM&R (Public Responsibility in
Medicine and Research), 153n. 13
Prisoners, research, 440, 475-78, 506
historical abuses of, 6
Privacy. *See* Confidentiality
Professional ethics. *See* Medical, professional ethics
Proxy consent. *See also* Mentally infirm and/or institutionalized persons; Nonconsenting/assenting
subjects; Parental permission
by legally authorized advocate/
guardian/representative, 411,
482
by next of kin, 242, 285
Psychiatry, 49, 406
Public bioethics. *See also* Ethics advisory boards; History of; Politics,
influence of on research
ad hoc ethics advisory boards. *See*
Ethics advisory boards
alternative ways of organizing,
debates and proposals, 169-75,
376-77
defined, 155
ethics of/rationales for, 155-57
history of, 159-66
need of/proposals for new public
forums, 156-58, 166-75, 371,
376-77
promise and perils of, 155-58
Public Health Service. *See under* U.S.A.
Public Health Service Syphilis Study,

7, 9-10, 120-21, 159-60, 178n. 11.
See also under Minority groups
effect on enrollment of black Americans in clinical trials, 121
Publicity as a test of morality of research projects, 54
Publishers/publications
ethics of publishing genetics research
results, 416-19
International Council of Biology
Editors, 422

Quality of life, 323

Racial discrimination. *See* Discrimination
Radiation experiments, 11, 171
Ramsey, Paul, 65, 307, 339-45
Randomized clinical trials. *See also under* Cancer; Multicenter clinical
trials
design of as ethical concern. *See*
Research, design of
and equipoise principle, 55
ethical justifications for. *See* Research, justifications
inclusion/exclusion of subjects. *See*
Research, inclusion/exclusion
Rawls, John, 61, 70-71, 84-85
Recruitment of subjects. *See* Selection/
recruitment of subjects
Regulations. *See also* Children; Embryo; Fetal tissue; Fetus; Institutional review boards; Research,
regulation of
Code of U.S. Federal Regulations,
[Reprinted as Appendix D], 10-
11, 37, 40. *See also* Regulations,
United States
as Common Federal Rule for federal departments, 132-34
challenges to implementation
of, 133-34
criticisms of, 308, 345-47, 356
ethical assumptions of, 89-91
in contrast to *Nuremberg Code*
and the *Declarations of
Helsinki*, 91

costs of, 171
and ethics. *See* Ethics, and regulation(s)
noncompliance with, 131-32, 468-69
research in
Canada
Royal Commission on New Reproductive Technologies, 382, 385, 393, 395
Israel, 25n. 49
Scandinavia, 25n. 49
United Kingdom
embryo and oocyte, 394
fetal tissue research, 382, 385
post-marketing research, 213
United States. *See also Regulations, Code of U.S. Federal*
components of, 10
disputes over effectiveness of self-regulation, 131
history of. *See* History
Office for Protection from Research Risks (OPRR), functions of. *See* Office for Protection from Research Risks
predicated on self-regulation and mutual trust, 130
of U.S.A. Food and Drug Administration (FDA). *See under* U.S.A.
Religion, 67-69, 309
Research
AIDS. *See* HIV/AIDS
behavioral, 164-66
HIV/AIDS, 165
violent behavior, 166
as beneficial/useful to society. *See* Research, justifications for
benefits and burdens of, for subjects, 37. *See also under* Justice
on body fluids/specimens, 50, 100. *See also* Tissue, human
cancer. *See* Cancer
children. *See* Children, research
cognitively impaired and institutionalized subjects. *See* Mentally

infirm and/or institutionalized persons
community-based, 114-16
conflict of interest. *See* Conflict of interest
costs, 11, 203. *See also* Financial issues
cross-cultural. *See* Cross-cultural research
deceptive, 9-10, 42n. 11, 120-22. *See* Wrongs, of deception
justification of, 100-101
definitions and terminology, 19n. 17, 434-36, 438-39, 455-56, 501-3
design. *See also under* Cancer; Multicenter clinical trials
inclusion/exclusion criteria, 331-35
ethical significance of, 307, 331-36
disclosure of results to subjects. *See* Genetics research
distribution of burdens and benefits. *See* Justice
embryos. *See* Embryo, research
epidemiological. *See* Epidemiological
ethics case examples. *See* Ethics, case studies
extent of in the U.S. at present, 11-14, 198-200
fetal. *See* Fetus, research
freedom of researchers and subjects. *See* Freedom
gametes. *See* Gametes, research
genetics. *See* Genetics research
harms. *See* Harms, of research
as hazardous or not. *See* Harm(s), of research
healthcare and healthcare policy, 167
history of. *See* History of
inclusion/exclusion criteria as ethically significant, 110-16, 331-35
industry/biotech industry, sponsorship. *See* Sponsorship
informed consent for. *See* Informed

consent
injuries, compensation for. *See* Compensation for research-caused injuries
injuries, extent of. *See* Harm(s), of research
justifications for, 14, 64-66. *See also* Beneficence; Benefits; Risk(s), justification of
benefits to society, 7-11, 14, 86, 91, 333, 343
constrained by ethical duties to subjects, 45-57, 83-84, 344
as justifying compromises to subjects' interests, 93-94
benefits to subjects/as therapeutic, 199, 320-21
and equipoise principle, 55, 332-33
reduction of medical injuries/ harms, 93-96
medical records, 48-49, 92-93
in medical schools/institutions, 12. *See also* University hospitals
minorities. *See* Minority groups
morality of. *See* Ethics; Research, justifications for
multicenter trials. *See* Multicenter clinical trials
nonconsenting/assenting. *See* Non-consenting/assenting subjects
nontherapeutic. *See* Nontherapeutic research
participation in
as a duty or moral obligation, 35-36, 91
inducements. *See* Subjects, inducements
phases of. *See* Phases of clinical trials
placebos, use of. *See* Placebos
and politics. *See* Politics, influence of on research; Public bio-ethics
pregnant women. *See* Women, pregnant
prisoners. *See* Prisoners, research
quality of life, 323

regulation, 10-11. *See also* Regulations
results
as beneficial/useful to society. *See* Research, justifications
disclosure of to subjects in genetics research, 412-15
as varying with researchers' interests, 152n. 12
review committees. *See* Institutional review boards
review of. *See* Expedited review; Institutional review boards; Regulations
risk-free, 47
risks of. *See* Risk(s)
scientific integrity of. *See* Researchers, scientific integrity
scientific merit of, 331-35, 432, 434, 445-47, 496-97
without scientific merit, 6
social benefits of. *See* Research, justifications for
sponsorship, disclosure of. *See* Disclosure of
termination of, 136
vaccine, 140, 168, 286-88, 508
women. *See* Women
Research committees. *See* Institutional Review Boards
Researchers. *See also* Bias(es), researchers
competency of, 432, 434
conflict of commitment/loyalty, 152n. 10, 434
conflict of interest. *See* Conflict of interest
ethical rights of, 56
moral character/integrity/virtues. *See* Ethics, virtue ethics
public scrutiny of, 185-86
reputation of, 23n. 39, 129-33
scientific integrity/objectivity of, 130-32, 148-49, 288, 434
Respect for Persons. *See also* Ethics, rights, human; Freedom; Informed consent, ethical and legal basis; Persons/personhood

and autonomy, 439-40. *See also*
  Autonomy
children. *See under* Children
as ethical principle, 34, 38, 48, 248,
  281-82, 439-40
as foundation for subjects' rights,
  323-25
historical background, 324-25
in non-Western cultures, 248, 255,
  282, 286-88
and self-worth of subjects. *See* Worth
Rifkin, Jeremy, 130, 361-62
Rights, ethical and legal. *See* Freedom;
  Respect for persons
Risk(s). *See also* "Do no harm"/non-
  maleficence; Harm(s)
assessments of, 349-50
  as subjective, 350
and benefits (probable or anticipated) to subjects. *See also under* Beneficence; Selection/re-
  cruitment of subjects
balancing/weighing of, 42n. 13,
  89-91, 98-99, 435, 445-47, 462
estimates as subjective, 55-56
ethical basis of harm/benefit
  analysis, 34, 445-47
terminology involving, 445
to children. *See* Children, research
classification of, 64-66, 74. *See also*
  Minimal risk
definitions, 445
description/disclosure of. *See* Informed consent, information
in genetics research. *See* Genetics
  research
justification of, 65-66, 76-80, 89-90,
  446. *See also* Research, justifications for
of maximum tolerated dose (MTD)
  agents. *See under* Informed consent
minimal. *See* Minimal risk
minimization of, 89, 98-99, 462
  ethical basis for, 89. *See* "Do no
    harm"/nonmaleficence
negligible, 47, 85
psychological and social. *See* Genet-

ics research, risks
unforeseen, 464
to women. *See* Women
Robertson, John, 383-84
Roe v. Wade, 371-72
Rules, ethical. *See* Ethics, duties/ob-
  ligations; Ethics, principles of

Scientific integrity/objectivity. *See*
  Researchers
Selection/recruitment of subjects. *See
  also* conscription of persons into
  research; Financial issues; Justice
criteria/ethical bases for, 34, 39, 447-
  48, 462. *See also* Autonomy;
  Beneficence; Justice; Risk(s)
inclusion/exclusion criteria. *See*
  Research, inclusion/exclusion
  criteria
and informed consent. *See* Informed
  consent
and justice. *See* Justice
minorities. *See* Minority groups
non-Western. *See* Cross-cultural
  research
women. *See* Women
Self-determination. *See* Autonomy;
  Respect for persons
Self-interest. *See* Conflict of interest
Smoking and substance abuse, 168
Social
  risks. *See* Genetics research, risks
  stigmatization. *See* Stigmatization
Specimens, use of. *See* Tissue
Sperm research, 391-92. *See also* Gametes, research
Sponsorship of research, extent of, 13,
  193-95. *See also under* Disclosure
  of
Staging of research. *See* Phases of clinical trials
Stigmatization, social, 108, 406, 409-
  10, 447. *See also* Genetics research,
  risks; Minority groups
Stopping clinical trials. *See* Research,
  termination
Subject(s). *See also* Patients
  abuse of. *See* Abuses

awareness/unawareness of research
    involvement, 9-10, 47-49, 120-
    21, 207-8
coercion of, 6-8, 275. See also Codes/
    codifications, Nuremberg Code
competence. See Competence
dependent populations. See Vulner-
    able persons
disclosures to. See Disclosure of;
    Genetics research, ethics
inducements to participate, 504. See
    also Financial issues
informed consent of. See Informed
    consent
misinforming of. See Wrongs, of
    deception
numbers involved in research, 12-13
protection as a moral priority, 84-
    87, 283, 323-25, 440-41, 445-47.
    See also "Do no harm"/non-
    maleficence
rights of. See Freedom; Respect for
    persons
selection of. See Selection of sub-
    jects
vulnerable. See Vulnerable persons
Sullivan, Louis B., 165, 374
Surgery, 175n. 2, 387-88
Surrogate consent. See Proxy consent
Surveillance of institutional review
    boards, 10, 12-13, 127-36. See also
    Office for Protection from Re-
    search Risks (OPRR)
Syphilis research. See Public Health
    Service Syphilis Study

Terminal illness,
    ethical issues regarding care of, 162,
    168
    as subjects of research, 21n. 27. See
    also under Cancer
Thalidomide research, 118-20, 159
    as discouragement of research in-
    volving women and children,
    118-19
Theories, ethical. See Ethics
Third-party payers. See Insurance
    companies' payments

Tissue, human, 47-49. See also Research,
    on body fluids/specimens; Fetal
    tissue/tissue transplant
Touching, unconsented or wrongful.
    See Wrongs, ethical
Transplantation. See also Fetal tissue/
    tissue transplant
    organs, human, 175n. 2
    xenografts. See Xenografts/trans-
    plant research
Trust. See also Distrust; Researchers,
    scientific integrity
    as basis for U.S. regulatory review,
    130-31
Tuskegee Syphilis study. See Public
    Health Service Syphilis Study

Uncomprehending subjects. See Sub-
    jects, awareness
Unethical research. See Harm(s), of
    research; Wrongs
Uniform Anatomical Gift Act, 265,
    372, 380
United Kingdom. See Regulations, of
    research
University hospitals. See also Research,
    in medical schools
    interests/possible conflicts of inter-
    ests, 197-98
    involvement in research, extent of,
    12, 197
U.S.A. See also National
    Department of Health and Human
        Services (DHHS), 10-11, 129-
        33, 163-66, 374
    Department of Health, Education
        and Welfare (DHEW), 10
    Federal regulation of research. See
        Regulations, Code of U.S. Fed-
        eral
    Food and Drug Administration
        (FDA), 10, 12-13, 112-13, 119,
        203-4
    National Institutes of Health. See
        National, Institutes of Health
    Office of Technology Assessment,
        167-68, 372, 375, 377
    Public Health Service, 9, 120-21, 128,

159, 243
Utilitarianism. *See* Ethics, utilitarianism

Vaccine research. *See* Research, vaccine
Values/goods, types of. *See also under* Ethics; Moral/morality
conflicts between, 67-69, 148, 157, 162-66
cultural/social. *See also* Autonomy, cultural; Cross-cultural research, ethics; Persons/personhood
non-Western, 264-65, 287-89
Western
autonomy, 264-66
individualism, 67-68, 264
financial, 13. *See also* Financial issues, increasing significance
human worth. *See* Worth
medical professionals, well-being and power of, 157, 160, 168
medicine. *See* Medical
moral, 3. *See also* Ethics
national/political, 6-7, 69, 160-66
during wartime, 6-7
non-moral, 3, 6-11
prudential/practical, 3, 81
racial. *See* Minority groups
religious, 67-69
of technological/scientific discoveries, 7-11, 14, 59, 160-70, 174-75, 193. *See also* Benefits, of biomedical research
Veatch, Robert M., 92, 98-99
Venipunctures. *See* Children, research, venipunctures
Veracity. *See* Ethics, *prima facie* ethics; Ethics, principles, truth-telling
Volunteer. *See* Autonomy
Vulnerable persons/subjects, 462. *See also* Fetus; Justice; Poverty/research on poor persons
abuses of, 6-10, 120-21, 159-60
changing views of, 106-22
children. *See* Children, research
exclusion/inclusion of, 37-38, 44n.

25, 447-48
justice and, 39. *See* Justice
mentally infirm and/or institutionalized. *See* Mentally infirm and/or institutionalized persons
poor/disadvantaged, 9-10, 23n. 37, 120-21, 441-42
pregnant women. *See* Women, pregnant
prisoners. *See* Prisoners, research

Waiver of consent. *See* Informed consent, waivers
Willowbrook State School Studies, 9, 159, 341
Withdrawal from research or therapy. *See* Freedom
Women. *See also* Justice
access to/inclusion in clinical trials, 11, 37, 111-16, 120, 484-88
justice and, 37-38, 106-7
active recruitment of, 492, 496-500
emancipation/improved status, 292, 294
health needs, 112-13, 120, 505-7
loss of privacy over fetal tissue donation, 383
pregnant, 44n. 25, 113, 121-23, 389-90, 473, 507
underrepresented in research, 111-13, 487-88, 498-500
as vulnerable or not, 39, 118-20
Wong, David, 229
World Health Organization (WHO). *See* Codes/codification, Council for International Organization of Medical Sciences (CIOMS) and World Health Organizaton
Worth
of persons, 98, 292
sense of/self-esteem, 292
Wrongs. *See also* Abuses of research subjects; Harm(s), of research
of deception, 9-10, 42n. 11, 120-22
ethical, 35

Xenograft/transplant research, 168, 386